Patellofemoral Disorders

Patellofemoral Disorders

Diagnosis and Treatment

Edited by

Roland M. Biedert

Institute of Sports Sciences,
Magglingen, Switzerland

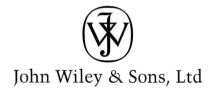

John Wiley & Sons, Ltd

Other Wiley Editorial Offices

John Wiley & Sons Inc., 111 River Street, Hoboken, NJ 07030, USA

Jossey-Bass, 989 Market Street, San Francisco, CA 94103-1741, USA

Wiley-VCH Verlag GmbH, Boschstr. 12, D-69469 Weinheim, Germany

John Wiley & Sons Australia Ltd, 33 Park Road, Milton, Queensland 4064, Australia

John Wiley & Sons (Asia) Pte Ltd, 2 Clementi Loop #02-01, Jin Xing Distripark, Singapore 129809

John Wiley & Sons Canada Ltd, 22 Worcester Road, Etobicoke, Ontario, Canada M9W 1L1

Wiley also publishes its books in a variety of electronic formats. Some content that appears
in print may not be available in electronic books.

Library of Congress Cataloging-in-Publication Data

Patellofemoral disorders : diagnosis and treatment/edited by Roland M. Biedert.
      p. ; cm.
   Includes bibliographical references and index.
   ISBN 0-470-85011-6 (cloth : alk. paper)
  1. Patellofemoral joint–Diseases–Diagnosis. 2. Patellofemoral joint–Diseases–Treatment. I. Biedert, Roland M.
   [DNLM: 1. Patella–physiopathology–Case Reports. 2. Knee Joint–Case Reports. 3. Pain–diagnosis–Case Reports.
   4. Pain–therapy–Case Reports. WE 870 P2948 2004]
   RD561.P376 2004
   617.5′82–dc22
                                                                                          2004011337

British Library Cataloguing in Publication Data

A catalogue record for this book is available from the British Library

ISBN 0-470-85011-6

Typeset in 10.5/13pt Sabon by Laserwords Private Limited, Chennai, India
Printed and bound in Italy by Conti Tipocolor, SpA., Florence, Italy
This book is printed on acid-free paper responsibly manufactured from sustainable forestry
in which at least two trees are planted for each one used for paper production.

*The intention to understand a problem
is the first step toward resolving the problem.*

Contents

Foreword

Roland Biedert is well known in Sports Medicine and is also an outstanding expert in the field of pathology of patellofemoral disorders and their diagnosis and treatment. He is a leading contributor to the knowledge of proprioceptive function and sensorimotor control of our musculoskeletal system. To compile this eminent book, *Patellofemoral Disorders: Diagnosis and Treatment,* he gathered an excellent team of specialists to bring all the recent advances to you.

The names of the contributors – Scott Dye, Niklaus Friederich, Hans Ulrich Stäubli, Andrew Amis, Alan Merchant, Philippe Neyret, Robert Teitge and Roland Biedert himself – guarantee the best information available. They share their expert knowledge of the basics, functional and cryosectional anatomy, biomechanics, patellofemoral joint replacement, case studies, and the importance of physical therapy in the care of patients with patellofemoral disorders or injuries.

The work in this book is so important because the so-called 'patellofemoral joint' is not a joint in the classic anatomical sense but is instead a unique functional unit in the system of the decelerating–accelerating knee–quadriceps mechanism. There are many publications about the static anatomomorphological aspects and instability problems of the patellofemoral joint. However, many other factors – especially aspects of the dynamics and sensorimotor control of which the patellofemoral joint is capable – are not generally known. This book by a distinguished group of authors is a valuable addition to the growing field of knowledge about the patellofemoral joint.

The patella is just a sesamoid bone in the tendon complex of the quadriceps system. This multidirectional system absorbs tremendous tension forces, e.g. when a Triple Sault athlete jumps, lands, decelerates with his quadriceps, and accelerates again with his quadriceps for the next jump. Dampening the forces of the first landing in eccentric function and continuing the action with an extreme concentric quadriceps action exposes the patella to extremely high-tension forces and to a high-pressure load. No wonder that the patella will be deformed by this action.

To function with ease and without pain, the patellotendon mechanism must be elastic. Its mechanical construction is similar to a biplane with two hard layers, one in front and one behind, facing the femur. This construction resists pressure on the back and tension forces on the front. In spite of the fact that the mechanical strength of the bone tissue itself is relatively weak against tension, the tension resistance of the patella is surprisingly high because of its location in a strong network of an important ligamentous tension-band system.

Consider the soccer player who could not resist immense tension forces for 4 weeks after receiving a kick to the front of the patella. Only the tendinous galea aponeurotica was ruptured. The radiographs at time of injury did not show any bony lesion. But the patella needed the protective help of the tension-absorbing collagenous tendon fibres, which have their origin in the quadriceps tendon, running to the front of the patella, into the patellar tendon and on to the tibia. Additionally, the medial superior femoropatellar ligament and the vastus medialis obliquus tendon join this tension-band sling system from the medial side. On the lateral side, the sling system is joined by the strong vastus lateralis and the lateral retinaculum. All of this mechanism is created anatomically to absorb and neutralize a critical amount of tension force. In the transverse retinaculum, longitudinal lateral parapatellar retinaculum fibres and fibres from the iliotibial tract are also included. Together they function as an antivarus restraint that includes the patella. This anatomical fact leads to the question, 'How benign is the lateral retinacular release?'

On the medial side we find the proximal patellofemoral ligament (medial transverse retinaculum), which connects the patella with the medial femoral epicondyle, close to the cross-point of the adductor tendon and the medial collateral ligament. These medial and lateral transverse retinacular components form the transverse tension band, which becomes an important restraint in progressive flexion and full flexion of the knee.

Active and passive forces must act together for optimal function. In a dislocation, the medial patellofemoral ligament ruptures at its weakest medial part, where it no longer has enough support from the actively protecting vastus medialis obliquus. The longitudinal retinaculum itself is the longitudinal part of the vastus medialis tendon reaching the tibia just proximal to the pes anserinus tendon's insertion.

Everything seems to be clear, *but do we know all about*:

♦ What is painful in 'anterior knee pain'?

♦ How do Hoffa's fat pad and the plicae around the patella and above the trochlea interact with the decelerator–extensor mechanism?

♦ Is the ligamentum mucosum a possible sensor to limit the quadriceps-extension action in preventing active hyperextension?

♦ How do the patellar positions – normal, alta, infera and baja – affect the corresponding contact areas of the thick cartilage layers on the femur and on the patella?

♦ How should we describe the innumerable individual morphological varieties of the trochlea and the patella, and the biomechanical consequences for their function? Are some knee constructions mechanically weaker than others?

♦ How should we manage symptomatic patellar instability and subluxation?

♦ What is the solution for an individual's treatment?

These are all still burning questions.

I am sure this book by Roland Biedert and his outstanding team of authors will help us find answers to all these questions and show us new ways to understand and treat patellofemoral disorders.

Werner Müller
Basel, Switzerland
May 2003

Preface

I was encouraged to write this book in response to the high number of unsuccessfully treated patients suffering from patellofemoral problems. During the last two decades I have tried to analyse these unsuccessful clinical outcomes with minute carefulness. I was astonished to learn that in numerous cases the treatment performed was not the result of a clear diagnosis with correct analysis of the underlying pathology, but only a treatment for unspecific patellofemoral pain or chondropathia patellae (whatever this means). Such procedures did not resolve the initial problem, but often created a second pathology with impairment over the long term. Surgical interventions on children and adolescents caused the most severe secondary complications, with multiple operations as the patients grew older. Besides the psychological factors, these treatments ended too often with an escalation of irreparable structural damage and chronic disability.

Together with the invited authors – all experts on the topic of the patellofemoral joint (and most of them members of the International Patellofemoral Study Group) – I faced up to the challenge of gaining more insight into patellofemoral disorders and consolidating the present knowledge. In the first part of the book I have tried to present a clear and structured overview with consensus to facilitate the handling of patellofemoral joint problems. This was an extremely challenging task and I am probably the person who learned most, by reading all the literature, discovering unsuccessful treatments and proposing better ones on the proven base of secured knowledge. The daily clinical work, precise analyses – especially of the 'bad cases' – and ears and mind open for the ideas of my colleagues helped me to realize the fulfilment of consolidating the finest of present knowledge into this book. As Professor Erwin Morscher from Basel once said: 'Good results come from experience, experience from bad results'.

The second part of the book presents typical case studies as we see them in our offices every day. An axial view and some questions briefly show the main problems at the beginning of each of the cases described. As Professor John Feagin illustrated in the second edition of his book, *The Crucial Ligaments* (1994), these selected cases represent my philosophy of diagnosis and decision making. The cases are structured from simple nonoperative treatment to multioperated patients with salvage procedures.

Although the majority of patients with patellofemoral disorders should be treated nonoperatively, in the case studies I focused on the surgical interventions because the negative secondary effects following surgery may be disastrous and the structural damage is often irreparable. Treatment of patellofemoral problems must initially be in the conservative domain. Surgical interventions must be performed in a response to a clear underlying pathology and only after nonoperative treatment fails.

Roland M. Biedert
Magglingen, Switzerland
August 2003

Contributors

Andrew A. Amis
Department of Mechanical Engineering,
Imperial College of Science, Technology and
Medicine,
London SW7 2BX, UK

Tarik Aït Si Selmi
Centre Livet,
Clinique de Chirurgie du Genou,
8 Rue de Margnolles,
F-69300 Caluire, Lyon, France

Roland M. Biedert
Institute of Sports Sciences, Orthopaedics and
Sports Traumatology,
Federal Office of Sports,
CH-2532 Magglingen, Switzerland

Mario Bizzini
Schulthess Clinic,
Lengghalde 2,
CH-8008 Zürich, Switzerland

Anthony M. Bull
Department of Bioengineering,
Imperial College of Science, Technology and
Medicine,
London SW7 2AZ, UK

Scott F. Dye
University of California San Francisco,
Davies Medical Center,
Medical Office Building, Suite 117,
45 Castro Street,
San Francisco, CA 94114, USA

Farzam Farahmand
Department of Mechanical Engineering,

Sharif University of Technology,
Azadi Avenue,
Tehran, Iran

Niklaus F. Friederich
Department of Orthopaedic Surgery,
Kantonsspital Bruderholz,
CH-4101 Bruderholz, Switzerland

Vroni Kernen
Department of Rheumatology and Rehabilitation,
Bethesda Hospital,
CH-4020 Basel, Switzerland

I. A. Kramers-de Quervain
Laboratory for Biomechanics,
Department of Materials,
ETH Zurich,
Wagistrasse 4,
8952 Schlieren, Switzerland

Alan C. Merchant
Stanford University School of Medicine,
2500 Hospital Drive, Bldg. 7,
Mountain View,
CA 94040, USA

Stephan Meyer
Department of Physical Therapy,
Institute of Sports Sciences,
Federal Office of Sports,
CH-2532 Magglingen, Switzerland

Jean-Luc Meystre
Rue du Panorama 16,
CH-1800 Vevey, Switzerland

Werner Müller
Spechtweg 10,
CH-4125 Riehen, Switzerland

Philippe Neyret
Orthopaedic Department Centre Livet,
Clinique de Chirurgie du Genou,
8 Rue de Margnolles,
F-69300 Caluire, Lyon, France

Wongwit Senavongse
Department of Mechanical Engineering,
Imperial College of Science, Technology and
Medicine,
London SW7 2BX, UK

Elvire Servien
Centre Livet,
Clinique de Chirurgie du Genou,
8 Rue de Margnolles,
F-69300 Caluire, Lyon, France

Yi-Fen Shih
Department of Mechanical Engineering,
Imperial College of Science, Technology and
Medicine,
London SW7 2BX, UK

Hans Ulrich Stäubli
Salem Spital,
CH-3013 Bern, Switzerland

Robert A. Teitge
Hutzel Health Center,
4050 East 12 Mile Road, Suite 110,
Warren,
MI 48092, USA

René De Vries
Sports and Orthopaedic Rehabilitation,
University of New Zealand,
NZ-5001 Wanganui, New Zealand

Acknowledgements

I wish to express my gratitude to many people who helped in the realization of this book.

Special help and author's assistance

Lottie B. Applewhite, author's editor, helped me from the initial idea of this proposal through the final realization of *Patellofemoral Disorders*. She gave me all the necessary support, from structural formula to language assistance. Her 'PCLs' (Please Clarify for Lottie) forced me throughout the book to write the text in an understandable form for everybody. Her outstanding experience and personality were an indescribable support for me personally and for the book.

Manuela Pflugi has done the majority of the work preparing the manuscripts and the final preparation of the figures for electronic transmission. She was assisted by Hedi Winkelmann, Esther Puma, Klaus Hübner and Stefan Rickli.

Contributing authors

They gave personal inputs and experience – most valuable gifts.

Medical illustrations

Jean-Luc Meystre, orthopaedic surgeon, provided all graphics and drawings for the chapters and case studies. The precise and wonderful artworks are the result of his special orthopaedic knowledge. They show that he is an expert in the patellofemoral joint.

Photographs

Daniel Käsermann provided photographs for several chapters.

Financial support

Financial support for this book was provided by the Institute of Sport Sciences, Federal Office of Sports, Magglingen, Switzerland.

Exemplars

Professor Werner Müller and Professor John A. Feagin Jr.

Special friends

Numerous co-workers of the Institute of Sport Sciences at Magglingen, and Riana Egli.

Publisher's staff

Members of John Wiley & Sons, Ltd, in particular Celia Carden, were helpful from the beginning, with suggestions and guidance throughout.

Most of all, I am grateful to **my family.**

Roland Biedert

PART I

INTRODUCTION

Reflections on Patellofemoral Disorders

Scott F. Dye

Patellofemoral pain: a tissue homeostasis perspective

Despite recent advances in the treatment of many musculoskeletal conditions, patients with anterior knee pain remain an orthopaedic enigma. Unfortunately, the worst cases of patellofemoral pain are often in patients who have had multiple surgical procedures for symptoms that initially were only mild anterior knee discomfort[1] (Figure I.1). With the possible exception of operative treatment for low back pain, no other area of orthopaedic surgery has an iatrogenic failure rate as great as that for patients with chronic anterior knee pain. The lack of a safe and predictable approach for patients with anterior knee pain represents a genuine orthopaedic concern, and implies a profound lack of understanding of the causative factors associated with the genesis of patellofemoral pain. The current treatment approach to patients with patellofemoral pain is based on the concept that observable structural and biomechanical factors are primarily responsible for the symptoms, and thus that treatment addressing those factors should be curative.[2,3]

Two main factors have traditionally been thought to be of causal significance in the genesis of anterior knee pain – the presence of chondromalacia and/or malalignment of the patellofemoral joint. This common belief in the structural and biomechanical origin of anterior knee pain has served as a justification for treatment that has resulted in worsening of symptoms. These treatments include aggressive physical therapy with extension of the knee against resistance to strengthen the vastus medialis obliquus to correct 'maltracking'. Further, the use of various surgical procedures, such as the lateral release, aggressive chondroplasties and major proximal and distal realignments, have not infrequently resulted in further injury, including medial patellar dislocation and reflex sympathetic dystrophy.

Patellofemoral Disorders: Diagnosis and Treatment. Edited by Roland M. Biedert
© 2004 John Wiley & Sons, Ltd ISBN: 0-470-85011-6

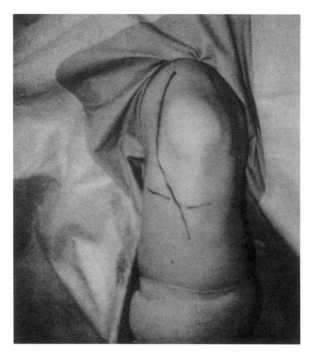

Figure I.1 Patient with multiple failed surgical procedures for patellofemoral pain. Each procedure was based on 'correcting patellofemoral malalignment'. All resulted in worsening of the patient's symptoms. Reproduced with permission from Dye, 2001[30]

Chondromalacia

The presence of chondromalacia was once thought to be so commonly associated with anterior knee discomfort that it became the accepted clinical diagnosis for symptoms of patellofemoral pain.[4–6] Studies[7–9] have shown, however, that even advanced chondromalacic changes can be asymptomatic, and that patients with normal-appearing articular cartilage can experience substantial patellofemoral pain. Despite these observations, aggressive surgical approaches to chondromalacia are still being performed on the patellofemoral joint, including drilling of bone, mosaicplasties and autogenous chondrocyte transplantations. However, such operative procedures have not demonstrated long-term benefit, and have resulted in worsening patellofemoral symptoms in many patients. The presence of observable chondromalacia in a patient with

patellofemoral pain does not prove that the structural damage of articular cartilage is causing the discomfort. For example, this author has patellae with documented grade III chondromalacia that are totally asymptomatic even to direct probing without intraarticular anaesthesia[8] (Figure I.2).

It is known by histological examination that articular cartilage is aneural. Therefore, the absence of sensation to palpation should not be surprising. However, despite this intellectual understanding, the absence of sensation in the region of advanced chondromalacia of my own patellar articular cartilage was a personal revelation. This finding has guided my own subsequent operative approach to the presence of chondromalacia in patients with patellofemoral pain. I am now much less aggressive regarding surgical debridement of observed chondromalacic damage than in the past. The presence of chondromalacia may be at least indirectly involved in the genesis of anterior knee pain, however. Thinning of articular cartilage can lead to excessive loading of subchondral bone, which, because it is richly innervated, can be a potential source of pain, as noted by Radin.[10] Further, the breakdown products of

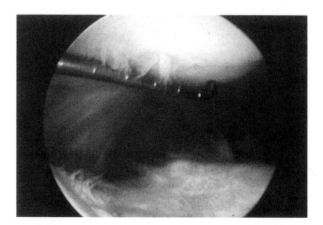

Figure I.2 Probing of the author's unanaesthetized right patella, showing grade III chondromalacia. No sensation was experienced during palpation of the articular cartilage. Reproduced with permission from Dye et al, 1998[8]

fibrillated cartilage can stimulate cytokine production and inflammatory biochemical processes within the innervated synovium, leading to chemical irritation of nerve endings and ultimately to the perception of pain.[11] Swelling of the peripatellar synovial tissues can also lead to increased susceptibility to mechanical impingement.

Malalignment

At present, the most widely accepted concept for the genesis of chronic anterior knee pain is that some form of malalignment between the patella and femur exists, even though it may be subtle.[2,12] Although this view is biomechanically appealing to many physical therapists and orthopaedic surgeons, it has not, in my experience, held up to close scientific scrutiny or thorough logical analysis. Worse, the belief in the concept of malalignment as a necessary but not always sufficient condition for the genesis of anterior knee pain has served as the justification for the unwary orthopaedic surgeon to perform operative procedures designed to correct the supposed underlying malalignment. Proponents of the malalignment concept also believe that if such a malalignment-orientated procedure fails, it may be due to over-correction or under-correction, further encouraging additional surgical perturbation of an already iatrogenically injured joint. Such an approach has led to well-meaning but ill-considered multiple surgical attempts to get the patellofemoral position 'just right', only to further traumatize this region of the knee.

Lack of importance of variable indicators of patellofemoral malalignment was confirmed in research performed at Letterman Army Medical Center in San Francisco in the 1980s. At that time, we performed a clinical evaluation which included imaging patients with patellofemoral pain compared to control subjects. Several putative indicators of malalignment, including a high Q angle, high congruence angle, and the presence of a meniscus of osseous sclerosis of the lateral facet of the patella on axial radiographs were not found with a statistically greater frequency in the symptomatic population than in the asymptomatic control population.[13]

More recent work by Thomee et al[14] substantiates this view that factors other than malalignment (i.e. overuse of anatomically normal patellofemoral components) are most likely the cause of symptoms of anterior knee pain.[2] Groundbreaking anatomical research by Stäubli et al[15] has thrown into question the primary method of determining the presence of malalignment, which for decades has been based on the measurement of osseous landmarks of the patellofemoral joint. These authors have shown that the articular cartilage morphology does not necessarily match the osseous morphology. Thus, when one determines that tilting of the patella is present by measuring osseous landmarks, the cartilage surfaces may in fact be mating perfectly. If one then performs a surgical procedure to 'untilt' the patella to achieve osseous radiographic normalcy (thus supposedly correcting the malalignment), one may in fact be creating an iatrogenic malalignment which results in worsening of symptoms.

Logical analysis

If the presence of malalignment is crucial in the genesis of anterior knee pain, why does one find patients with bilateral radiographically determined patellofemoral malalignment (i.e. patellar tilts) with only unilateral symptoms? Why do more than 90% of patients with patellofemoral pain who have a diagnosis of malalignment as the cause have a successful response to conservative therapy, even though there has been no 'correction' or restoration of the supposed underlying indicators of malalignment (e.g. a high Q angle or a shallow trochlea)? Patients have lived and adapted to their unique biomechanical factors their entire lives before the onset of anterior knee pain. Just because one examines them at a time when symptoms are present does not mean that these so-called indicators of malalignment are important in the genesis of anterior knee pain. The success of conservative treatment, such as the pain-relieving patellofemoral taping technique of McConnell, does not necessarily work by 'correcting malalignment', but may in fact decrease patellofemoral pain by unpinching and thus mechanically relieving swollen and irritated peripatellar tissues. These tissues may eventually heal, resulting in long-term pain relief, without a permanent change in patellofemoral alignment characteristics.

Furthermore, the supposed secondary indicators of the so-called 'excessive' lateral-pressure facet syndrome (purported to be the most common form of malalignment), including the radiographic findings of perpendicularization of lateral facet trabeculae and a meniscus of osteosclerosis of the lateral patellar facet, were not present at a greater frequency in the symptomatic group than in the asymptomatic control group in our study.[13] The malalignment theory also does not explain the variability of anterior knee symptoms in the same patient at different times, including the presence of sharp pain on one occasion and dull aching pain on another, as well as the possible absence of pain. The so-called 'movie sign', patellar aching with prolonged knee flexion, is also not explained by the malalignment theory.

What, then, can provide a better explanation? During the past 20 years, our research group in San Francisco has been attempting to address these questions. One of the confusing variables regarding patellofemoral pain is that some patients *do* have clinically significant malalignment that responds to malalignment-orientated treatment, including a lateral release. In my experience, however, the number of these patients is relatively small. An alternative perspective to the malalignment and chondromalacia theory must also address several issues, including the following. What is the source of the anterior knee pain? What tissues are involved? What are the pathophysiological factors relative to the nociceptive neurological output? Why do some patients have

patellofemoral pain with no observable structural abnormalities? Why do unilateral symptoms exist in patients with similar structural characteristics of both knees? What accounts for the variability of symptoms in the same patient from sharp to dull, to absence of pain? What accounts for the presence of the 'movie sign'?

What are the potential sources of discomfort? I have experienced sharp lancinating pain secondary to transiently increased intraosseous pressure produced experimentally within the right patella through a 15-gauge Jamshidi needle (placed painlessly within the medial facet under local anaesthesia).[16,17] In a separate study, I noted that even a light touch to unanaesthetized peripatellar synovium was quite painful[8] (Figure I.3). Histological observations revealed the distribution of nerves in all peripatellar tissues, with the exception of articular cartilage.[18] This was documented by Biedert and Kernen.[18,19]

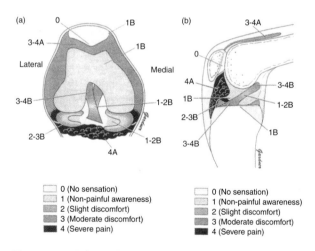

Figure I.3 Schematic representation of a neurosensory map of the human knee obtained by palpation of intraarticular structures of the author's knees without anaesthesia. Perceived pain ranged from 0 (no sensation) to 4 (severe pain) and either (a) accurate spatial localization or (b) poor spatial localization. Palpation of synovium elicited severe localized pain (4a) and similar palpation of patellar articular cartilage was completely without sensation (0). (a) Coronal representation; (b) sagittal representation. Reproduced with permission from Dye et al, 1998[8]

In addition, Wojtys et al[20] have shown the presence of the neuroactive peptide associated with pain perception (substance P) within the nerves of symptomatic peripatellar synovium.

Summarizing the above, one can logically assume that the perception of patellofemoral pain, in most instances, is a function of nociceptive neurological output of any combination of innervated patellar and peripatellar tissues. The most likely candidates for the genesis of nociceptive output resulting in the perception of anterior knee pain, in this author's view, are peripatellar synovium and related soft tissues, as well as the intraosseous environment of the patella. In addition, it is important to assess whether the anterior knee pain may be emanating from a non-patellofemoral source, such as referred pain from an injury to the saphenous nerve or degenerative arthrosis of the ipsilateral hip. Andrish (J.T. Andrish MD, Cleveland Clinic, Cleveland, Ohio, personal communication, 2001) has made the astute observation that in some teenage females the perception of anterior knee pain may represent somatization secondary to possible physical or sexual abuse.

Tissue homeostasis

Pain denotes irritation of peripheral nerves, either mechanically, such as through pinching of the synovium and increased interosseous pressure, or chemically, such as with the presence and production of cytokine enzymes. Pain connotes loss of tissue homeostasis.[21] Normal asymptomatic living structures, such as bone and ligaments, can be described as having the characteristic of tissue homeostasis with constant maintenance of normal physiological processes at the cellular and molecular level, as well as the capability of restoring normal physiological processes after injury (i.e. healing).[22–24] Tissue homeostasis is perhaps best manifested currently in living bone through the use of technetium scintigraphy.[16,17]

The perception of pain evolved throughout hundreds of millions of years of evolution.

The perception of pain is as a type of negative feedback-loop system designed to detect the presence of dangerous conditions and noxious stimuli. Pain alerts the central nervous system of these adverse conditions. Posttraumatic inflammation after tissue overload (e.g. strain, contusion) results in production of a complex biochemical cascade, which includes the fabrication of cytokines that irritate nerve endings and result in the perception of pain. Without this negative feedback-loop system, musculoskeletal components are at constant risk of supraphysiological overload that can lead to permanent structural damage. Patients born with congenital insensitivity to pain exemplify just such cases. Such patients often experience advanced degenerative changes of their joints at a young age.[25] The destructive changes of Charcot joints, following certain conditions that affect the neurological system in adults, also reflect failure of the negative feedback-loop system by decreasing the perception.[26]

A method to manifest sensitively the metabolic characteristics of living bone (technetium 99m methylene diphosphonate scintigraphy) to our clinical and radiological evaluation of patients with anterior knee pain led to the concept of the loss of tissue homeostasis as an important, yet covert, factor in the genesis of symptoms. It was noted that about one-half of our patients with patellofemoral pain demonstrated increased patellar uptake, compared with only 4% of the control subjects ($p < 0.001$).[17] The increased osseous metabolic activity of the patella manifested by the technetium bone scan was proven by biopsy to represent increased remodelling activity of bone, compared with controls without evidence of tumour or infection. Many patients with intensely positive scintigraphic activity had histological findings identical to the findings one sees in the early stages of a stress fracture, manifested by cutting cones and Howship's lacunae.[16] Individuals with anterior knee pain and a positive bone scan were treated conservatively and followed-up clinically. When these patients underwent

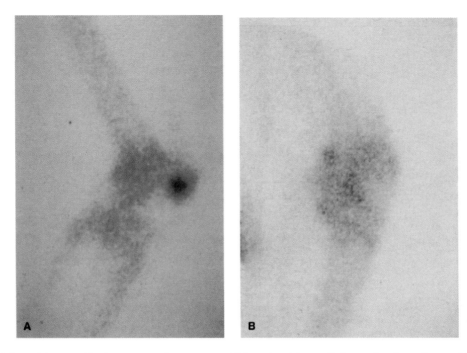

Figure I.4 (a) Positive patellar bone scan of a 32 year-old female with patellofemoral pain and no evidence of malalignment, representing loss of osseous homeostasis. (b) Repeat bone scan of the same patient 4 months later, at the time of symptom resolution, showing restoration of osseous homeostasis. Reproduced with permission from Dye, 2001[32]

follow-up imaging, it was often noted that many who experienced resolution of painful symptoms also demonstrated resolution of the bone scan activity to normal levels[27] (Figure I.4a and b). Therefore, the findings of a positive patellar bone scan came to be interpreted as representing a loss of osseous tissue homeostasis, and that a subsequent normal bone scan demonstrates restoration of osseous homeostasis. The use of technetium scintigraphy was thus viewed as a method to manifest sensitively the presence or absence of tissue homeostasis of the osseous aspect of the patellofemoral joint, which often correlated with the presence of pain and its resolution.[16] Technetium scintigraphy illuminated well the osseous metabolic tile of the mosaic of possible pathological processes accounting for the genesis of patellofemoral pain. Because only one-half of the patients with patellofemoral pain manifested an abnormal bone scan, it was clear that other factors were present to account for the

genesis of symptoms in many patients, in addition to the loss of osseous homeostasis.[17] The innervated peripatellar soft tissues were the obvious nonosseous potential sources of pain. The importance of these peripatellar soft tissues in the genesis of pain can be inferred clinically by the presence of tenderness to palpation of, for example, the patellar tendon, retinaculum or synovium/capsule. It was also logical to interpret the presence of pain and tenderness of the peripatellar soft tissues as representing the symptomatic loss of homeostasis of these tissues. This concept was later proved in synovium with biopsy specimens compared to those of control subjects[22] (Figure I.5a and b).

The *tissue homeostasis perspective* appears to explain, with much greater clarity, the often variable nature of patellofemoral pain from patient to patient that is clearly lacking in the malalignment theory. The variable nature of a given patient's symptoms on a particular day can be viewed, in

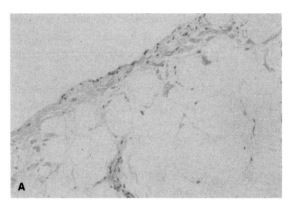
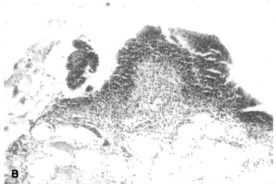

Figure I.5 (a) Biopsy of normal peripatellar synovium and fat pad showing a thin layer of synovial cells and deeper oval fat cells. (b) Biopsy of peripatellar synovium of a patient with patellofemoral pain showing thickening, inflammation and lymphocyte infiltration of the synovium. Reproduced with permission from Dye, 2001[32]

essence, as a function of the variable mosaic of loss of tissue homeostasis of innervated patellar and peripatellar tissues.[22] The presence of sharp pain most often represents mechanical pinching of peripatellar synovium – a tissue that is documented to be well innervated.[8] Such mechanical pinching episodes occur frequently in knees without any evidence of patellofemoral malalignment. The presence of an effusion is also consistent with synovitis as one of the tiles of the mosaic of pathophysiological processes that can account for patellofemoral pain. The dull aching that patients often experience after exercise is understandable as overload and subsequent irritation of innervated tissues. The absence of pain reflects loading that is non-irritating to those innervated tissues. The 'movie-sign', theoretically, is best explained by possible transient increases in intraosseous pressure, as a function of slight venous outflow obstruction that may resolve rapidly with extension or ambulation. One should also be aware of seemingly confounding variables not directly related to patellofemoral loading, such as the perception of patellar pain secondary to changes of barometric pressure. This phenomenon may be attributable to barosensitivity of the intraosseous environment of the sensitized patella.[21] Furthermore, the presence of painful neuromas, as demonstrated by Fulkerson and Hungerford[3] and Sanchis-Alfonso and colleagues[28] in the retinacula

and other peripatellar tissues, can also play a role in the genesis of patellofemoral symptoms.[28,29] These painful neuromas represent a direct neural pathophysiological source of nociception. Small neuromas are unimageable by any current technique, including MRI, and are often diagnosed

Table I.1 Factors influencing patellofemoral nociceptive output

Mechanical environment
   Direct patellofemoral trauma
   Excessive intrinsic compressive and tensile
     forces
     Normal alignment
     Malalignment (load shifting)
   Impingement of intraarticular structures
   Increased intraosseous pressure
   Barometric pressure changes
Chemical environment
   Presence of cytokines
   Altered pH of damaged tissues
Localized peripheral neuropathy
   Painful neuroma
Nonpatellofemoral sources
   Referred pain (such as hip arthrosis)
   Phantom limb pain in above-the-knee amputee

Reproduced by permission from Dye and Vaupel (1994)[21]

only clinically by tenderness to palpation and a positive Tinel's sign, and ultimately by histological analysis following surgical excision. The possible pathological factors that are likely to induce patellofemoral pain are listed in Table I.1. Patellofemoral malalignment can be a factor in the genesis of patellofemoral symptoms, representing, in essence, an internal load-shifting. Its importance, however, is properly put into perspective in a more diminished role than is currently espoused.

Knee as transmission

Since the primary goal of orthopaedic treatment is restoration of joint or musculoskeletal function, what then is the function of the knee? The knee can be thought of as a type of biological transmission system whose purpose is to accept, redirect and ultimately dissipate biomechanical loads.[23] The patellofemoral joint can be seen as a large slide bearing within this living self-maintaining self-repairing transmission system. Ligaments can be viewed as sensate adaptive linkages, with the menisci viewed as mobile sensate bearings. The muscles in this analogy act as living cellular engines, which, in concentric contraction, provide motive forces across the

knee (transmission) and, in eccentric contraction, act to absorb and dissipate shock loads.

The functional capacity of a joint to accept and transfer a range of loads and yet maintain tissue homeostasis can be represented by a load/frequency distribution termed the 'Envelope of Function' (or, alternatively, the 'Envelope of Load Acceptance')[24,25,30] (Figure I.6a). If too little load is placed across a joint for an extended period of time, exemplified by prolonged bed rest, loss of tissue homeostasis can ensue, manifested by muscle atrophy and disuse osteopenia (Figure I.6b). This region of diminished load is termed 'the zone of subphysiological underload'. If excessive loads are placed across a joint, beyond the range of acceptable limits but insufficient to cause macrostructural damage, loss of tissue homeostasis can ensue, manifested in bone by a positive technetium scintigraph before radiographic changes, as exemplified by a stress fracture of the tibia in a long-distance runner. This region of excessive loading is termed the *'zone of supraphysiological overload'*. If sufficiently great loads are placed across a joint or musculoskeletal system, overt macrostructural damage can occur, exemplified by a fracture of bone or a rupture of a ligament. This region of excessive loading

Figure I.6 (a) Graph representing the Envelope of Function for an athletically active young adult. The letters represent loads associated with different activities. All of the loading examples, except *, are within the Envelope of Function for this particular knee. The shape of the Envelope of Function represented here is an idealized theoretical model. The actual loads transmitted across an individual knee under these different conditions are variable and are due to multiple complex factors, including the dynamic centre of gravity, the rate of load application and the angles of flexion and rotation. The limits of the Envelope of Function for the joint of an actual patient are probably more complex. Reproduced with permission from Dye, 1996[23] (b) Graph showing the four different zones of loading across a joint. The area within the Envelope of Function is the zone of homeostasis. The region of loading greater than that within the Envelope of Function but insufficient to cause macrostructural damage is the zone of supraphysiological overload. The region of loading great enough to cause macrostructural damage is the zone of structural failure. The region of decreased loading over time resulting in a loss of tissue homeostasis is the zone of subphysiological underload. Reproduced with permission from Dye et al, 1999[33] (c) Supraphysiological loads outside the Envelope of Function: a dashboard injury, running uphill for 1 hour, and hiking downhill for 2000 m. Reproduced with permission from Dye et al, 1999[22] (d) Diminished Envelope of Function after supraphysiological patellofemoral loading, showing that activities of daily living and activities such as climbing four flights of stairs and pushing a clutch in a vehicle for 2 hours have become supraphysiological loads, leading to recurrent loss of tissue homeostasis and continuance of peripatellar symptoms. Reproduced with permission from Dye et al, 1999[22] (e) Incremental expansion of the diminished Envelope of Function by restricting patellofemoral loading to within the Envelope. Reproduced with permission from Dye et al, 1999[22]

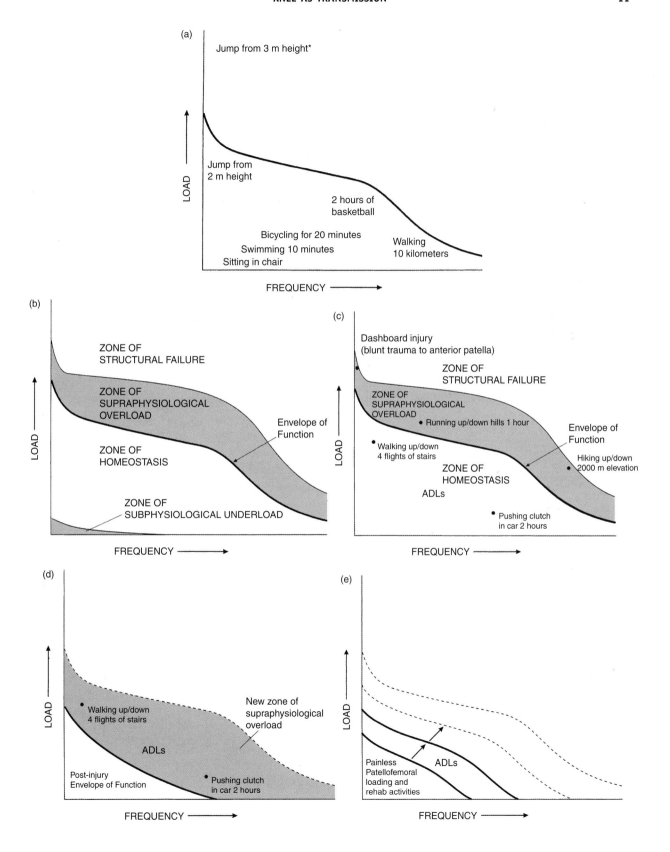

resulting in overt structural damage is termed the *'zone of structural failure'*.

In my opinion, the most common loss of tissue homeostasis, important in the genesis of patellofemoral pain, is in the patient with normal patellofemoral alignment who sustains loading into the region of supraphysiological overload through either a single event or with repetitive loading[21,22] (Figure I.6c). The tissues of the patellofemoral joint sustain the highest loading of any joint, and often function at or near the limits of biological load acceptance and transference capacity.[31] Therefore, these tissues are often the first about the knee to be loaded to the point of supraphysiological failure leading to symptomatic loss of tissue homeostasis, indicated by the perception of anterior knee pain. The Envelope of Function, with a safe range of painless loading, frequently diminishes after an episode of injury to the level where many activities of daily living that previously were once well-tolerated become symptomatic (out of the Envelope of Function) leading to the prolongation of symptoms (Figure I.6d). Decreasing loading to within the newly diminished Envelope of Function allows normal tissue healing processes to proceed to homeostasis most rapidly without recurrent subversion (Figure I.6e). This restriction of loading to pain-free levels is the clear purpose of the evolution-designed negative feedback-loop system; it also corresponds to common sense. Recurrent painful loading out of the Envelope by participating in previously well-tolerated activities, such as stair climbing and arising from or sitting in chairs, only subverts normal healing processes and is a hallmark of chronic patellofemoral pain in many patients.

Therapeutic implications of a tissue homeostasis approach to patellofemoral pain

The goal of any orthopaedic treatment should be to maximize the Envelope of Function for a given joint or musculoskeletal system as safely and predictably as possible. This therapeutic approach emphasizes restoration of tissue homeostasis with the associated resolution of painful symptoms over the achievement of certain measurable structural or biomechanical characteristics of the patellofemoral joint. The tissue homeostasis perspective is inherently empirical, and thus fundamentally safer than many current therapies that are based solely on correction of structural and biomechanical factors thought to be of causal significance. Such structurally and biomechanically orientated treatments can, and often do, result in worsening of anterior knee pain symptoms. An example of these treatments would include an aggressive physical therapy programme solely emphasizing vastus medialis obliquus strengthening to 'correct maltracking' by extension of the knee against resistance. Such an exercise programme can result in increased anterior knee pain. The narrow emphasis on muscle strengthening at the expense of increased patellofemoral symptoms is inherently illogical and violates the medical principle of *primum non nocere*.

In addition, many currently accepted operative approaches to patients with anterior knee pain – based solely on structural and biomechanical characteristics – can inadvertently result in worsening of symptoms. Such procedures would include excessive use of the lateral release, aggressive chondroplasties for findings of chondromalacia, and major proximal and/or distal realignment surgeries.[30] The worst cases of patellofemoral pain and dysfunction that this author has witnessed are in patients who have had multiple surgical procedures for an initial problem of only modest patellofemoral discomfort.

Before the initiation of treatment, a diagnosis should be established. The assessment of patients with patellofemoral pain should concentrate on the history and physical examination, rather than imaging studies. Frequently, a careful history will often elicit an underlying supraphysiological loading event or series of events that preceded the development of symptoms. However, it is not unusual for patients to be unable to identify a specific occurrence of causal significance. Patients may simply report that certain activities of daily living associated with high patellofemoral loading, such as stair climbing, squatting, kneeling or sitting in or arising from chairs, have now become symptomatic. One must also exclude mechanical instability as a cause of symptoms, exemplified by a patellar dislocation or subluxation. Such patients are treated differently.

The clinical examination should be orientated to determine the anatomical site of pain and tenderness, and to assess which loading activities are of importance in the genesis of anterior knee pain. Specific sites of tenderness often lead to specific diagnoses, such as patellar tendinitis, synovitis or retinacular strain. It is also important to have the patient reproduce, if possible, the activities that induce anterior knee pain, e.g. one should assess the knee under load by having the patient step up onto and down from a foot stool. It is important that the exact activities associated with the initiation of and persistence of anterior knee symptoms be identified, so that they can be rigorously controlled. Such painful loading activities are, by definition, out of that patient's Envelope of Function. In addition, one should observe physical characteristics, such as muscle bulk and patellar tracking, and should assess the overall alignment of the limb. One should also assess whether a nonpatellofemoral source may play a role in the genesis of symptoms, such as tight hamstrings or referred pain from an arthritic hip or from saphenous nerve irritation.

There are two basic categories of imaging of the patellofemoral joint: structural imaging [radiographs, computed tomography (CT) and magnetic resonance imaging (MRI)]; and metabolic imaging [technetium scintigraphy and positron emission tomography (PET scanning)]. Standard screening radiographs, including a Merchant's or Laurin's view (axial patellofemoral radiographs), should be obtained to rule out overt structural causes of pain, such as fractures or osseous loose bodies. Minor degrees of patellofemoral tilting and subluxation on axial

radiographs do not, in my experience, reveal much regarding the genesis of anterior knee pain. We noted that degrees of patellar tilting and subluxation did not correlate with the presence or absence of anterior knee pain.[27] In addition, MRI is poor at identifying which of the patellofemoral tissues may be producing pain.[32] As has been shown, even identified structural damage of articular cartilage may not necessarily play a role in the genesis of anterior knee symptoms.[8] A careful examination of MRI of the patellofemoral joint often manifests low-grade effusions associated with symptomatic peripatellar synovitis. This finding frequently goes unreported by radiologists because of their focus on the structural characteristics of joints. Therefore, it is important for the treating orthopaedic surgeon to look at the images directly. I believe peripatellar synovitis to be one of the most common under-diagnosed conditions of clinical significance about the knee. Technetium scintigraphy, which manifests loss of osseous homeostasis, often corresponds well with patellar pain and its resolution.

Treatment of patients with patellofemoral pain from a tissue homeostasis perspective is a logical empirically-based programme aimed at expanding the Envelope of Function for a given patient's knee to its maximum as safely and predictably as possible.[22,23] One must help create, in that patient's joint, the internal biological environment most conducive to restoration of tissue homeostasis, with the associated resolution of pain. Each patient's condition (mosaic of pathophysiological processes and healing potential) is unique. Therefore, the treatment of each case must be individualized. It is the principles of treatment that are most important for healing to occur. In my experience, most patients with patellofemoral pain will respond to the application of three basic principles: (a) correcting the pathokinematics, principally the temporary conditions, but with scrupulous adherence to load restriction within the patient's reduced Envelope of Function; (b) an antiinflammatory programme; and (c) rehabilitation. Loads across the symptomatic patellofemoral joint must be diminished to the point where no new tissue damage or irritation is being created. Simply, the patient must decrease the loading across the symptomatic joint to within its current Envelope of Function, i.e. the range of loading that is clinically painless and most conducive to tissue healing. The patient must be made aware that continuing painful loading activities reflect a subversion of the normal tissue-healing processes. Analogies can be helpful in this instruction to the patient. I believe an extremely common aspect of the mosaic of pathophysiological events associated with anterior knee pain is patellofemoral synovitis. I often liken this process to biting the inside of one's cheek. If one repetitively bites the inside of one's swollen cheek, the painful loss of homeostasis represented by the irritated tissues can persist indefinitely.

Frequently, the activities that are associated with the persistence of patellofemoral pain are readily identified and controllable, resulting in rapid diminution of pain. Simple modifications of the activities of daily living can often be sufficient to achieve such a range of painless patellofemoral loading. The restriction of these loading activities can often be accomplished by the limitation of excessive stair climbing, squatting and kneeling, and similar pain-inducing activities that are currently out of the Envelope of Function for the patellofemoral joint. Modifying the manner in which one sits in and arises from a chair is another activity of daily living that should be addressed. Sitting in a higher chair to keep the knees in a more extended position is often helpful. For women, the temporary use of an elevated toilet seat can also help ameliorate anterior knee pain symptoms. When resting, patients should be instructed to keep the knee in an extended position, which can prevent the deep aching of the 'movie sign'.

An inflammatory component underlies most chronic anterior knee pain, in my opinion. Chronic synovial irritation and cytokine production of various innervated tissues can respond well to simple antiinflammatory treatment, no matter what the specific tissue source. Such an antiinflammatory approach would include tissue cooling and the use of oral nonsteroidal antiinflammatory medications of the therapist's choice. Patients often report improvement of patellofemoral pain with a repetitive tissue cooling programme of icing for 15–20 minutes, two or three times/day. The symptomatic benefit of tissue cooling reflects both a temporary decrease of swelling in inflamed peripatellar tissues, not unlike the use of an ice pack in a patient with a symptomatic swollen cheek. The decrease in metabolic activity results in a temporary decrease in cytokine production within inflamed innervated tissues. One must caution patients against over-cooling the joint, so as not to create a new iatrogenic hypothermal injury.

Rehabilitation, to include *painless* muscle strengthening, stretching and patellofemoral taping, is often beneficial in combination to help create the biomechanical environment most conducive to maximal tissue healing. Some degree of muscle atrophy is common in patients with chronic anterior knee pain. This sign often is interpreted as a primary factor in the genesis of symptoms, when in fact it may represent a secondary phenomenon of disuse. Nonetheless, muscle strengthening, including the vastus medialis obliquus, is considered beneficial. Such strengthening exercises, however, must be performed in a painless manner, i.e. within the Envelope of Function. It does little good to force patients to strengthen the quadriceps musculature in such a way, e.g. painful extension of the knee against resistance, so as to aggravate already sensitive and inflamed peripatellar tissues. What may be beneficial for the muscles/molecular engines may be bad for the knee tissues/biological transmission. Stretching of tight structures, such as the hamstrings and retinacula, often is beneficial, and also should be performed in a slow, measured fashion, so as not to create new tissue damage. The absence of pain is the best indicator that the involved structures are not being injured.

Patellar taping, often termed 'McConnell taping' after the Australian physical therapist who developed it,[2] can be of great benefit if it results in noticeable pain reduction. I believe the often dramatic improvement of patellofemoral discomfort with this technique reflects a decrease in mechanical irritation of the peripatellar tissue (not unlike using a finger to pull away the swollen cheek tissue from the teeth), rather than representing a correction of patellofemoral malalignment. Patellofemoral taping may also increase the beneficial proprioceptive characteristics of the joint. This frequently successful technique is best used temporarily to protect the symptomatic joint while tissue homeostasis/healing occurs. It is not designed for long-term use. Patients who use prolonged taping can experience other problems, such as skin irritation.

The mosaic of loss of tissue homeostasis leading to patellofemoral pain is often one of crisis and resolution. I am unaware of any physical therapy technique that has resulted in documented permanent correction of indicators of malalignment (e.g. high Q angle and shallow femoral trochlear sulcus) after successful nonoperative treatment. The knowledge of the concepts of safe patellofemoral loading, as exemplified by the Envelope of Function, can be a powerful tool in the resolution of symptoms in and of itself. Using these concepts, patients have a much better understanding of the biomechanical environment that induced their symptoms. With regards to bracing, an elastic knee sleeve with a patellar relief zone can be helpful in many patients. Some patients report improvement with braces designed to correct maltracking. The use of bracing is a logical choice if the symptoms are controlled. Nonrigid orthotics can also be beneficial to many patients.

The treatment programme must be individualized and empirical, meaning that the patient must be helped to find his/her Envelope of Function, antiinflammatory therapy, and exercise programme that results most reliably in pain reduction. It is not unlike trying to find the numbers to a combination lock. The solution is unique and the patient must be helped to find it from inherently safe treatment choices. The patient should persist in the treatment principles long enough for healing to occur. Once the painful symptoms have resolved, the patient may gradually and incrementally increase patellofemoral loading. Our experience with technetium scintigraphy, with documented resolution of patellofemoral pain along with restoration of osseous homeostasis, revealed that a period of 6–9 months of conservative therapy is often required for a successful nonoperative treatment programme.[17] However, many patients can experience resolution of their patellofemoral symptoms much sooner. One often must be diligent and persevere with the principles of this programme to be successful. The first pain-free moment does not mean that the Envelope of Function has been fully restored, but instead that healing is most likely occurring. The tissue homeostasis approach is inherently safe, in that any treatment factor that results in increased symptoms of patellofemoral pain is stopped immediately. When in doubt, go to the safe region of the Envelope of Function by decreasing loading. No one programme will work for all patients, because the underlying mosaic of pathophysiology and tissue healing potential are unique to the individual patient.

Patellofemoral surgery

Patellofemoral surgery can be beneficial as part of a tissue homeostasis approach to anterior knee pain, but it must be approached rationally and cautiously.[9] As noted previously, the worst cases of patellofemoral pain and dysfunction are often in patients who have had multiple operative procedures in an attempt to correct supposed chondromalacia or malalignment. The initial surgery is often a lateral release, with or without an aggressive chondroplasty, followed by additional attempts at improving the alignment characteristics of the symptomatic joint. Reversing the high rate of failure after surgery for patellofemoral pain is one of the greatest orthopaedic challenges that remain in this century. In this author's opinion, the high rate of failure results almost entirely from the belief that patellofemoral malalignment or chondral injury is the primary cause for patellofemoral pain.

Surgery performed from a tissue homeostasis perspective must be logically aimed at those aspects of the mosaic of pathophysiology responsible for the genesis of anterior knee pain most amenable to operative intervention. Not all 'tiles' of the mosaic can be addressed with surgery, so improvement rather than complete resolution to painless function after surgery is most common. Operative procedures must be done in a manner that respects patellofemoral tissues by being as gentle as possible, so as not to create an additional injury to the joint. In this author's experience, most patients with chronic peripatellar pain that does not resolve with the conservative treatment principles outlined above, have peripatellar synovitis as a substantial aspect of their problem. Careful arthroscopic removal of swollen and inflamed peripatellar synovium can be helpful[32] (Figure I.7a and b). However, through the years, I have learned that one must follow certain basic principles to help achieve improvement with the use of such surgery. The inflamed synovium must

be carefully removed so that one can visualize the inferior articular cartilage surface of the patella. There are few occurrences more metabolically irritating to a living knee than a substantial haemarthrosis. Thus, the avoidance of a postoperative haemarthrosis is *essential*. This is achieved most often by meticulous interoperative haemostasis following the arthroscopic debridement of impinged synovium. I always drain the knee with an 1/8 inch (3.2 mm) diameter haemovac for at least a few hours following surgery and occasionally overnight, depending on the output. Approximately 40 ml of 1% lidocaine with 1:100 000 epinephrine is injected in the synovium and fat pad tissues deep to the region of the synovectomy. In addition, 50 ml of 0.25% marcaine with 1:200 000 epinephrine and 10 mg of morphine is often injected into the knee through the haemovac tube, which is then clamped for a period of at least 15 minutes to 1 hour to allow the epinephrine and morphine to have an ameliorative effect. This is followed by application of a compressive dressing. The patient is then instructed to remain at a low level of activity for several days following surgery (I liken this temporary restriction of loading after surgery as similar to letting a souffle set without banging the oven door). Following the operative procedure, the patient must help create the internal

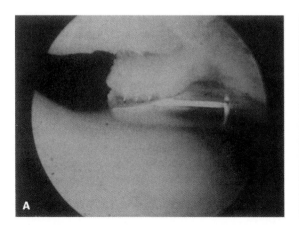 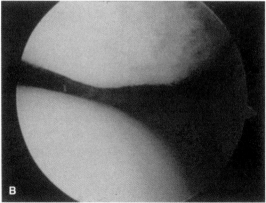

Figure I.7 Peripatellar synovectomy in a patient with patellofemoral pain. (a) Before synovectomy; (b) after synovectomy. Reproduced with permission from Dye et al, 1999[22]

conditions to allow healing to occur most rapidly. In my experience, this is accomplished most often by icing five or six times/day for 15–20 minutes, the use of painless straight-leg raising, and the initiation of an appropriate careful, reasoned and painless postoperative rehabilitation programme the week following the surgery. In addition, a gentle conservative chondroplasty may be beneficial to stabilize a region of chondral damage. I disagree that aggressive drilling, picking procedures, mosaicplasties or cartilage transplantation techniques in the patellofemoral region are indicated in most cases. The biomechanical environment in this region is often just too severe for long-term success of most cartilage replacement techniques. Removal of loose bodies can also be helpful.

A lateral release should be performed only in the setting of a documented tight lateral retinaculum, as described by Fulkerson and Hungerford.[3] Personally, I rarely perform this procedure, despite seeing a large number of symptomatic patellofemoral pain cases. The rate of performance of the lateral release within the International Patellofemoral Study Group has dramatically decreased during the past decade, as it has been recognized that this operation is not a panacea and has inherent dangerous characteristics. Major proximal and distal realignments for patellofemoral pain are more dangerous because they often involve extensive tissue dissection and osteotomy of innervated osseous structures. The long-term results of such procedures are inherently unpredictable, no matter how well the patellofemoral joint may appear to be tracking at the time of surgery. The unpredictability is attributable to factors beyond the surgeon's control, including the development of differential postoperative muscular atrophy and possible alteration of cerebellar sequencing of motor-unit firing. In most cases, such major surgery should be contemplated only for a demonstrated recurrent symptomatic patellofemoral instability or for established patellofemoral arthrosis.

Restoration of tissue homeostasis (healing) of perturbed highly loaded tissues involved in the genesis of patellofemoral pain is a result of billions of years of molecular and cellular evolutionary refinements. Respecting the special nature of the patellofemoral joint through a careful empirical treatment programme designed to maximize healing as predictably and safely as possible is best in most cases. Failing this, a careful analytical surgical approach may be warranted.

References

1. Hillsgrove DC, Paulos L (1995) Complications of patellofemoral surgery. In: *The Patella*. Berlin, Springer-Verlag, pp 277–290
2. Grelsamer RP, McConnell J (1998) *The Patella. A Team Approach*. Gaithersburg, MD, Aspen
3. Fulkerson JP, Hungerford DS (1990) *Disorders of the Patellofemoral Joint*, 2nd edn. Baltimore, MD, William & Wilkins
4. Bentley G (1970) Chondromalacia patellae. *J Bone Joint Surg Am* **52**: 221–232
5. Bentley G, Dowd G (1984) Current concepts of etiology and treatment of chondromalacia patellae. *Clin Orthop* **189**: 209–228
6. Insall J, Falvo KA, Wise DW (1976) Chondromalacia patellae. A prospective study. *J Bone Joint Surg Am* **58**: 1–8
7. DeHaven KE, Collins HR (1975) Diagnosis of internal derangements of the knee. The role of arthroscopy. *J Bone Joint Surg Am* **57**: 802–810
8. Dye SF, Vaupel GL, Dye CC (1998) Conscious neurosensory mapping of the internal structures of the human knee without intraarticular anesthesia. *Am J Sports Med* **26**: 773–777
9. McGinty JB, McCarthy JC (1981) Endoscopic lateral retinacular release: a preliminary report. *Clin Orthop* **158**: 120–125
10. Radin EL (1979) A rational approach to the treatment of patellofemoral pain. *Clin Orthop* **144**: 107–109
11. Kimball ES (1991) *Cytokines and Inflammation*. Boca Raton, FL, CRC Press
12. Grelsamer RP (2000) Patellar malalignment. *J Bone Joint Surg Am* **82**: 1639–1650

13. Dye SF, Boll DH (1985) An analysis of objective measurements including radionuclide imaging in young patients with patellofemoral pain. *Am J Sports Med* **13**(abstr): 432

14. Thomee R, Renstrom P, Karlsson J, Grimby G (1995) Patellofemoral pain syndrome in young women. I. A clinical analysis of alignment, pain parameters, common symptoms, and functional activity level. *Scand J Med Sci Sports* **5**: 237–244

15. Stäubli HU, Dürrenmatt U, Porcellini B, Rauschning W (1999) Anatomy and surface geometry of the patellofemoral joint in the axial plane. *J Bone Joint Surg Br* **81**: 452–458

16. Dye SF, Chew MH (1993) The use of scintigraphy to detect increased osseous metabolic transmission with an envelope of function. *J Bone Joint Surg Am* **75**: 1388–1406

17. Dye SF, Boll DA (1986) Radionuclide imaging of the patellofemoral joint in young adults with anterior knee pain. *Orthop Clin North Am* **17**: 249–262

18. Biedert RM, Stauffer E, Friederich NF (1992) Occurrence of free nerve endings in the soft tissue of the knee joint. A histologic investigation. *Am J Sports Med* **20**: 430–433

19. Biedert RM, Kernen V (2001) Neurosensory characteristics of the patellofemoral joint: What is the genesis of patellofemoral pain? *Sports Med Arthrosc Rev* **9**: 295–300

20. Wojtys EM, Beaman DN, Glover RA, Janda D (1990) Innervation of the human knee joint by substance-P fibers. *Arthroscopy* **6**: 254–263

21. Dye SF, Vaupel GL (1994) The pathophysiology of patellofemoral pain. *Sports Med Arthritis Rev* **2**: 203–210

22. Dye SF, Stäubli HU, Biedert RM, Vaupel GL (1999) The mosaic of pathophysiology causing patellofemoral pain: therapeutic implications. *Operative Tech Sports Med* **7**: 46–54

23. Dye SF (1996) The knee as a biologic transmission with an envelope of function: a theory. *Clin Orthop* **325**: 10–18

24. Guyton AC, Hall JE (1986) *Textbook of Medical Physiology.* Philadelphia, PA, WB Saunders

25. Hirsch E, Moye D, Dimon JH III (1995) Congenital indifference to pain: long-term follow-up of two cases. *South Med J* **88**: 851–857

26. Koshino T (1991) Stage classifications, types of joint destruction, and bone scintigraphy in Charcot joint disease. *Bull Hosp Jt Dis Orthop Inst* **51**: 205–217

27. Dye SF, Peartree PK (1989) Sequential radionuclide imaging of the patellofemoral joint in symptomatic young adults. *Am J Sports Med* **17**: 727

28. Sanchis-Alfonso V, Roselló-Sastre E, Monteagudo-Castro C, Esquerdo J (1998) Quantitative analysis of nerve changes in the lateral retinaculum in patients with isolated symptomatic patellofemoral malalignment. A preliminary study. *Am J Sports Med* **26**: 703–709

29. Sanchis-Alfonso V, Roselló-Sastre E (2000) Immunohistochemical analysis for neural markers of the lateral retinaculum in patients with isolated symptomatic patellofemoral malalignment. A neuroanatomic basis for anterior knee pain in the active young patient. *Am J Sports Med* **28**: 725–731

30. Dye SF (2001) Therapeutic implications of a tissue homeostasis approach to patellofemoral pain. *Sports Med Arthritis Rev* **9**: 306–311

31. Dye SF (1994) Functional anatomy and biomechanics of the patellofemoral joint. In: Scott JE (ed), *The Knee.* St. Louis, Mosby, pp 381–389

32. Dye SF (2001) Patellofemoral pain current concepts: an overview. *Sports Med Arthritis Rev* **9**: 264–272

33. Dye SF, Wojtys EM, Fu FH et al (1999) Factors contributing to function of the knee joint after injury or reconstruction of the anterior cruciate ligament. *Instr Course Lect* **48**: 185–198

PART II

1 Anatomy

Roland M. Biedert and **Niklaus F. Friederich**

The patellofemoral joint consists of multiple components that function in a complex synergistic functional interplay. The asymmetrical design and functional morphology reflect the requirements of high biomechanical loading.

Patellofemoral articulation

Patella

The central structure of the patellofemoral articulation is the patella. The patella, a sesamoid bone, possesses the thickest articular cartilage of all human joints and provides a central point of attachment for ligaments and tendons. The patella exists at the centre of numerous static and dynamic vector forces. The proximal part of the patella is embedded in the quadriceps tendon, lies extraarticularly and has no articular surface[1] (Figure 1.1). The intraarticular part extends from the quadriceps tendon to the inferior patellar pole. It partially forms the anterior suprapatellar pouch. The inferior articular surface of the patella does not have full contact with the trochlea during the range of motion. The medial patellar facet, with a thick articular cartilage, is poorly

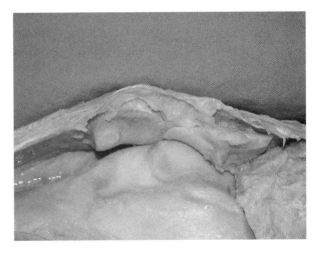

Figure 1.1 Sagittal anatomy of the patella in relation to the quadriceps tendon, the suprapatellar pouch, the patellar ligament and the Hoffa fat pad (view from medial side, left knee)

congruent with the medial trochlea, whereas the lateral articular patellar facet is reasonably congruent with the lateral part of the trochlea.[1] Also, the distal end of the patella (patellar apex) is embedded in ligamentous tissue, the patellar ligament. Directly posterior to the patellar apex and the patellar ligament is the infrapatellar fat pad (Hoffa's fat pad).

Patellofemoral Disorders: Diagnosis and Treatment. Edited by Roland M. Biedert
© 2004 John Wiley & Sons, Ltd ISBN: 0-470-85011-6

Infrapatellar fat pad (Hoffa)

The anterior intraarticular space of the knee joint is filled with the infrapatellar fat pad (Figure 1.2). The fat pad lies in an extrasynovial and intracapsular space. It has direct contact to the patellar ligament, the medial and lateral longitudinal retinacula and the anterior head of the tibia. It is held in place by the alar plicae, projecting into the sides of the joint space, and in most of the cases by the infrapatellar synovial plica. The fat pad has a rich nerve supply and is well-vascularized. Knee flexion and maximal knee extension cause compression of the fat pad by the patellar ligament.

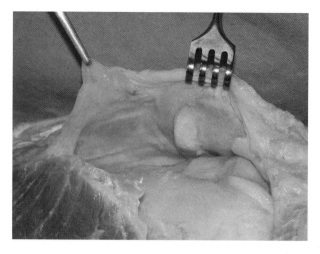

Figure 1.3 Suprapatellar synovial pouch

Suprapatellar synovial pouch and plica fold

The suprapatellar synovial pouch (recess) is the most proximal part of the intraarticular cavity with a relation to the patellofemoral joint (Figure 1.3). Proximally, the articularis genus muscle attaches to the pouch; anteriorly, the synovial folds are attached to the most posterior deep layer (vastus intermedius muscle) of the quadriceps and medial and lateral to the retinacula.[2-4] The posterior wall of the suprapatellar pouch is formed by the femur, covered

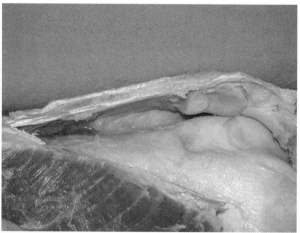

Figure 1.4 Suprapatellar pouch with supratrochlear fat pad on the anterior side of the femur

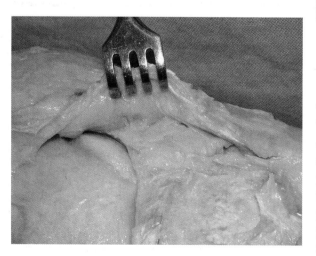

Figure 1.2 Infrapatellar fat pad in relation to the bordering structures (view from medial side, left knee)

with the supratrochlear fat pad (Figure 1.4). The suprapatellar plica originates laterally at the oblique portion of the vastus lateralis muscle and attaches to the rectus intermedius at the proximal part of the patella.[3] It continues distally around the medial patella to connect to the medial infrapatellar fat pad (Figure 1.5). A medial plica fold parallels the vastus medialis obliquus and the medial patellofemoral ligament. Both the suprapatellar pouch and the plica folds are dynamically controlled by the articularis genus muscle.

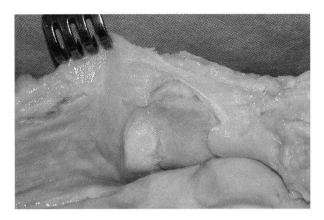

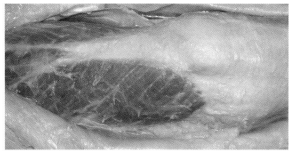

Figure 1.7 Insertion of the vastus medialis and obliquus muscles on the medial patella

Figure 1.5 Supra- and mediopatellar plica in relation to the infrapatellar fat pad

In knee flexion, a normal and free suprapatellar pouch guarantees the unrestricted movements of the quadriceps tendon, the patella and the plica. With these, the patellofemoral joint moves smoothly and unrestricted.

Quadriceps muscle

The quadriceps muscle consists of different muscle groups – the vastus lateralis and obliquus,[5] vastus intermedius, rectus femoris, and vastus medialis and obliquus muscles[3] (Figure 1.6).

The rectus femoris lies on the vastus intermedius centrally and parallel to the femur.[6] The vastus medialis consists of two muscle groups according to their orientation to the patella and inserts on the superomedial third of the patella, the medial retinaculum and the patellofemoral

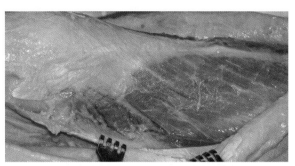

Figure 1.8 Insertion of the vastus lateralis and obliquus muscles

ligament (Figure 1.7). The vastus lateralis muscle fibres insert on the superolateral corner of the patella and some of the fibres insert more proximally[6] (Figure 1.8). The tendinous insertion of the vastus lateralis obliquus may show different anatomical patterns: origin beneath the main muscle belly of the vastus lateralis and then circling inferiorly and anteriorly to insert obliquely on the quadriceps tendon; interdigitation with the superficial oblique retinaculum and not completely with the quadriceps tendon; or interdigitation with the superficial oblique retinaculum receiving the vastus lateralis obliquus muscle without contributing to the patellar tendon.[5] The tendinous fibres of the vastus intermedius insert directly into the proximal patella deeper than the remaining three tendons.[6]

The separate muscle groups have different insertional patterns and dynamic vectors: vastus lateralis 30–40°; vastus lateralis obliquus

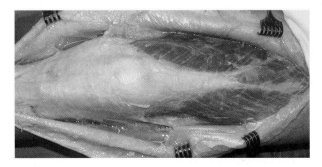

Figure 1.6 Quadriceps muscle group

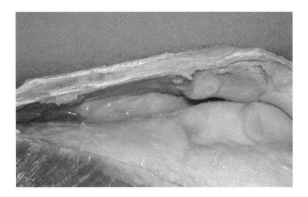

Figure 1.9   Different layers of the quadriceps tendon in relation to the patella and suprapatellar pouch

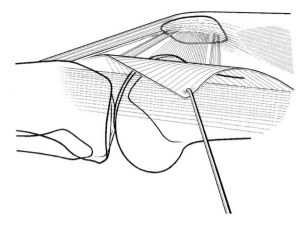

Figure 1.10   Anatomy of the lateral retinaculum – superficial and deep layers

38–48°; vastus medialis 15–25°; and vastus medialis obliquus 50–65°[3–5,7] (Figure 1.6).

The quadriceps tendon inserts on the proximal pole of the patella and continues distally as a tendinous expansion over the anterior patella (galea aponeurotica) to merge with the patellar tendon[6] (Figure 1.9). Most of the fibres anterior to the patella are in continuation of the rectus femoris tendon.[6] The quadriceps tendon consists of different layers: the superficial layer of the rectus femoris, the middle layers of the vastus medialis and lateralis, and the deep layer of the vastus intermedius.[2,8] The superficial anterior layer of the rectus femoris is extraarticular; the deepest posterior layer of the vastus intermedius is lined with articular synovium.[2]

Lateral side

Lateral retinaculum

The lateral retinaculum is a fibrous connective tissue structure on the lateral side of the knee. It is composed of two anatomical layers – superficial and deep[9–11] (Figure 1.10).

The superficial oblique retinaculum

The superficial oblique retinaculum fibres originate from the iliotibial tract and interdigitate with

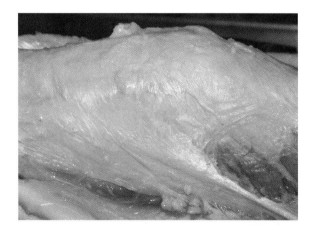

Figure 1.11   Lateral retinaculum in relation to the iliotibial tract, the patella and the patellar tendon

longitudinally orientated fibres of the vastus lateralis tendon on the lateral border of the patella and the patellar tendon[9,11] (Figure 1.11). Most fibres of the superficial retinaculum proceed into the anterior part of the patellar tendon; some deep fibres go to the patellar tendon to overlap the capsule anteriorly.[10] The thickness of this superficial retinaculum decreases distally[10] (Figure 1.12).

The deep transverse retinaculum

Deep into the layer of the superficial oblique retinaculum are the fibres of the deep transverse

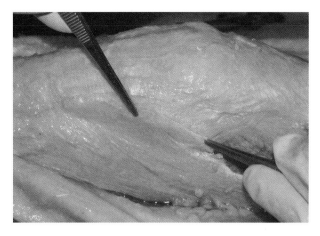

Figure 1.12 Superficial oblique retinaculum after longitudinal parapatellar incision

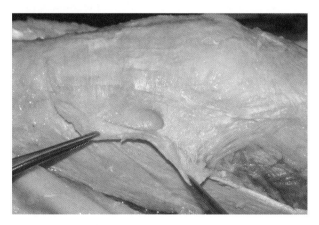

Figure 1.13 Deep transverse retinaculum after separation from the superficial layer (hold with forceps)

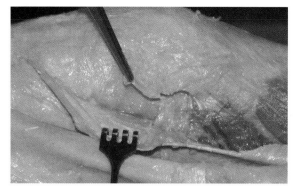

Figure 1.14 Capsulosynovial layer after incision of the deep transverse retinaculum (hold with forceps)

retinaculum.[10,11] It runs from the deep part of the fascia lata directly to the lateral patella (Figure 1.13). In contrast to the superficial layer, these fibres do not extend distal to the patella and do not insert into the patellar tendon. Hence, at the level of the patellar tendon there exists only the superficial oblique retinaculum with no underlying deep transverse fibres.[10] In the lower border of the deep transverse retinaculum, a distinct patellotibial ligament can be found. Its fibres may proceed directly out of the distal patella or from the iliotibial band to insert obliquely in the lateral meniscus and tibia (Figure 1.10).[10] At the superior border of the deep transverse retinaculum, the epicondylopatellar ligament runs from the lateral intermuscular septum and the lateral epicondyle to the lateral patella.[10] The patellotibial and epicondylopatellar ligaments tether the patella to the anterolateral tibia and the lateral epicondyle (Figure 1.1).

Both the superficial and the deep retinaculum are dynamized by the vastus lateralis, tensor fasciae latae (iliotibial tract) and gluteus maximus muscles (iliotibial tract). Through the contributions of the iliotibial tract and the fascia lata in the formation of the lateral retinacula, a posterolateral force is exerted on the patella during knee flexion.[9] The main function of the lateral retinacula is to control patellofemoral tracking and to equalize compressive loads between the medial and lateral facets of the patella.[1] These anatomical findings and connections must be considered when performing any kind of surgical interventions on the lateral retinacula.

Beneath the deep transverse retinaculum is a thin capsulosynovial layer[10] (Figure 1.14). Although capsule and synovium could be separated into two distinct layers, they are quite adherent and also, as combined structures, relatively thin.

Medial side

The medial soft tissue stabilizers of the patella include the medial retinaculum and the medial

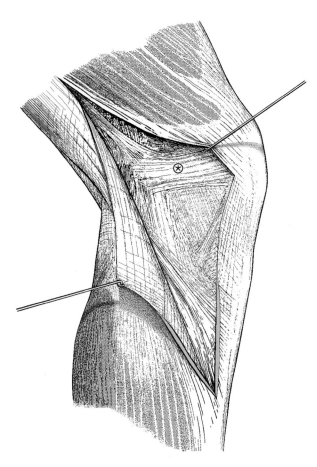

Figure 1.15   Graphic of the medial structures (★, medial patellofemoral ligament)

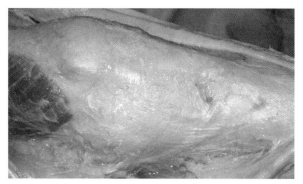

Figure 1.16   Medial patellar retinaculum

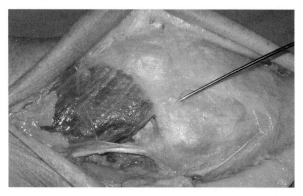

Figure 1.17   Medial patellofemoral ligament (running over the hook) with the insertion sites and the 'bare spot'

patellofemoral and patellomeniscal ligaments (Figure 1.15).

Medial retinaculum

The medial patellar retinaculum arises broadly between the patella, vastus medialis and medialis obliquus and passes distally to the medial head of the tibia, where it inserts posterior to the pes anserinus and anterior and proximal to the medial collateral ligament[1] (Figure 1.16).

Medial patellofemoral ligament

The medial patellofemoral ligament is an extracapsular structure.[12] The ligament is variable in size and thickness and consists of a proximal and distal bundle; the width has been described to be on average 1.9 cm and the length 5.3 cm.[13,14] The medial patellofemoral ligament is a continuation of the deep retinacular surface of the vastus medialis obliquus muscle fibres.[12] The middle part of the ligament joins the undersurface of the musculus vastus medialis obliquus.[14] Proximally, the ligament extends to the distal muscle fibres of the vastus medialis obliquus and is adherent to the deep fascia of the vastus medialis obliquus[15] (Figure 1.17). Laterally, the ligament extends from the proximal two-thirds of the patella, both as a direct insertion and with fibres joining the suprapatellar quadriceps fibres.[14] The majority of the medial patellofemoral ligament fibres originate with a firm bony attachment on the

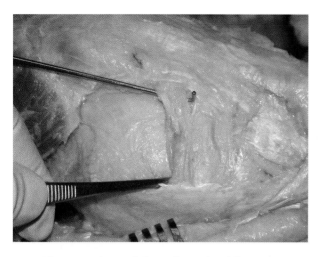

Figure 1.18 Medial patellomeniscal ligament

medial epicondyle.[6,14] The ligament originates just anterior to the insertion of the medial collateral ligament and distal to the insertion of the adductor magnus tendon.[12] Some superficial fibres of the medial patellofemoral ligament may cross over the adductor tubercle and blend into the posterior soft tissue. The adductor tubercle is the insertion site for the adductor magnus tendon.[12] The superior edge of the medial patellofemoral ligament, the adductor magnus tendon and the vastus medialis form a constant triangle ('bare spot') (Figure 1.17).

Patellomeniscal ligament

The medial patellomeniscal ligament extends from the inferior medial margin of the patella through and in close relation to the infrapatellar fat pad[14] (Figure 1.18). It has a wide distal insertion to the anterior horn of the medial meniscus. The medial patellomeniscal ligament is the second most important restrictor (after the medial patellofemoral ligament) to lateral patellar dislocation, contributing 13–22% of the total force.[14,16,17]

References

1. Hunziker EB, Stäubli HU, Jakob RP (1992) Surgical anatomy of the knee joint. In: Jakob RP, Stäubli HU (eds), *The Knee and the Cruciate Ligaments*. Heidelberg, Springer-Verlag, pp 31–47

2. Stäubli HU, Bollmann C, Kreutz R et al (1999) Quantification of intact quadriceps tendon, quadriceps tendon insertion, and suprapatellar fat pad: MR arthrography, anatomy, and cryosections in the sagittal plane. *Am J Roentgenol* **173**: 691–698

3. Terry GC (1989) The anatomy of the extensor mechanism. *Clin Sports Med* **8**: 163–177

4. Hughston JC, Walsh WM, Puddu G (1984) *Patellar Subluxation and Dislocation. Saunders Monographs in Clinical Orthopaedics*, Volume V. Philadelphia, PA, WB Saunders

5. Hallisey MJ, Doherty N, Bennett WF, Fulkerson JP (1987) Anatomy of the junction of the vastus lateralis tendon and the patella. *J Bone Joint Surg Am* **69**: 545–549

6. Panni AS, Biedert RM, Maffulli N et al (2002) Overuse injuries of the extensor mechanism in athletes. *Clin Sports Med* **21**: 483–498

7. Malone T, Davies G, Walsh WM (2002) Muscular control of the patella. *Clin Sports Med* **21**: 349–362

8. Zeiss J, Saddemi SR, Ebraheim NA (1992) MR imaging of the quadriceps tendon: normal layered configuration and its importance in cases of tendon rupture. *Am J Roentgenol* **159**: 1031–1034

9. Ford DH, Post WR (1997) Open or arthroscopic lateral release. Indications, techniques, and rehabilitation. *Clin Sports Med* **16**: 29–49

10. Fulkerson JP, Gossling HR (1980) Anatomy of the knee joint lateral retinaculum. *Clin Orthop* **153**: 183–188

11. Nonweiler DE, DeLee JC (1994) The diagnosis and treatment of medial subluxation of the patella after lateral retinacular release. *Am J Sports Med* **22**: 680–686

12. Arendt EA, Fithian DC, Cohen E (2002) Current concepts of lateral patella dislocation. *Clin Sports Med* **21**: 499–519

13. Conlan T, Garth WP Jr, Lemons JE (1993) Evaluation of the medial soft-tissue restraints of the extensor mechanism of the knee. *J Bone Joint Surg Am* **75**: 682–693

14. Tuxoe JI, Teir M, Winge S, Nielsen PL (2002) The medial patellofemoral ligament: a dissection study. *Knee Surg Sports Traumatol Arthrosc* **10**: 138–140

15. Feller JA, Feagin JA Jr, Garrett WE (1993) The medial patellofemoral ligament revisited. An anatomical study. *Knee Surg Sports Traumatol Arthrosc* **1**: 184–186

16. Sallay PI, Poggi J, Speer KP, Garrett WE (1996) Acute dislocation of the patella. A correlative pathoanatomic study. *Am J Sports Med* **24**: 52–60

17. Desio SM, Burks RT, Bachus KN (1998) Soft tissue restraints to lateral patellar translation in the human knee. *Am J Sports Med* **26**: 59–65

Suggested reading

Ford DH, Post WR (1997) Open or arthroscopic lateral release. Indications, techniques, and rehabilitation. *Clin Sports Med* **16**: 29–49

Fulkerson JP, Gossling HR (1980) Anatomy of the knee joint lateral retinaculum. *Clin Orthop* **153**: 183–188

Tuxoe JI, Teir M, Winge S, Nielsen PL (2002) The medial patellofemoral ligament: a dissection study. *Knee Surg Sports Traumatol Arthrosc* **10**: 138–140

2 Cross-sectional Anatomy with Regard to CT and MRI Geometry

Roland M. Biedert and **Hans Ulrich Stäubli**

Osseous anatomy

The anatomy and geometry of the patellofemoral joint show numerous variations.[1-3] Anatomical dissections have revealed differences of the osseous contours of the femur and patella.[3] The variations of the form of the distal femur are important for the patellofemoral contact area. Müller and Wirz[3] described great differences in the size of the trochlea in the craniocaudal and mediolateral dimensions (Figures 2.1, 2.2,

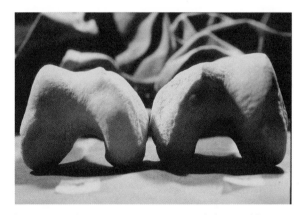

Figure 2.2 Convex osseous contour of the trochlea (left) and normal concave form of the trochlea (right) (view from distal). Reproduced with permission from Müller and Wirz[3], © 2000 Steinkopff-Verlag

2.3 and 2.4). The trochlea can vary in length, width, depth and shape. These variations in anatomy and geometry can be documented by CT (Figures 2.5, 2.6 and 2.7) or MRI (Figures 2.8, 2.9 and 2.10). Müller[2] also described a different configuration and length of the medial and lateral femoral condyle. The medial condyle is longer than the lateral. There exists a difference in the length of the annular sector of the femoral

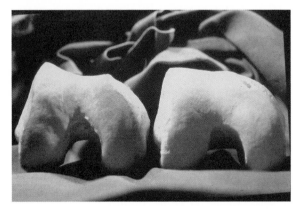

Figure 2.1 Flat trochlea (right) and normal trochlea (left) (view from distal). Reproduced with permission from Müller and Wirz[3], © 2000 Steinkopff-Verlag

Patellofemoral Disorders: Diagnosis and Treatment. Edited by Roland M. Biedert
© 2004 John Wiley & Sons, Ltd ISBN: 0-470-85011-6

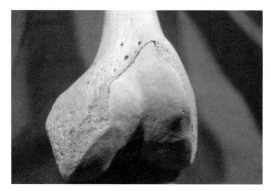

Figure 2.3   Normal trochlea with longer articular surface on the lateral side (view from ventral). Reproduced with permission from Müller and Wirz[3], © 2000 Steinkopff-Verlag

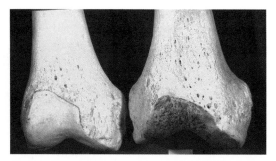

Figure 2.4   Very short trochlea (right) and hypoplastic medial trochlea (left) (view from ventral). Reproduced with permission from Müller and Wirz[3], © 2000 Steinkopff-Verlag

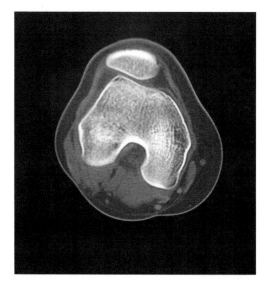

Figure 2.5   Dysplastic trochlea with flat lateral condyle (CT, axial view, extension)

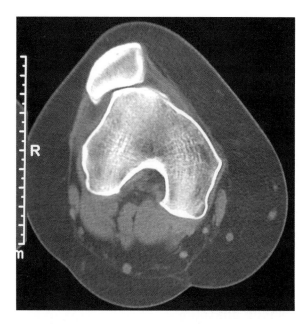

Figure 2.6   Central bump with convex osseous contour of the trochlea (CT, axial view, extension)

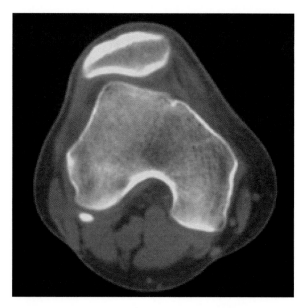

Figure 2.7   Dysplastic trochlea with flat lateral condyle and hypoplasia of the medial trochlea (CT, axial view, extension)

condyle between the trochlea and the medial condyle, the annular sector which determines the amount of the automatic final rotation.[2,3]

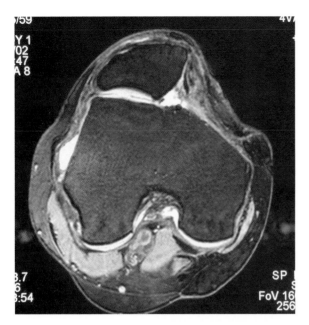

Figure 2.8 Flat lateral condyle with dysplastic trochlea (MRI, axial view, extension)

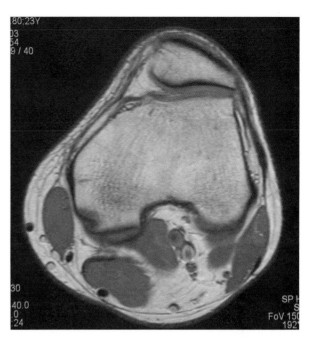

Figure 2.10 Hypoplasia of the trochlea (MRI, axial view, extension)

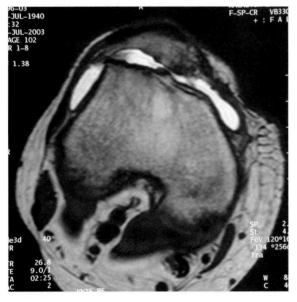

Figure 2.9 Central bump with convex form of the trochlea. Severe osteoarthritis of the patellofemoral joint (MRI, axial view, extension)

The automatic rotation at the beginning of flexion or the end of extension between the tibia (external) and the femur (internal) has great influence on the position of the patella in the trochlea.[2] Therefore, it is important to image precisely any existing variations of configuration and congruence of the articular cartilage and the subchondral bone of the patellofemoral joint.

Cryosections and MRI

Axial plane

Cross-sections (cryosections) from cadaver knees and magnetic resonance (MR) arthrotomograms reveal surface differences of the articular cartilage of the trochlea and patella.[1] The shape and geometry of the articular cartilage and subchondral bone vary, depending on the level of the section in the axial plane. There is gradual shifting of the articular cartilage contact zone from proximal–lateral (Figure 2.11) to central (Figure 2.12) to distal–medial (Figure 2.13). Considerable intraspecimen and interspecimen variations have been documented.[1] Stäubli et al[1] showed that the ridge of the articular cartilage of the patella

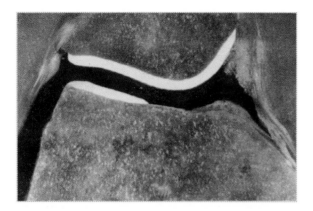

Figure 2.11 Axial cryosection through the proximal part of the joint. The articular cartilage surface and the subchondral osseous prominence of the patella match, whereas the asymmetry of cartilage cover of the intercondylar sulcus is obvious. The contact zone of the patellofemoral cartilage is located on the lateral part of the trochlea. Reproduced with permission from Stäubli et al,[1] © 1999 *J Bone Joint Surg Br*

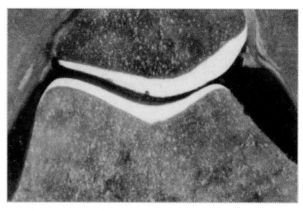

Figure 2.13 Axial cryosection through the distal part of the joint. The patellofemoral contact area is asymmetrical medially. Intercondylar cartilage and osseous part of the trochlea match, whereas asymmetry is noted on the patella. Reproduced with permission from Stäubli et al,[1] © 1999 *J Bone Joint Surg Br*

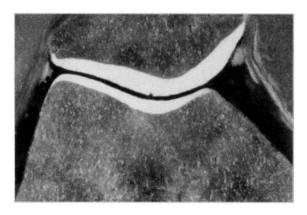

Figure 2.12 Axial cryosection through the middle of the joint. The deepest part of the intercondylar cartilage sulcus is medial to the deepest part of the femoral trochlea. The articular cartilage surfaces match perfectly, but asymmetry of the subchondral osseous contours is present. Reproduced with permission from Stäubli et al,[1] © 1999 *J Bone Joint Surg Br*

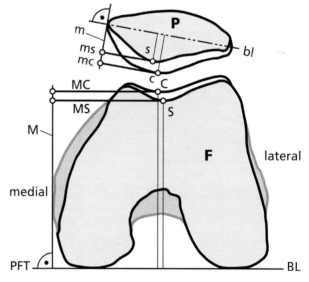

Figure 2.14 Asymmetrical medial ridge with respect to the osseous contour of the patella (P). The deepest part of the intercondylar cartilage sulcus (C) is medial to the deepest part of the femoral trochlea (S). The articular cartilage surfaces match perfectly. Osseous contours do not match. m, Medial tangent patella; M, medial tangent femur; s, subchondral bony prominence; c, cartilage ridge. Reproduced with permission from Stäubli et al,[1] © 1999 *J Bone Joint Surg Br*

was more often lateral to the corresponding subchondral osseous prominence than medial or coincident (Figure 2.14). They also examined the concavities of the deepest part of the surface of the articular cartilage of the intercondylar sulcus and the corresponding deepest point of the femoral groove. They found that in most cases the deepest part of the articular cartilage of the intercondylar sulcus is lateral to the corresponding deepest point of the femoral trochlea[1] (Figure 2.15). The points can correspond or be more medial. In conclusion, the osseous anatomy of the patellofemoral joint often does not match with the corresponding surface geometry of the articular cartilage, but individual intraspecimen matching of opposing articular cartilage surfaces in the contact area is evident. Therefore, imaging modalities reflecting the opposing surface geometry of the articular cartilage are recommended in cases where subtle pathoanatomy requires more precise analysis.[1,4] Accurate insight into the congruence of the articular surfaces is possible using intraarticular injection of a contrast medium for double-contrast arthrography, axial CT arthrotomography or MR arthrotomography.[1]

Sagittal plane

Standard sagittal radiographs in 30° knee flexion are used to document patellar height, degenerative joint disease, patella bimultipartita, osseous fragments, patellar tilt and trochlear dysplasia.[5-14] Standard radiographs document the osseous contour of the patella and distal femur and the position of the patella in reference to the trochlea.[10-12,15] Thickness and condition of the articular cartilage can only be measured using MR arthrotomography[1,16] (Figure 2.16). Bosshard et al[16] measured the contour congruence of the articular cartilage surface and the corresponding subchondral bone of the patellofemoral joint in the sagittal plane. They documented contour incongruence of the articular cartilage surfaces and the corresponding subchondral bone in all knees. The subchondral bone

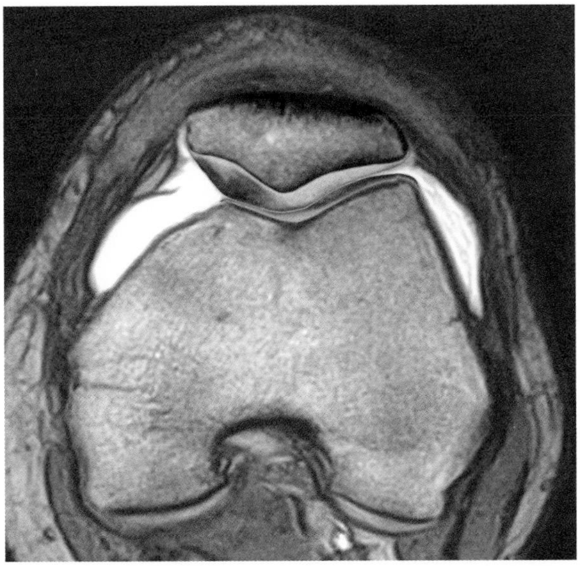

Figure 2.15 Asymmetry between the cartilage ridge and the osseous prominence of the patella. The intercondylar cartilage sulcus and the osseous part of femoral trochlea have a symmetrical shape. The patellofemoral contact zone is asymmetrical medially. There exists a medial patellofemoral contact area distally. Reproduced with permission from Stäubli et al,[1] © 1999 *J Bone Joint Surg Br*

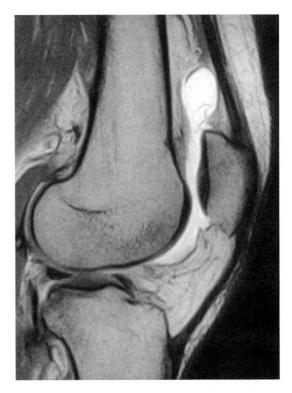

Figure 2.16 Sagittal MR arthrotomography documenting the incongruence between cartilage and osseous contours in the patellofemoral joint

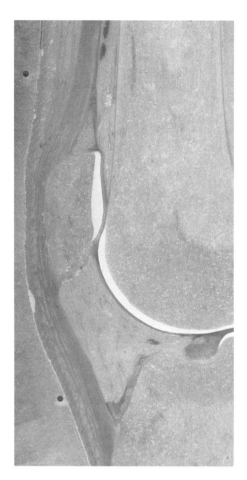

Figure 2.17 Articular cartilage surface of the patella with the corresponding subchondral bone in the sagittal plane. Reproduced with permission from Bosshard et al, 1997,[16] © 1997 Springer-Verlag

exhibited an anterior convexity, whereas the corresponding articular cartilage contour exhibited a posteriorly convex contour[16] (Figure 2.17). The articular cartilage was thickest close to the zone of anterior convexity of the subchondral bone. Therefore, this finding of the osseous contour has no significance for the condition of the articular cartilage. Bosshard et al[16] also found no contour congruence of the articular cartilage surface and subchondral bone of the patellofemoral joint. In conclusion, the osseous anatomy in the sagittal plane of the patellofemoral joint does not correspond with the articular cartilage surface.

Statements about dysplasia of the patellofemoral joint using only standard radiographs must be interpreted with caution and awareness of this fact.

Summary

The anatomy and geometry of the distal femur are individually different. Variations of the osseous and articular joint surface morphology can be easily identified. There exists a significant lateral-to-central-to-medial shift in the contact zone of the patellofemoral articular cartilage contact area from proximal to distal. Exact analysis of the joint congruence and the complex surface geometry is needed to depict any pathology of the patellofemoral joint and to tailor the necessary treatment.

Radiographs and CT scans are helpful as screening methods or in specific cases. CT arthrotomography or MRI arthrotomography may offer an accurate insight into the functional congruence of the articular surfaces. Knowledge about the anatomy and geometry as well as precise evaluation is necessary for successful treatment.

References

1. Stäubli HU, Dürrenmatt U, Porcellini B, Rauschning W (1999) Anatomy and surface geometry of the patellofemoral joint in the axial plane. *J Bone Joint Surg Br* **81**: 452–458

2. Müller W (1982) *Das Knie*. Heidelberg, Springer-Verlag

3. Müller W, Wirz D (2000) Anatomie, Biomechanik und Dynamik des Patellofemoralgelenks. In: Wirth CJ, Rudert M (eds), *Das patellofemorale Schmerzsyndrom*. Darmstadt, Steinkopff-Verlag, pp 3–19

4. Witonski D (2002) Dynamic magnetic resonance imaging. *Clin Sports Med* **21**: 403–415

5. Blackburne JS, Peel TE (1977) A new method of measuring patellar height. *J Bone Joint Surg Br* **59**: 241–242

6. Walch G, Dejour H (1989) [Radiology in femoro-patellar pathology]. *Acta Orthop Belg* **55**: 371–380

7. Insall J, Salvati E (1971) Patella position in the normal knee joint. *Radiology* **101**: 101–104

8. Hughston JC, Walsh WM, Puddu G (1984) *Patellar Subluxation and Dislocation. Saunders Monographs in Clinical Orthopaedics*, volume V. Philadelphia, PA, WB Saunders

9. Macnicol MF (1986) *The Problem Knee*. London, William Heinemann Medical Books

10. Dejour H, Walch G, Nove-Josserand L, Guier C (1994) Factors of patellar instability: an anatomic radiographic study. *Knee Surg Sports Traumatol Arthrosc* **2**: 19–26

11. Dejour H, Walch G, Neyret P, Adeleine P (1990) [Dysplasia of the femoral trochlea]. *Rev Chir Orthop Reparatrice Appar Mot* **76**: 45–54

12. Nove-Josserand L, Dejour D (1995) [Quadriceps dysplasia and patellar tilt in objective patellar instability]. *Rev Chir Orthop Reparatrice Appar Mot* **81**: 497–504

13. Caton J, Deschamps G, Chambat P et al (1982) [Patella infera. Apropos of 128 cases]. *Rev Chir Orthop Reparatrice Appar Mot* **68**: 317–325

14. Wiberg G (1941) Roentgenographic and anatomic studies on the femoropatellar joint. *Acta Orthop Scand* **12**: 319–410

15. Goutallier D, Beaufils P, Bernageau J et al (1999) Pathologie fémoro-patellaire. In: *Le Cahiers d'Enseignement de la SOFCOT 1999 Concernant la Pathologie Fémoro-patellaire.*

16. Bosshard C, Stäubli HU, Rauschning W (1997) Konturinkongruenz von Gelenkknorpeloberflächen und subchonralem Knochen des Femoropatellargelenks in der sagittalen Ebene. *Arthroskopie* **10**: 72–76

Suggested reading

Bosshard C, Stäubli HU, Rauschning W (1997) Konturinkongruenz von Gelenkknorpeloberflächen und subchonralem Knochen des Femoropatellargelenks in der sagittalen Ebene. *Arthroskopie* **10**: 72–76

Stäubli HU, Dürrenmatt U, Porcellini B, Rauschning W (1999) Anatomy and surface geometry of the patellofemoral joint in the axial plane. *J Bone Joint Surg Br* **81**: 452–458

3 Patellofemoral Joint Biomechanics

Andrew A. Amis, A. M. J. Bull, F. Farahmand, W. Senavongse and **Y. F. Shih**

From the viewpoint of a bioengineer, it is easy to see why there are so many clinical problems associated with malfunction of the patellofemoral joint. It is also clear that this is related to a complex and subtle set of interacting variables, some of which, such as torsional alignment of the leg, are not clearly associated with the patellofemoral joint itself. It does not require detailed examination to realize that this is a joint that has rather incongruent articular surfaces that are not configured to ensure great stability. The patella is a small bone that has a large range of motion around the distal femur, and it acts as the focus for a set of powerful muscles that converge onto it from a range of directions. The medial and lateral retinacular structures that help to guide the patella along its path of motion, and stabilize it against leaving that normal path, appear to be small and weak when compared to the size of the muscles.

The description above shows that normal function of the patellofemoral joint relies on many interactions between the different mechanisms. These can be classified under three main headings:

♦ Static stability factors – the geometry of the joint surfaces.

♦ Active stability factors – the muscle tensions.

♦ Passive stability factors – the retinaculae.

Although there is an extensive literature relating to the patellofemoral joint and this is not the first book devoted entirely to this small joint, the fact remains that there is little quantitative data available on how all the different stability factors compare in importance, or how they relate to each other. It seems, therefore, that we are still lacking much of the fundamental objective scientific knowledge that will be needed to set out a rational derivation of how to treat this joint. One of the aims of this chapter is to show how knowledge of the different factors that influence the mechanical workings of the patellofemoral joint is being gained by scientific work, both in the laboratory and *in vivo*.

Geometry and contact areas of the patellofemoral joint

While the overall shapes of the joint surfaces are described in the anatomy chapters, it is worthwhile to examine them in greater detail from the mechanical viewpoint.

Patellofemoral Disorders: Diagnosis and Treatment. Edited by Roland M. Biedert
© 2004 John Wiley & Sons, Ltd   ISBN: 0-470-85011-6

There have been a number of studies that have made detailed measurements of the articular geometry, relating to both the alignment and shape of the joint. In them, these aspects then relate to patellar tracking kinematics and to joint stability, respectively. From the clinical viewpoint, patellofemoral stability is a major concern. This will be examined in the section on Patellofemoral joint forces, below. For now, however, it is sufficient to note that stable tracking of the patella along the patellar groove of the femoral trochlea will be aided by deepening the groove. This will lead to the slopes of the medial and lateral trochlear facet being both higher and steeper – they are more difficult for the patella to climb up and over, if there is any tendency towards dislocation.

There have been different descriptions of the orientation of the trochlear groove in relation to the femur. The mechanical axis of the femur passes from the centre of the knee to the centre of the hip, while the anatomical axis passes along the shaft of the femur. These diverge by approximately 6°. Many knee prostheses have been made with the trochlear groove perpendicular to the joint space, aligned to the mechanical axis.[1] However, many geometric studies in the past were based on either dry bones or radiographs that did not include the articular cartilage. Stäubli et al [2] noted that the articular cartilage has variable thickness across the joint surfaces, and so the real articular surfaces are not the same shapes as the underlying bones. This is a good reason for examining MR images, rather than CT radiographs. When measuring the cartilage surfaces, Shih et al (YF Shih and colleagues, Mechanical Engineering Department, Imperial College London, UK; manuscript submitted for publication) found that the trochlear groove deviated laterally by 19° from the femoral axis (13° from the sagittal plane, perpendicular to the transepicondylar axis) as it passed distally/posteriorly. This should be related to patellar tracking kinematics.

Measurements of trochlear groove geometry are often based on the transepicondylar axis as the measurement datum. If 'skyline' views are examined in relation to this axis,[3] it is seen that the lateral facet of the trochlea is both wider and higher than the medial facet anteriorly, in a skyline view that is looking proximally, parallel to the femur. As the femur flexes, the skyline moves distally and then posteriorly. As this view changes, so the lateral facet becomes less prominent and the medial facet becomes more prominent (Figures 3.1 and 3.2). The large lateral facet in extension is the feature that must 'capture' the patella when the knee starts to flex, to ensure that it is guided into the trochlear groove. The larger the lateral facet is, the more the laterally acting resultant joint force provides a relatively uniform level of contact pressure across the width of the patella.[4] In the section on Patellar joint forces, below, these forces are discussed.

The sulcus angle measures how deep or shallow is the trochlear groove. It is defined as the angle joining the most prominent points of the medial and lateral edges of the trochlea to the deepest point to the groove, in a skyline view (Figure 3.1). A smaller sulcus angle means a deeper groove and, hence, a more stable joint. The sulcus angle is typically 140° in extension, range 116–151° in normal knees;[3,5] the range varies a small amount with knee flexion.

A transverse skyline section of the trochlear sulcus shows that it is not just two straight lines, as implied by the sulcus angle measurement. The two facets are linked by a rounded concave central groove. This merges into convex condylar outlines medially and laterally. The convex outline means that the slope of the facets increases towards the centre of the groove, and so a congruent patella will be located stably there. It also means that, if the initial stability has been overcome and the patella subluxes laterally, it will also tilt laterally.

The articular surface of the patella has a complex geometry that is described approximately by dividing it into two slightly concave facets that are congruent with those of the trochlear surfaces when the knee is flexed. These facets are separated

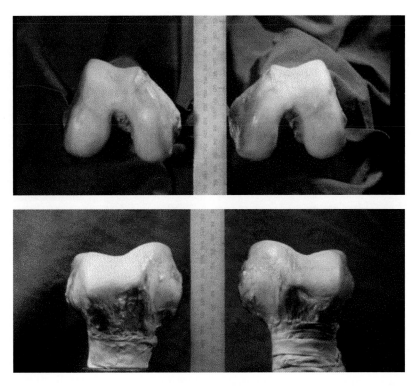

Figure 3.1 The lateral trochlear facet is most prominent anteriorly, engaging the patella in the extended knee (top). The medial facet becomes more prominent as the knee flexes (bottom)

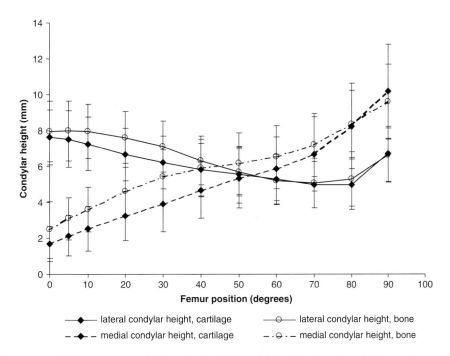

Figure 3.2 Graph showing the variation of the height of the lateral and medial trochlea with flexion

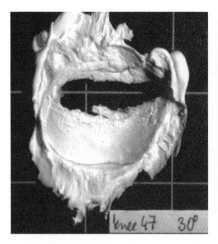 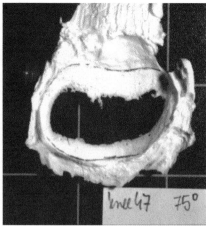

Figure 3.3 As the knee flexes, so the contact area spreads across the width of the patella, increases and migrates proximally. The contact areas shown were obtained by silicone rubber moulding of the joint at 30° and 75° of knee flexion

by a convex ridge that runs proximal–distal. The lateral facet is larger, so that it can resist the larger forces applied by the Q-angle effect. More detailed analyses of the geometry have subdivided these facets into variable numbers of articulations. These 'subarticulations' have limited functional significance, apart from the 'odd' facet on the extreme medial edge of the patella, which articulates against the medial femoral condyle in deep knee flexion when the patella is bridging across the intercondylar notch.[6]

If the patellar articular geometry is studied in the sagittal plane, it is convex distally and concave proximally. This shape is different from that of the underlying bone, which is slightly concave from proximal to distal on a lateral view radiograph. If the cartilage is imaged, we see that the thickness is not constant and that the distal convexity of the articular surface corresponds to localized cartilage thickening.

The contact area of the patellofemoral joint is important because a small contact area, which arises from incongruent joint surfaces, leads to large articular cartilage contact stresses caused by the joint forces. When the knee starts to flex, the initial contact area on the patella is on the distal end of the central ridge, as the convex surface

starts to meet the sulcus. As the patella engages the trochlea at approximately 20° of knee flexion, so the contact areas spreads rapidly across the width of the distal patella (Figure 3.3). In deeper knee flexion, the contact area migrates proximally to the concave area. This allows the patella to fit congruently to the femur, and so the joint force is spread over a large contact area. This pattern of increasing contact area, to reduce the stresses, fits perfectly to the way that the joint forces increase with knee flexion, and also to the way that the knee kinematics control the location of the contact area (see the next section on Patellar kinematics). Finally, with the knee flexed beyond 90°, there are two separate contact areas: the lateral facet of the patella rests on the distal aspect of the lateral femoral condyle, while the 'odd' medial facet wedges against the lateral-facing slope of the medial femoral condyle, at the edge of the intercondylar notch.

Patellar kinematics

A review of published work on patellar kinematics[7] shows that there have been many measurement methods, both *in vitro* and *in vivo*, that many different patellar tracking patterns have been

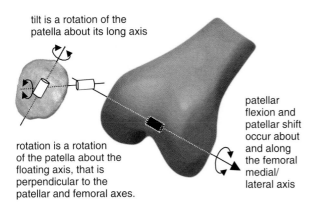

tilt is a rotation of the patella about its long axis

patellar flexion and patellar shift occur about and along the femoral medial/lateral axis

rotation is a rotation of the patella about the floating axis, that is perpendicular to the patellar and femoral axes.

Figure 3.4 Measurement of patellar motion is shown using a fixed femoral axis and a 'floating' axis within the patella. Reproduced with permission from Bull et al, 2001[14]

described, and that few data have been obtained from analyses of real load-bearing dynamic activities *in vivo*.[8–13]

All three-dimensional movements require the measurement of six degrees of freedom of motion to describe them fully. These are three linear translations and three rotations that occur around mutually perpendicular axes. The most useful system of measurements is defined in Figure 3.4.[14] In this system, which is known as a 'floating axes' system,[15] some of the axes about which measurements are taken remain fixed in the femur (e.g. the medial–lateral axis) while others move with the patella (e.g. the proximal–distal axis of the patella, around which the patella tilts). This system corresponds most closely to readily understandable clinical meanings and measurements. Because clinical measurements are most often made in cases of suspected patellar maltracking, when the patella may tend to leave the trochlear groove, the most important of the six degrees of freedom are patellar medial–lateral translation and patellar tilt, which were recognized as a form of malalignment by Laurin et al.[16] The largest motions, of course, are those due to knee flexion, when the patella translates distally and posteriorly, from the anterior to the distal aspect of the distal femur, while rotating in flexion.

In early knee flexion, the patella translates distally, before it starts to flex around the femoral articulation. Because of this, patellar flexion lags approximately 30% behind tibiofemoral (knee) flexion. It should be remembered that not all authors have used this system in their reports. The most common alternative is to define the patellar motion in relation to the femur. However, this can be confusing because the physical meanings of the rotations can change as the knee flexes, e.g. a rotation around the femoral axis in the extended knee corresponds to patellar tilt, whereas that same measured rotation in a flexed knee is now measuring what is defined as medial–lateral rotation (Figure 3.4).

Patellar medial–lateral tracking during knee flexion has most often been described as having an initial phase of medial patellar translation, as the patella engages the trochlear groove in the first 20° of knee flexion, followed by a progressive lateral translation from 20° to 90° of knee flexion. Figure 3.5 shows the range of patellar tracking measurements that have been published, among which is seen the predominant pattern just described. Figure 3.6 shows the range of patellar tilting measurements that have been reported. With measurements of such small

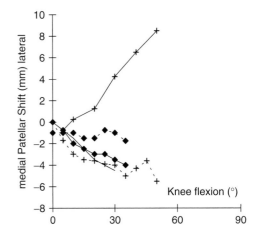

Figure 3.5 Variation of patellar medial–lateral translation during knee flexion, obtained from a review of published data. Reproduced with permission from Katchburian et al, 2003[7]

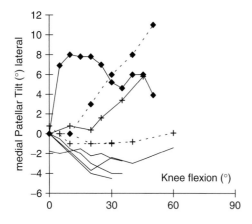

Figure 3.6 Variation of patellar medial–lateral tilting rotation during knee flexion, obtained from a review of published data. Reproduced with permission from Katchburian et al, 2003[7]

rotations, it is clear that the results will depend sensitively on the exact definition of the axes of motion, and on how the measurements are made. Beyond noting the differences in the studies, it seems that the only conclusion to be reached is that patellar tilt is over a relatively small arc of motion and is probably not far from zero in many knees. The remaining degree of freedom is patellar medial–lateral rotation, which occurs around an axis embedded in the patella, i.e. perpendicular to the plane of the patella. This is influenced by tibial internal–external rotation because the tibial tubercle moves medial–lateral during these rotations; this alters the direction in which the patellar tendon is pulling the distal pole of the patella. Although this may have some effect on the patellofemoral joint contact areas, especially in tibial torsion, the patellar rotation movement is believed to have little clinical significance.

Patellofemoral joint forces

The most important joint-force characteristics do not require sophisticated engineering analysis for them to become clear. It is obvious that the strength of the quadriceps muscles will cause large tensile forces in the extensor apparatus,

and that this muscle force tends to pull the patella onto the femur most strongly in the flexed knee.

The contact area between the patella and the femur is at the distal part of the patella when the knee is in extension and moves proximally across the patella as the knee flexes. This mechanism is a direct result of the pattern of forces acting. If the forces acting on the patella are examined in the sagittal plane, they may be simplified into three force vectors – the quadriceps and patellar tendon tensions and the compressive joint force. This is, of course, a simplification – the quadriceps tension is the single resultant force obtained by allowing for all the muscle heads, and the joint force is the resultant force obtained by allowing for contributions across the width of the trochlea. It is assumed that other forces, such as retinacular tensions, are small enough to be neglected here. If an object has three forces acting on it, then it can be proved that the force vectors must intersect at a point if the object is in equilibrium. Knowing the lines of action of the muscle and tendon forces, this intersection rule allows us to predict the line of action of the joint force. Also, because the articulation has low friction, the joint force will be almost entirely compressive and have no significant shearing component. Therefore, the joint force vector must act perpendicular to the surfaces. Figure 3.7 shows the configuration of the knee at two angles of flexion. The lines of muscle and tendon tensions were added, and then the joint-force vector was drawn in accordance with the rules described. It shows how the contact force is distal on the patella with the knee near extension, and proximal in the flexed knee.

The relative magnitudes of the forces can also be derived, based on a further rule of equilibrium – that the three force vectors must combine to zero resultant force. This means that we can construct a force vector triangle, starting from a chosen value of patellar tendon tension (Figure 3.7). If the quadriceps tension and joint-force vectors are added in the correct directions,

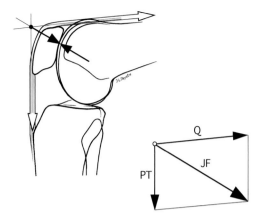

Figure 3.7 Near knee extension, the patellar tendon (*PT*) tension and quadriceps (*Q*) tension oppose each other and result in a small joint force, *JF*. In the flexed knee, *PT* and *Q* combine to cause a much larger joint force, *JF*, for the same value of *PT*. The quadriceps tension *Q* is also much larger, for the same *PT*, in the flexed knee. The joint force *JF* is distal on the patella in the extended knee, and proximal in the flexed knee, because it must be directed at the intersection of the lines of *PT* and *Q*

then their lines of action will intersect to form a triangle. The magnitudes of the three forces are in proportion to the lengths of the three force vectors in each triangle. This allows us to find further information.

When the knee is near extension, the patellofemoral contact force is seen to be much smaller than the patellar tendon force or quadriceps tendon force. In the flexed knee, for the same magnitude of patellar tendon tension, the joint contact force is now much larger and exceeds the patellar tendon tension (Figure 3.7). This is the underlying mechanism that explains the 'movie sign', when an arthritic patellofemoral joint is painful in the flexed knee. The rise in patellofemoral contact force that accompanies knee flexion does not inevitably lead to increased contact pressure to be borne by the articular cartilage. This is because, as already noted, the contact area rises significantly as the knee flexes, and so the ratio of force per unit contact area does not rise in the same way as the joint force. This is the underlying reason why the

patella is concave in the sagittal plane and, hence, congruent with the femur, in the proximal part of the articular surface.

As the knee flexes, so the angle between the quadriceps and patellar tendon tensions reduces. This means that their tensions add vectorially to give a larger resultant force that pulls the patella onto the femur. This effect does not continue to increase beyond approximately 70° of knee flexion, because the central part of the quadriceps tendon rests on the femoral trochlea and wraps around the bone as flexion increases further.[17] Thus, the angle of the quadriceps to the patella does not increase beyond 70° of knee flexion.

A further effect is also visible in the force vector triangles in Figure 3.7, i.e. the ratio between the quadriceps and patellar tendon tensions changes as the knee flexes. Near knee extension, the quadriceps and patellar tendon tensions are approximately equal, and so the output force (the patellar tendon tension) is nearly the same as the input force (the quadriceps tension). This is not the case in the flexed knee. The quadriceps tension is clearly larger than the patellar tendon tension, and so the output force is only approximately 70% of the input force. Thus, in the flexed knee, a given extension force at the foot or ankle will require approximately 50% more muscle tension than if the knee is near extension (neglecting other effects that will be described in following paragraphs).

This variable force ratio effect has only been recognized comparatively recently. Before the 1970s it was thought that the patellar tendon tension would always be the same as the quadriceps tension, because the patellofemoral joint has low friction and the distal femur would act like a low-friction pulley. This argument is an approximation to the truth following a patellectomy, when the tendons do simply wrap and slide around the end of the femur, but does not hold up in the face of the equilibrium analysis.

A simplified model explains the changing patellar tendon:quadriceps tension ratio. Figure 3.8 shows a block, which represents the patella,

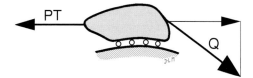

Figure 3.8 Representation of forces acting on the patella in the flexed knee. To ensure left–right equilibrium, the horizontal components must be equal and so *Q* has to be larger than *PT*

resting on a flat surface, which represents the femur, via low-friction rollers. It is being pulled left and right by the patellar tendon and quadriceps tensions. These are shown acting in approximately their correct physiological directions, relative to the body of the patella, for a flexed knee. To maintain equilibrium, the opposing left–right tension components must be equal and opposite, as drawn. It is clear that the quadriceps tension has to be larger than that in the patellar tendon to ensure equilibrium.

A number of investigators[17–19] have measured the patellar tendon and quadriceps tensions *in vitro* and have thus proved the engineering analysis. The general trend of all of these results followed the analysis – a tension ratio of unity near extension, falling to 0.7 at 90° of knee flexion and maintaining that ratio thereafter. Some of these experiments revealed that the patellar tendon tension was actually *larger* than the quadriceps tension (1.1 times) with the knee approaching full extension. Our initial thought was that this must be an error. However, there is a rational explanation for this result. Close to full extension, the initial patellofemoral contact is between the distal end of the patella, where it is convex and domed, and the proximal-facing edge of the trochlea. This geometry causes the joint reaction force to angle proximally, thus augmenting the quadriceps tension.

For people with a sedentary lifestyle, the patellofemoral joint is loaded most heavily when rising from a chair, and the elderly may find that this activity demands their maximum knee extension strength. The mechanical reason for

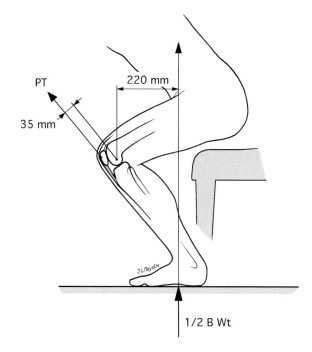

Figure 3.9 Static analysis of forces when rising from a chair. The foot must be on the line of the body weight, posterior to the knee, so there is a large flexing moment that must be overcome by the extension moment, so *PT* × 35 mm = 0.5 *BW* × 220 mm. If *BW* = 750 N, *PT* tension = 2343 N, *Q* = 3347 N and *JF* = 40084 N (5.45 *BW*)

this is seen in Figure 3.9. The knee is a long way anterior to the line of action of body weight when sitting. The foot–floor contact must be on the line of action of the body weight, and so the knee has to be flexed more than 90°. The maximum isometric knee extension moment in this situation is 82 Nm in males, and 59 Nm in females.[20] This corresponds to half of the body weight of 750 N acting on a line 220 mm posterior to the centre of rotation of the knee (Figure 3.9). The patellar tendon (PT) tension must produce an equal and opposite knee extension moment: with a PT moment arm of 35 mm, the PT tension must equal 2343 N (3.12 body weight). Knowing that the PT:Q ratio = 0.7 in the flexed knee, the quadriceps tension Q will be 3347 N (4.46 body weight). If PT and Q act at 90° to each other (Figure 3.7), then the patellofemoral joint force =

4084 N (5.45 BW). While these forces seem large, another study[21] has reported knee extension moments 50% larger than these, leading to correspondingly higher joint forces. Note that this was a simple 'static' force analysis – the movement was slow enough to neglect the inertial effects that arise from the accelerations of the limb segments during gait.

As the knee extends, so the flexing action of the body weight reduces, because the knee moves posteriorly, closer to the line of action of the body weight. In full extension, or hyperextension, the centre of rotation of the knee passes posterior to the line of body weight, and so a standing posture allows the quadriceps to relax completely.

A final factor relating to the mechanics of the extensor mechanism, which can be found in Figure 3.7, relates to the changing orientation of the patellar tendon as the knee flexes. When the knee is near extension, the patellar tendon is directed anteriorly, away from the tibia. As the knee flexes, this anterior angulation reduces to zero, beyond which the patellar tendon has a posteriorly directed component of its tension. In this situation, the anterodistal aspect of the femur acts like a cam, and the patella is the cam follower. Although this phenomenon is often referred to as 'femoral roll-back', the centres of the circular femoral condyles do not move far posteriorly in relation to the tibia as the knee flexes, but the distance from these points to the patella on the sagittal outline of the femur decreases greatly and the patellar tendon swings posteriorly by approximately 35° as the knee flexes.[22]

There are two practical effects arising from the alteration of the direction of the patellar tendon tension, that relate to the cruciate ligaments and to the efficiency of knee extension. First, the changing angle means that a knee extension effort will tend to sublux the tibial plateau anteriorly when the knee is in an extended posture, thus tensing the anterior cruciate ligament. Conversely, the posterior slope of the patellar tendon when the knee is in a flexed posture means that an extension effort will then tense the posterior

cruciate ligament.[23] The effects of various knee rehabilitation exercises on anterior cruciate ligament strains have been measured by Beynnon and Fleming,[24] who confirmed the 'quads neutral' angle of approximately 60° of knee flexion when the patellar tendon is parallel to the tibia. This mechanism may also contribute to posterior cruciate ligament ruptures in falls onto the flexed knee. Not only does the tibia get displaced posteriorly when the body weight impacts onto the tibial tubercle, but the rapid stretching of the quadriceps before impact will have led to a high tension that also will have tended to pull the tibia posteriorly, and therefore load the ligament before the impact.

The second effect arising from the changing patellar tendon angle with knee flexion is that this reduces the moment arm of the extensor mechanism. If a knee extension effort is analysed, the patellar tendon tension needed rises as the moment arm about the centre of rotation reduces. In a simplified sagittal plane model, this moment arm approximates to the perpendicular distance from the patellar tendon to the intersection of the cruciates (Figure 3.10).

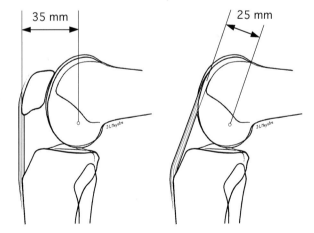

Figure 3.10 The knee extension moment is the product of the tension PT and the moment arm, the distance between the line of action of PT and the centre of rotation of the joint. Patellectomy reduces the moment arm, and so a larger PT is needed to have the same knee extension strength

The effect described above shows why patellectomy causes the knee to be disadvantaged mechanically. Figure 3.10 shows how the loss of the patella means that the line of action of the patellar tendon drops back further, until it is tangential to the patellar groove. Therefore, to obtain the same knee extension moment, the patellar tendon tension may have to rise 30–40% after a patellectomy.[25] This effect is so important that the main function of the patella has been described as being its role in elevating the line of the patellar tendon tension away from the front of the femur.[26]

While the effect described may be true when the knee is near extension, the picture is rather more complex in deep flexion, and not necessarily as bad as suggested by the analysis above. This is important because it affects the ability of a weak patient to rise from a seated posture, when the body weight must be raised from a position with more than 90° of knee flexion. That is necessary to bring the feet back to a position coincident with the line of action of the body weight. In this posture with an intact knee, an earlier analysis (Figures 3.7 and 3.8) showed that the quadriceps tension was approximately 1.5 times the patellar tendon tension, due to the directions of the force vectors acting on the patella. This does not apply following a patellectomy; the tendons now simply slide around the femoral trochlea. The low friction coefficient of the tendofemoral contact means that the quadriceps tension following patellectomy will not be much larger than the patellar tendon tension, perhaps 5–10% if the friction coefficient is 0.05–0.1 and the tendon wraps 60° around the femur. Putting all this together, it appears that the effect caused by the loss of patellar tendon moment arm is partly counterbalanced by the absence of the patellar tendon:quadriceps tension ratio in the flexed knee.

There is, however, a further weakening effect caused by patellectomy, because of its effect on the quadriceps muscles. The architecture of muscles is adapted to each joint. In particular, the change in muscle length caused by active contraction of the muscle fibres is limited – there is a point beyond which the muscle cannot shorten any further, when the muscle fibres have contracted to 0.6 of their resting length.[27] A patellectomy causes the tendinous remnant of the extensor mechanism to wrap closely around the end of the femur, which slackens the quadriceps. The result of this is known as an 'extensor lag', in which the muscles do not shorten sufficiently to extend the knee in a normal way during gait. Because of this phenomenon, if a patellectomy is really necessary, the resulting defect should be closed end-to-end, in order to shorten the extensor mechanism and maintain quadriceps length and tension.

Patellofemoral joint stability

In the introduction to this chapter, we stated that the patella is a small bone that is acted on by large muscles and that the underlying patellofemoral joint is not sufficiently congruent to ensure stability. In addition, there are interactions with the passive retinacular stabilizing structures on either side of the patella. All of this adds up to a joint that is predisposed to problems with instability, and this is, of course, a major clinical problem. 'Instability' can mean different things to different people; in this chapter on biomechanics we are not concerned with the subjective sensation of instability that patients complain about. Instead, we are concerned with instability in the classical engineering sense i.e. the tendency of an object to resist being displaced away from a position of equilibrium, or the strength with which that object (the patella in this case) tries to return to its equilibrium position. This is an objective measurement that can be used to quantify the effectiveness of surgical procedures that realign the patella.

If the patella is unstable, this implies that the patella can either be moved out of its stable position of congruent articulation in the trochlear groove relatively easily, or else that it does so spontaneously. This usually manifests itself as a transient episode of patellar maltracking during knee flexion–extension. The tendency to move out of the groove occurs in a transverse plane relative to the patella, and so maltracking is normally measured in terms of patellar medial–lateral translation parallel to the femoral transepicondylar axis, plus patellar tilt, when the patella rotates around its own proximal–distal axis. It is believed that different pathologies can cause different amounts of patellar medial–lateral translation and tilt, but this is largely conjectural, due to lack of objective data and the complexity of the extensor mechanism. Lateral patellar tilt, for example, is sometimes related to an abnormally tight lateral retinaculum, which is thought to tether the lateral edge of the patella.[28] This may sometimes be true, but is not necessarily true. We have watched 'dynamic' MRI sequences of knee flexion–extension with laterally tilted patellae and lateral retinaculae that were clearly slack.

The geometry of the articular surfaces provides a static contribution to patellofemoral joint stability; this is principally due to the prominence and slope of the lateral facet of the femoral trochlea, which resists the common tendency for the patella to move laterally if it is unstable. Some authors have confused incongruity of the joint with a lack of stability, with the Wiberg classification[29] for the shape of the patella being cited in this context, for example. The shape of the patella is not important – it is the slope of the lateral facet of the trochlea that resists lateral patellar movement, like trying to roll a ball up an inclined plank, where the 'articulation' has no congruity yet the situation is stable. The Lyon school[30,31] has found that lateral trochlear dysplasia was present in 96% of the cases of 'objective patellar instability', and Davies et al[32] found that a shallow trochlear sulcus angle was the best predictor of patellar instability.

Surgical procedures that aim to steepen the slope of the lateral facet of the femoral trochlear surface are logical from the mechanical viewpoint. The Albee procedure,[33] which raises the lateral edge of the trochlea, has the desired effect, but this additional bony prominence may then cause problems by over-tightening the lateral retinacular structures. The alternative is femoral trochleoplasty, in which the central area of a dysplastic trochlea is undermined and the resulting osteochondral shell is depressed to form a new central trochlear groove.[30]

The importance of the slope of the lateral facet of the trochlea has been shown recently by work in vitro. A protocol was developed that allowed the patellar lateral stability to be measured during controlled lateral displacements imposed by a materials testing machine (Figure 3.11).[34] We have also studied biomechanically in vitro the effects of articular, retinacular or muscular deficiencies on patellofemoral joint stability (W. Senavongse and A. Amis, Mechanical Engineering Department, Imperial College London, UK; manuscript submitted for publication). The different parts of the quadriceps were loaded physiologically and the force required to cause 10 mm of patellar lateral displacement was measured, from 0° to 90° of knee flexion. After doing this with the joint intact, a wedge was removed from the lateral femur, allowing the trochlea to be flattened (Figure 3.12). This was a 'reversed Albee procedure'. When the patellar stability tests were repeated, the force needed to cause 10 mm of lateral displacement had fallen by up to 70% (Figure 3.12). Despite the limitations of work in vitro, this was clearly a major effect.

As the patella moves along the trochlear groove during knee flexion–extension, it is guided by the retinacular structures on either side. These are passive tensile restraints that are akin to extraarticular ligaments. The soft tissues around the patella have been described in a series of layers.[35,36] The medial retinaculum, that resists patellar lateral subluxation, includes well-defined bands that pass from the patella to the tibia, meniscus and femur, in addition to fascial layers and capsule. The contributions of each of these structures to resisting patellar lateral displacements have been shown by 'sequential

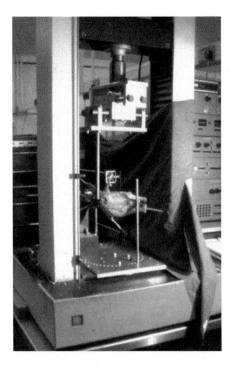
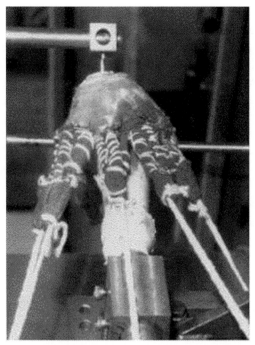

Figure 3.11   Patellar stability measurement *in vitro*. The knee is mounted on the base of the test machine and the quadriceps are tensed. The bar in front of the tibia holds the knee at the chosen angle of flexion. The moving crosshead of the test machine connects to a ball joint within the patella, and force versus lateral patellar displacement graphs are drawn. The system of bearings at the top allows the patella to move freely during the tests

cutting studies'.[37–39] This method measures the force required to displace the patella a fixed distance. If a restraining structure is cut, the force required to produce the same displacement drops by an amount equal to the restraining action of the cut structure. This has shown that the medial patellofemoral ligament is the major passive restraint, contributing approximately 55% of the total passive resistance when the knee is near full extension.

Recent work *in vitro* has shown how the contribution of the medial patellofemoral ligament to patellar lateral stability varies across the range of knee flexion, using the same methods as for the trochlear flattening described above. The medial retinacular contribution rose rapidly as the knee extended from 20° to 0° (Figure 3.13), which suggests that the retinaculae are pulled tight as the knee reaches full extension and the patella moves proximally.

The medial patellofemoral ligament is a rather variable structure that can be transparently thin, yet it had a mean strength of 208 N in elderly cadaveric knees.[40] Realization of the role of the medial patellofemoral ligament, and its significant strength, is leading to greater interest in its reconstruction.

The different parts of the quadriceps approach the patella from different directions (Figure 3.14). In particular, both the vasti medialis and lateralis have distal oblique parts (vastus medialis obliquus and vastus lateralis obliquus) that have greater transverse components to their lines of action.[41] This means that, although they are comparatively small as a proportion of the total physiological cross-sectional area of the quadriceps,[42] they have a larger contribution to patellar medial–lateral equilibrium. In Figure 3.14, the lengths of the force vectors are in proportion to their physiological cross-sectional areas, and the

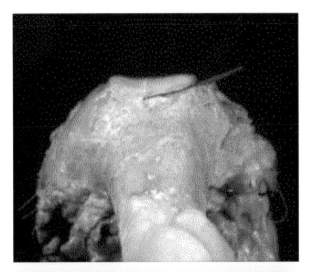

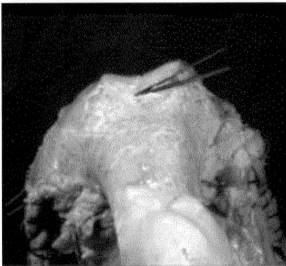

Figure 3.12 The lateral facet of the trochlea was flattened by removing a wedge of bone. This caused the force required to produce 10 mm patellar lateral displacement to fall significantly

directions were measured on cadaver limbs.[42] In addition, the vastus medialis obliquus and vastus lateralis obliquus approach the patella from relatively posterior origins. This means that they both act to pull the patella down onto the femur, helping to stabilize it. The measurements suggested that the vastus medialis obliquus acts equally in the proximal, medial and posterior directions.

It is accepted widely that the vastus medialis obliquus is the first part of the quadriceps to weaken in the face of patellofemoral pain and the last to regain its strength during rehabilitation, and so it is a major focus during physiotherapy. If all the muscle component force vectors in Figure 3.14 are added together, the resultant is parallel to the femur (Figure 3.15). If the vastus medialis obliquus action is absent, this causes the force resultant to deviate 9° laterally. The consequence of this was examined experimentally, using the method described above. It was found that the vastus medialist obliquus made a significant contribution to patellar lateral stability across the range of knee flexion examined, but its absence was not sufficient, with a normal trochlea, to cause patellar dislocation.

When all of the patellar stabilizing factors are put together, the work *in vitro* suggests that deficient trochlear geometry is the most important single factor. If patellofemoral stability is analysed in a transverse section (Figure 3.16), it is clear that the resultant force, which presses the patella against the trochlea, has components acting in both posterior and lateral directions. If the resultant force deviates from the sagittal plane by an angle greater than the slope of the trochlear surface, then the patella will sublux up the slope. Both of these force components are affected by knee flexion–extension.

The lateral component is caused by the Q angle, which is approximately 15° in the extended knee.[43] The Q angle is derived from the line of action of the patellar tendon and the resultant force of the quadriceps, in the coronal plane (Figure 3.17). Because knee flexion is accompanied by a coupled tibial internal rotation, the tibial tubercle moves medially. This reduces the Q angle, and so the patella is less likely to sublux laterally as the knee flexes. This description shows why medialization of the tibial tubercle is such a powerful procedure, because it realigns the entire effect of the extensor apparatus. This also explains why patellar medial instability

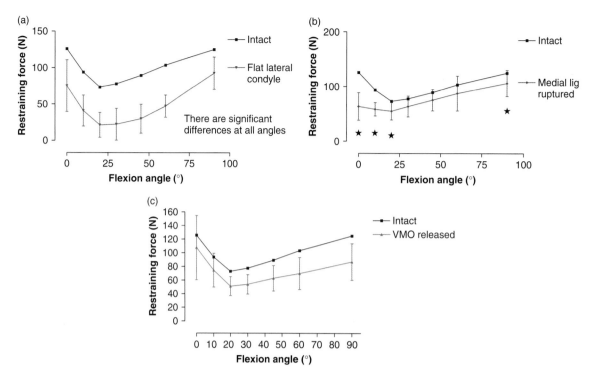

Figure 3.13   Comparison of the force required to displace the patella 10 mm laterally, between the intact knee and following rupture of the medial patellofemoral ligament (MPFL). The contribution of the MPFL rose rapidly as the knee extended from 20° of flexion

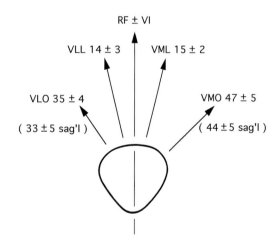

Figure 3.14   The force vectors show both the directions and magnitudes of the different components of the quadriceps. The figures in brackets show the direction posterior to the coronal plane of vastus medialis obliquus (VMO) and vastus lateralis obliquus (VLO)[42]

is usually iatrogenic, due to excessive tubercle medialization.[44]

The posterior force component arises from the angle between the quadriceps and patellar tendon tensions in the sagittal plane. It has already been shown how they combine vectorially to give a greater joint force as the knee flexes (Figure 3.6). Thus, knee flexion also increases the force component that pulls the patella down into the trochlear groove.

The descriptions above show that in the extended knee the lateral force component is at its largest and the posterior component is at its smallest; these trends combine to make the patella least stable in the extended knee. Conversely, in the flexed knee the lateral component is smaller while the posterior force is larger, and so the patella is stable. By allowing for these effects, Hvid[45] calculated that a Q angle of 20° would require a lateral trochlear slope of 35° near knee

NORMAL MUSCLE FORCES

VM INACTIVE

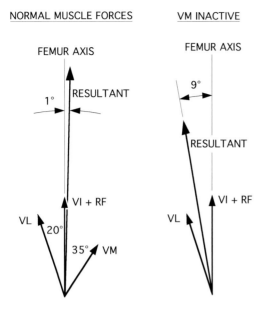

Figure 3.15 Addition of the quadriceps force vectors from normal limbs leads to a resultant force that is parallel to the shaft of the femur. If the vastus medialis obliquus is inactive, the force resultant acts 9° lateral to the femur

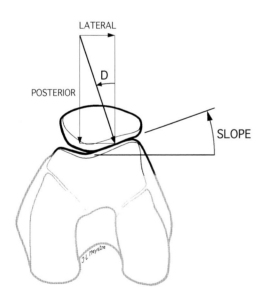

Figure 3.16 Patellar stability in a transverse plane. The resultant force *JF* derives from posterior (stabilizing) and lateral (displacing) force components. If the resultant deviates from the sagittal plane by an angle (*D*) greater than the slope of the lateral trochlear surface, the patella will tend to sublux laterally, up the slope

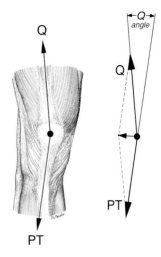

Figure 3.17 The Q angle arises from the difference in direction between the resultant quadriceps and patellar tendon tensions. Their effect is to cause a lateral force component to act on the patella. This decreases with knee flexion, when the tibia rotates internally, medializing the tibial tuberosity

extension, falling to a 20° slope at 50° of knee flexion to maintain patellar lateral stability.

Conclusions

Different mechanical factors interact to influence patellar kinematics and stability. Analysis of the muscle force vectors has shown that these large active tensions cause the patella to be least stable in the extended knee, and that the patella become more stable as the knee flexes. The changing directions of the patellar tendon and quadriceps tensions in the sagittal plane, as the knee flexes, explain why the contact area migrates proximally across the patella and why the forces rise. The patellar articular geometry is adapted to this, with large proximal concavities giving congruency and, hence, low cartilage contact stresses.

The medial patellofemoral ligament is the single most important structure among the passive restraints to patellar maltracking. The experimental evidence suggests that the role of the retinacula increases sharply as the knee approaches full extension. When this trend was added to that of the muscle forces, the overall result was that the patella was least stable in 20° of knee flexion.

The single most important factor for patellar stability has been shown to be the trochlear groove geometry. The procedures that aim to create a larger, steeper slope for the lateral trochlear facet are mechanically logical. If the trochlea is flat mediolaterally, then even a perfect soft-tissue balancing procedure will remain vulnerable to every minor lateral patellar perturbation.

References

1. Eckhoff DG, Burke BJ, Dwyer TF et al (1996) The Ranawat Award. Sulcus morphology of the distal femur. *Clin Orthop* **331**: 23–28

2. Stäubli HU, Dürrenmatt U, Porcellini B, Rauschning W (1999) Anatomy and surface geometry of the patellofemoral joint in the axial plane. *J Bone Joint Surg Br* **81**: 452–458

3. Merchant AC, Mercer RL, Jacobsen RH, Cool CR (1974) Roentgenographic analysis of patellofemoral congruence. *J Bone Joint Surg Am* **56**: 1391–1396

4. Hehne HJ (1990) Biomechanics of the patellofemoral joint and its clinical relevance. *Clin Orthop* **258**: 73–85

5. Aglietti P, Insall JN, Cerulli G (1983) Patellar pain and incongruence. I: Measurements of incongruence. *Clin Orthop* **176**: 217–224

6. Goodfellow J, Hungerford DS, Zindel M (1976) Patellofemoral joint mechanics and pathology. 1. Functional anatomy of the patellofemoral joint. *J Bone Joint Surg Br* **58**: 287–290

7. Katchburian MV, Bull AM, Shih YF, Heatley FW, Amis AA (2003) Review article: measurement of patellar tracking: assessment and analysis of the literature. *Clin Orthop* **412**: 241–259

8. Heegaard J, Leyvraz PF, Van Kampen A et al (1994) Influence of soft structures on patellar three-dimensional tracking. *Clin Orthop* **299**: 235–243

9. Kujala UM, Osterman K, Kormano M et al (1989) Patellar motion analyzed by magnetic resonance imaging. *Acta Orthop Scand* **60**: 13–16

10. Nagamine R, Otani T, White SE et al (1995) Patellar tracking measurement in the normal knee. *J Orthop Res* **13**: 115–122

11. Powers CM, Shellock FG, Pfaff M (1998) Quantification of patellar tracking using kinematic MRI. *J Magn Reson Imaging* **8**: 724–732

12. Reider B, Marshall JL, Ring B (1981) Patellar tracking. *Clin Orthop* **157**: 143–148

13. van Kampen A, Huiskes R (1990) The three-dimensional tracking pattern of the human patella. *J Orthop Res* **8**: 372–382

14. Bull AM, Katchburian MV, Shih YF, Amis AA (2002) Standardisation of the description of patellofemoral motion and comparison between different techniques. *Knee Surg Sports Traumatol Arthrosc* **10**: 184–193

15. Grood ES, Suntay WJ (1983) A joint coordinate system for the clinical description of three-dimensional motions: application to the knee. *J Biomech Eng* **105**: 136–144

16. Laurin CA, Levesque HP, Dussault R et al (1978) The abnormal lateral patellofemoral angle: a diagnostic roentgenographic sign of recurrent patellar subluxation. *J Bone Joint Surg Am* **60**: 55–60

17. Huberti HH, Hayes WC (1984) Patellofemoral contact pressures. The influence of Q-angle and tendofemoral contact. *J Bone Joint Surg Am* **66**: 715–724

18. Ahmed AM, Burke DL, Hyder A (1987) Force analysis of the patellar mechanism. *J Orthop Res* **5**: 69–85

19. Ellis MI, Seedhom BB, Wright V, Dowson D (1980) An evaluation of the ratio between the tensions along the quadriceps tendon and patellar ligament. *Eng Med* **9**: 189–194

20. Andriacchi TP, Natarajan RN, Hurwitz DE (1991) Musculoskeletal dynamics, locomotion, and clinical applications. In: Mow VC, Hayes WC (eds), *Basic Orthopaedic Biomechanics*. New York, Raven, pp 51–92

21. Mak MK, Levin O, Mizrahi J, Hui-Chan CW (2003) Joint torques during sit-to-stand in healthy subjects and people with Parkinson's disease. *Clin Biomech (Bristol, Avon)* **18**: 197–206

22. van Eijden TM, de Boer W, Weijs WA (1985) The orientation of the distal part of the quadriceps femoris muscle as a function of the knee flexion–extension angle. *J Biomech* **18**: 803–809

23. Zavatsky AB, O'Connor JJ (1993) Ligament forces at the knee during isometric quadriceps contractions. *Proc Inst Mech Eng [H]* **207**: 7–18

24. Beynnon BD, Fleming BC (1998) Anterior cruciate ligament strain *in vivo*: a review of previous work. *J Biomech* **31**: 519–525

25. Kaufer H (1971) Mechanical function of the patella. *J Bone Joint Surg Am* **53**: 1551–1560

26. Hungerford DS, Barry M (1979) Biomechanics of the patellofemoral joint. *Clin Orthop* **144**: 9–15

27. Elftman H (1966) Biomechanics of muscle with particular application to studies of gait. *J Bone Joint Surg Am* **48**: 363–377

28. Larson RL, Cabaud HE, Slocum DB et al (1978) The patellar compression syndrome: surgical treatment by lateral retinacular release. *Clin Orthop* **134**: 158–167

29. Wiberg G (1941) Roentgenographic and anatomic studies on the femoropatellar joint. *Acta Orthop Scand* **12**: 319–410

30. Dejour D, Nové-Josserand L, Walch G (1994) Patellofemoral disorders: classification and an approach to operative treatment for instability. In: Chan KM, Fu FH (eds), *Controversies in Orthopaedic Sports Medicine*. Hong Kong, Williams & Wilkins Asia-Pacific Ltd, pp 235–244

31. Dejour H, Walch G, Nove-Josserand L, Guider C (1994) Factors of patellar instability: an anatomic radiographic study. *Knee Surg Sports Traumatol Arthrosc* **2**: 19–26

32. Davies AP, Costa ML, Shepstone L et al (2000) The sulcus angle and malalignment of the extensor mechanism of the knee. *J Bone Joint Surg Br* **82**: 1162–1166

33. Keene GCR, Marans HJ (1993) Osteotomy for patellofemoral dysplasia. In: Fox JM, Del Pizzo W (eds), *The Patellofemoral Joint*. New York, McGraw-Hill, pp 169–175

34. Senavongse W, Farahmand F, Jones J et al (2003) Quantitative measurement of patellofemoral joint stability: force-displacement behavior of the human patella *in vitro*. *J Orthop Res* **21**: 780–786

35. Dye SF (1993) Patellofemoral anatomy. In: Fox JM, Del Pizzo W (eds), *The Patellofemoral Joint*. New York, McGraw-Hill, pp 1–12

36. Warren LF, Marshall JL (1979) The supporting structures and layers on the medial side of the knee: an anatomical analysis. *J Bone Joint Surg Am* **61**: 56–62

37. Conlan T, Garth WP Jr, Lemons JE (1993) Evaluation of the medial soft-tissue restraints of the extensor mechanism of the knee. *J Bone Joint Surg Am* **75**: 682–693

38. Desio SM, Burks RT, Bachus KN (1998) Soft tissue restraints to lateral patellar translation in the human knee. *Am J Sports Med* **26**: 59–65

39. Hautamaa PV, Fithian DC, Kaufman KR et al (1998) Medial soft tissue restraints in lateral patellar instability and repair. *Clin Orthop* **349**: 174–182

40. Amis AA, Firer P, Mountney J et al (2003) Anatomy and biomechanics of the medial patellofemoral ligament. *The Knee* **10**: 215–220

41. Bennett WF, Doherty N, Hallisey MJ (1993) Insertion orientation of terminal vastus lateralis obliquus and vastus medialis obliquus muscle fibers in human knees. *Clin Anat* **6**: 129–134

42. Farahmand F, Senavongse W, Amis AA (1998) Quantitative study of the quadriceps muscles and trochlear groove geometry related to instability of the patellofemoral joint. *J Orthop Res* **16**: 136–143

43. Insall JN (1984) *Surgery of the Knee*. New York, Churchill Livingstone

44. Hughston JC, Deese M (1988) Medial subluxation of the patella as a complication of lateral retinacular release. *Am J Sports Med* **16**: 383–388

45. Hvid I (1983) The stability of the human patellofemoral joint. *Eng Med* **12**: 55–59

4 Pathogenesis of Patellofemoral Pain

Roland M. Biedert

The patellofemoral joint includes a variety of tissues, such as cartilage, subchondral bone, synovial plicae, infrapatellar fat pad, retinacula, capsule and tendons (Figure 4.1). Each of these structures, alone or in combination, can be a source of patellofemoral pain.

The patellofemoral joint is a complex system that has to accept, transfer and dissipate loads.[1] The amount of load that can be applied across the patellofemoral joint in a given period without structural failure is individually different. Supraphysiological overload of most tissues is accepted over a short period. Unphysiological load over a longer duration or changed metabolic activities can lead to structural failure, with loss of homeostatic conditions and tissue damage.

Pain can be caused by a unique trauma or may be cumulative with time. The patellofemoral joint can become painful during periods of rapid growth in adolescence, after increased repetitive activity during sports, or with activities of daily living, like long sitting in a cinema with the knee flexed, or walking up and down the stairs.[2] This means that each level of activity or every specific use of the knee during various functions can cause patellofemoral pain. These considerations are essential in understanding the

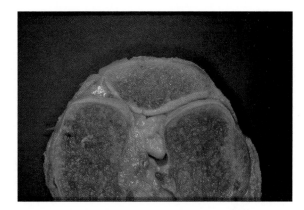

Figure 4.1 Axial dissection demonstrates the close relationship of the different structures

basics of this complicated topic. To determine the path to successful treatment, the underlying pathophysiology with respect to the specific involved structures and activities must be recognized. This presupposes an exact diagnosis, including mechanical, physiological and biochemical aspects.[3]

Physiology of pain

Pain results whenever tissues of the patellofemoral joint are irritated, inflamed, damaged or

Patellofemoral Disorders: Diagnosis and Treatment. Edited by Roland M. Biedert
© 2004 John Wiley & Sons, Ltd ISBN: 0-470-85011-6

overused – in other words, when they are injured in any way.[2,4] Pain is a protective mechanism for the body and causes the individual to react to eliminate the pain stimulus.[2] Two major types of pain are fast pain and slow pain. Fast pain, which is felt within 0.1 second after the stimulus is applied, is also described as 'sharp', 'acute' or 'electric' pain. Fast pain is not felt in most of the deeper structures of the body. Slow pain, also described as 'burning', 'aching' or 'chronic' pain, normally is present with tissue destruction. It can lead to prolonged suffering and occurs in the skin and the deep tissues, such as the structures of the patellofemoral joint.

Pain is elicited by different types of stimuli – mechanical, thermal and biochemical.[4,5] Fast pain is elicited by mechanical and thermal stimuli, whereas all three types of stimuli can cause slow pain. Some of the biochemical agents that excite pain include histamine, serotonin and bradykinin. Additionally, prostaglandins and substance P enhance the sensitivity of pain endings but do not directly excite them.[4] These biochemical substances are especially important in stimulating the slow type of pain (chronic, suffering pain) that occurs after tissue injury.

Pain receptors adapt very little and sometimes not at all. Under special conditions, excitation of pain fibres becomes progressively greater, resulting in chronic aching pain. The increase in sensitivity of the pain receptors is called hyperalgesia. This may explain the prolonged, unbearable suffering in patients presenting with chronic patellofemoral pain. The intensity of pain correlates with the rate of tissue damage from biochemical stimuli, tissue ischaemia, tissue contusion and increased or decreased pressure. These considerations play an important role in the general understanding of articular and periarticular pain.

Pain receptors are all free nerve endings (FNEs). These endings use two separate pathways for transmitting pain signals to the central nervous system – the fast–sharp pain pathway and the slow–chronic pain pathway. These pathways correspond to the two types of pain. The fast pain signals are transmitted in the peripheral nerves to the spinal cord with higher velocities (6 and 30 m/s) than the slow pain signals (0.5 and 2 m/s). This double system of pain innervation gives a double pain sensation – a fast pain that is transmitted to the brain (A fibres) followed by a slow pain (C fibres). The fast pain, e.g. impingement of a plica, makes the person react immediately to remove him/herself from the stimulus. The slow pain becomes more painful over time, eventually becoming the intolerable suffering of long-continued pain (e.g. chronic irritation of synovial membrane).

Nerve innervation of the knee joint

Current understanding of the specific pattern of innervation of the human knee is summarized best by Kennedy et al,[6] who describe two groups of articular nerves. The posterior group consists of the prominent articular nerve (as a branch of the tibial nerve) and a terminal branch of the obturator nerve. The anterior group consists of articular branches of the femoral, common peroneal and saphenous nerves. The posterior articular nerve supplies the posterior capsule and cruciate ligaments.[7] This nerve arises in the popliteal fossa and penetrates the posterior capsule.[8] The lateral articular nerve innervates the lateral and posterolateral parts of the knee, whereas the recurrent peroneal nerve supplies the middle and anterior portions of the lateral joint capsule. Anteriorly, the capsule is innervated by terminal branches of the femoral, common peroneal and saphenous nerves. The femoral nerve divides and innervates the vastus lateralis, medialis and intermedius muscles; it also contributes branches to the anterior medial joint capsule. The saphenous nerve contributes a branch to the anterior medial capsule and also provides sensory branches to the patellar tendon.[9]

The nerve supply of the patella was studied in detail by Fontaine.[10] He found that nerves travel to the entire medial side and to the proximal half of the lateral side. The medial branches are most important and originate from the nerve of the vastus medialis muscle. The lateral branches originate from the nerve of the biceps femoris muscle (caput breve) and the nerve of the vastus lateralis muscle.

The complex innervation of the structures of the patellofemoral joint may explain the variety of clinical findings in patients suffering from patellofemoral pain.

Anatomy of pain

Morphological studies reveal that joint receptors (mechanoreceptors) can be classified into four categories – Ruffini endings, Pacinian corpuscles, Golgi tendon organ-like endings, and free nerve endings (FNEs).[2,3,6,9,11]

Free nerve endings

Type IVa FNEs (Figure 4.2) detect crude touch, pressure, pain, heat and cold. Primarily, they constitute the articular nociceptive system. They transmit information on pain and inflammation and are therefore sources of patellofemoral pain.[6,12] They remain inactive during normal circumstances, but become active when they are subjected to abnormal mechanical deformation or special biochemical agents.[12,13] Type IVb FNEs function as efferent vasomotors.[12]

In a comprehensive histological study of neurological receptors in 19 static and dynamic knee structures, we recorded the qualitative and quantitative incidence of type IVa FNEs.[12] FNEs were stained by the haematoxylin–eosin and Masson's trichrome methods. The immunohistochemical tests were performed using S-100 and synaptophysin.[12]

Different structures of the patellofemoral joint showed high FNE counts (Figure 4.3). The tendon of the quadriceps muscle has the highest density, and the retinacula and patellar tendon have the second-highest FNE count. This is not surprising, because all three control acceleration, deceleration and rotation of the knee joint, and therefore they need a high proprioceptive capability for coordinating these conditions. It also indicates their importance in balancing the patella during the gliding mechanism. The correlation between these histological findings, patellofemoral pain and clinical pathology will be described later in this chapter.

Substance P

Substance P is considered one of the major neurotransmitters of painful stimuli by unmyelinated C fibres.[14] It has various inflammatory effects, such as vasodilatation,[15] activation of macrophages, B lymphocytes, polymorphonuclear cells, platelets, mast cells and synoviocytes.[14] It stimulates the secretion of interleukin 1 (IL-1) and potentiates the action of IL-1 on fibroblasts.[14]

Other studies[16–18] focus on the nociceptive afferent nerve supply about the knee joint using substance P or calcitonin gene-related peptide immunoreactivity. They suggest that substance P and calcitonin gene-related peptide are neurotransmitters of nociceptive sensation.[16–18]

Fibres containing substance P are isolated in the lateral retinaculum, the fat pad, synovial membrane, periosteum and the subchondral plate of patellae affected with degenerative

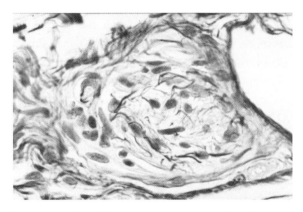

Figure 4.2 Type IVa free nerve ending stained by haematoxylin–eosin.[2,12] Reproduced by permission from Biedert et al, 1992[12]

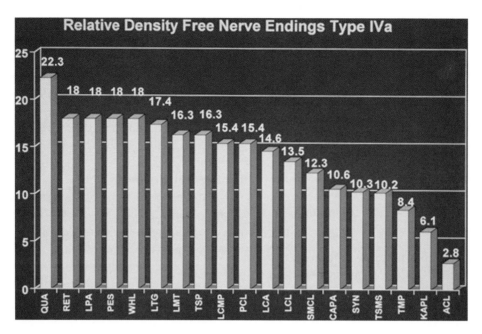

Figure 4.3   Distribution (relative density) of type IVa free nerve endings in the knee joint. QUA, quadriceps tendon; RET, medial and lateral retinacula; LPA, patellar tendon.[2,3,12] Reproduced by permission from Biedert et al, 2001[3]

disease.[16–19] Nerve fibres immunoreactive for substance P (Figure 4.4) are not observed in the articular cartilage of the patella.[15] Examination of subchondral bone, however, shows the presence of substance P-positive nerve fibres in the erosion channels, which are present in patients with degenerative joint disease.[15]

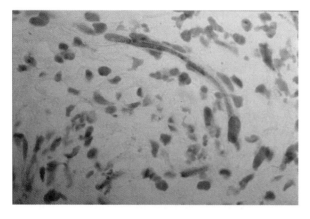

Figure 4.4   Substance P immunoreactive nerve fibre.[3,16,17] Reproduced by permission from Biedert et al, 2001[3]

The results of the studies by Witonski et al[15] and Sanchis-Alfonso and Roselló-Sastre[17] demonstrate that substance P-immunoreactive nerve fibres are widespread in the soft tissues around the knee joint. These tissues include especially the retinacula, synovium and fat pad. The investigators conclude that patellofemoral pain depends not only on mechanical factors (e.g. elevated subchondral pressure, jumper's knee), but also on neural factors (nerve damage in affected lateral retinaculum) that are involved in this process. Substance P-positive fibres are often associated with blood vessels.[15] Here, substance P functions as a vasodilator that can produce inflammation.[15]

Pathophysiological mechanisms

The evaluation of patellofemoral pain also includes pathophysiological mechanisms other than histological and immunological factors. These consist mainly of mechanical, neural and biochemical factors, which are often present in combination and can be cumulative. The mechanisms considered to be of causal significance are

Table 4.1 Patellofemoral pain: mechanisms and involved structures[3]

	Cartilage	Subchondral bone	Synovium, plicae	Retinaculae	Tendons
Neural		+	+	++	
Mechanical	++	++	++	++	+
Biochemical	(++)		++		

+, important; ++, very important; (++), indirect influence.

summarized in Table 4.1, with respect to the specific involved structures.

Mechanical mechanisms

A mechanical problem is present when the patellofemoral gliding mechanism is not normal. This can be caused by a variety of factors, such as lateral patellar displacement (Figure 4.5), patellar instability, lateral patellar tilt or lateral patellar compression syndrome, dysplastic lateral femoral condyle, and impinged plica or fat pad. The problem may also lead to defects in the articular surface and to an elevated subchondral bone pressure.[2]

The subchondral bone has a rich nerve supply, and so increased pressure can produce pain.[2,16,20–23] Dye and Boll[24] reported the

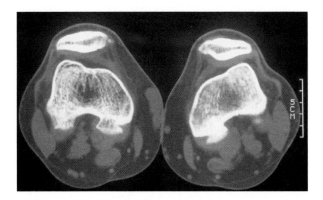

Figure 4.5 Axial CT scans showing lateral patellar displacement and pathological patellofemoral gliding mechanism on both sides

experience of sharp lancinating pain secondary to experimentally produced increased intraosseous pressure of the patella.

Increased intraosseous pressure may be caused by decreased energy absorption of articular cartilage, which in turn is caused by a smaller contact area.[3,21,25] Changes in the bone itself can also create pain because of abnormal patellar stress patterns with loss of bone stiffness.[26,27] Increased turnover and remodelling in the subchondral bone (patellar and femoral), caused by metabolic adaptations, can be painful.[20] Pain may originate from increased venous engorgement in the patella when abnormal patellofemoral rhythm and pressure are present.[28] Improvement of the patellofemoral contact area (osteotomies) and decrease of the subchondral pressure (retrograde drill holes) may relieve pain.[29,30]

Repetitive impingement of a synovial plica (Figure 4.6) or the fat pad are other mechanical factors that cause patellofemoral pain.[2,3,12,31] Synovium, plicae and fat pad have a rich nerve supply of FNEs and substance-P fibres.[3,12,15,18,32] Inflammation, thickening and scarring stimulate the FNEs and produce pain. Irritation of the synovium/plica with joint effusion leads to swelling of the fat pad, which is impinged behind the patellar tendon, especially during eccentric activities.[3,12,31,33] In addition, a tight lateral retinaculum may create fat pad impingement. McConnell[31,34] described different taping techniques to relieve patellofemoral pain, which may function primarily by mechanically relieving (unpinching) swollen and inflamed peripatellar tissues.

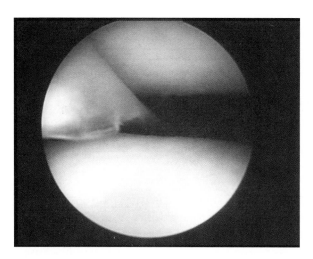

Figure 4.6   Arthroscopic view showing impingement of a synovial plica (left) between the patella (top) and femoral condyle (bottom)[3] Reproduced by permission from Biedert et al, 2001[3]

Neural mechanisms

A neural problem is present when an increased sensitivity of pain receptors causes chronic unbearable patellofemoral pain. The intensity of pain is in direct correlation with the rate of damage of the neural tissues. A neural genesis of patellofemoral pain can proceed only from structures with type IVa FNEs[12] or neuropeptide-containing nerve fibres.[15,17,19] Because hyaline (articular) cartilage is completely free of nerve fibres, it cannot be a direct source of patellofemoral pain (Table 4.1).[2,15,21,35] In contrast, nerve fibres were documented in the lateral and medial retinacula.[12,15,17,19] Fulkerson et al[36] described retinacular nerve injuries (neuromas) with patellofemoral malalignment, and Sanchis-Alfonso et al[16] found histological changes in the nerve fibres of the lateral retinaculum. We also documented neuromas as the source of pain in the lateral retinaculum of patients with chronic patellar subluxation (Figure 4.7).[2,3]

The aetiological factors of patellofemoral pain are a combination of a mechanical problem that results from the abnormal gliding mechanism of

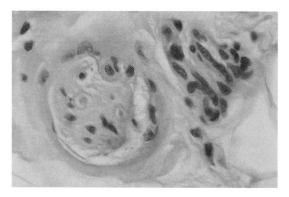

Figure 4.7   Nerve bundles with myxoid degeneration of the endoneurium in a chronically damaged lateral retinaculum caused by lateral patellar subluxation (haematoxylin–eosin staining). Reproduced with permission from Biedert et al, 2001[3]

the patella and histological changes with irreversible destruction in the nerves of the lateral retinaculum. Neural damage and subsequent hyperinnervation in the lateral retinaculum seem to be important in the pathophysiology of patellofemoral pain. Thus, unsuccessful conservative treatment in this chronic situation can be explained. Incisions in the lateral retinaculum for retinacular release or lengthening may cause denervation and therefore decrease pain. Painful patellar instability (primary or secondary) also can be partially explained by the loss of proprioception caused by damage of nerve fibres in the retinacula, both medial and lateral.[2,3,16] It has been shown that secondary patellar stabilization after lateral retinacular release improves both mechanical conditions and proprioception.[37] Although different studies have provided an improved understanding of the neuroanatomical basis for chronic patellofemoral pain, the exact mechanisms by which neural proliferation and damage of nerve fibres are produced remain unknown. However, patellofemoral malalignment may play a key role in the origin of this pain.[16,17,38] The peripatellar synovium, plicae and infrapatellar fat pad have a rich nerve supply.[12,15,16,32] Repetitive irritation or impingement lead to chronic inflammation of these tissues, with documented histological changes. They are a frequent source of patellofemoral pain as a result of mechanical (impingement, contusion) or biochemical irritation.[1,2,33]

Biochemical mechanisms

In normal articular cartilage, steady-state homeostasis exists through a fine balance of synthesis and degradation. This regulation can be disturbed by mechanical stress, initiating cartilage lesions by altering the chondrocyte–matrix interactions.[39–41] Cartilage destruction is a major characteristic of trauma injury (i.e. patellar dislocation) or mechanical malalignment (i.e. chronic patellar subluxation). The destructive process in the cartilage may release substantial amounts of cartilage matrix components and wear particles, which may then initiate and sustain a painful inflammatory reaction in the synovium.[42] Significant inflammation occurs in the synovial membrane, even at the earliest stages of cartilage damage.[43] Synovial microscopic changes include increased cellularity, vascularity and inflammatory (nonfollicular) infiltrates, depending on the amount of cartilage destruction.[3,43–45]

Numerous proinflammatory cytokines, such as the interleukins (ILs), tumour necrosis factors (TNFs), interferons (INFs) and colony stimulating factors (CSFs) are involved in the balance of cartilage degradation and synthesis. Although these factors were identified originally as secreted products of immune cells that modulate the function of other cells of the immunological system, many of them have effects on nonimmune cells, such as fibroblasts and chondrocytes.

The complex cytokine network influences the metabolic state of chondrocytes, which are responsible for synthesis and breakdown of the matrix (homeostasis).[42,46] The balance is also of great importance for the regulation of chronic inflammation. Elevated levels of proinflammatory cytokines have been measured in synovium and joint fluid with cartilage damage.[39] Synovial cells and articular chondrocytes are thought to be primary sources of cytokines in the synovial fluid, but cytokines may also originate from the infrapatellar fat pad.[47]

The catabolic cytokines such as IL-1 and tumour necrosis factor α (TNFα) appear to be responsible for inhibition of synthesis of the extracellular matrix. In contrast, anabolic factors, such as insulin-like growth factor (IGF), platelet-derived growth factor (PDGF), and transforming growth factor β (TGFβ) stimulate new cartilage formation. Of special interest are those cytokines that counteract or inhibit the catabolic cytokines.[48] TGFβ, IL-4 and IL-10 have been shown to prevent and reverse cartilage degradation in *in vitro* systems.[49] The effect of IL-6 and interferon γ (INFγ) on cartilage is not yet well-defined. IL-6 seems to play a key role in cytokine and growth-factor regulation. Cartilage pathology is the result of the balance of these mediators, and the expanding knowledge concerning these factors has led to greater understanding of the mechanisms involved in cartilage metabolism and chronic inflammation.

Because cartilage has a limited capacity to repair defects, lesions can remain in the affected structure for years, contributing to the ongoing process of synovial membrane inflammation. Here, the source of pain is not the aneural damaged cartilage, but the secondary inflammatory reaction in the synovium. To interrupt the chronic inflammation, homeostasis of the affected cartilage must be regained. This may be achieved, at least partially, by correction of the underlying mechanical pathophysiological cause.

Clinical implications

Patellofemoral pain can be experienced by the patient as sharp, acute or chronic pain. It can be aggravated by prolonged activity with increased patellofemoral compressive forces (e.g. climbing stairs, squatting or kneeling) or by prolonged periods of sitting in knee flexion (e.g. movie sign or driving).[21,50] Also, the duration of pain (seconds, hours or weeks) as it relates to specific activities or movements (e.g. patellar subluxation) is a diagnostic clue. A clear understanding of the localization, duration and type of pain is necessary for exact diagnosis and for determining the required therapy. This requires a precise clinical examination.

Cartilage

Patellofemoral pain is often present in patients with chondromalacia of the patella or trochlea. However, it is surprising that patients with normal-appearing cartilage can experience pain, and that others with extensive chondral damage can be pain-free.[35,51] Hyaline cartilage is completely free of nerve fibres,[15,21,35] therefore the aneural cartilage alone cannot be the source of pain. Also, defects in the surface are not believed to produce pain. Dye did not feel any pain during arthroscopic palpation of his extensive lesion of the patellar cartilage without intraarticular anaesthesia, as reported by Dye et al.[52]

Abnormal biomechanical configuration ('maltracking patella') is described as an important cause in the development of patellar chondromalacia.[15,53] Here, the sources of pain are the biochemical synovitis[3,25] with effusion and mechanical factors (Figure 4.8).[16,35]

Synovium

The synovium has a rich nerve supply of type IVa FNEs[12] and fibres containing substance P.[16] Synovium can be irritated and produce pain.[21,25] The primary function of the synovium as pain receptor has interested a number of clinicians and researchers, as noted by Biedert.[54] Kennedy et al[6] and de Andrade et al[55] reported irritation of FNEs in the synovium in Hoffa's disease and in symptomatic synovial plicae, with decreased quadriceps activity produced by only slight synovial effusion resulting from painful stimulation of FNEs. Repetitive impingement of a medio- or suprapatellar plica between patella and femur can also be the underlying cause of patellofemoral pain.[3,12] Often in such situations, the articularis genus muscle is unable to retract the synovial fold in the suprapatellar pouch whenever the plica is thickened, scarred or inflamed.[56] Peripatellar synovitis was described by Dye et al[33] as one of the most common causes of patellofemoral pain.

Destruction of articular cartilage (Figure 4.9) leads to a local tissue response with episodes of

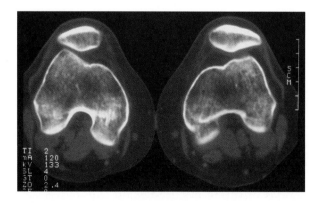

Figure 4.8 Axial CT scan with lateral patella subluxation causing damage to the retropatellar cartilage and the lateral retinaculum

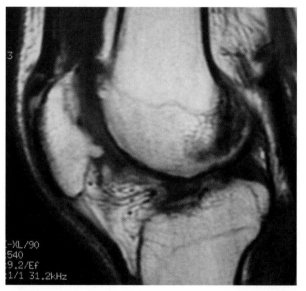

Figure 4.9 Sagittal MRI scan demonstrates retropatellar and trochlear damage of the articular cartilage, changed signal intensity in the patella, and degenerative changes

inflammation and synovitis.[57] Cartilage damage (e.g. maltracking) results not only from overuse, but also from active mechanisms in the metabolism of chondrocytes. During inflammation, there is decreased absorption of essential nutrients by the cartilage. Inflammation affects the integrity of the different components of the joint. Polymorphonuclear granulocytes, which are responsible for phagocytosis of damaged tissues, affect cartilage and joint structures.[21] The changes induced by inflammation cause painful stretching of the joint capsule by recurrent episodes of effusion.[57] Additionally, increased inflammation also may irritate the fibrous capsule's richly endowed nerve endings.[21] The increase in pain may be a result of synovitis or irritation of a synovial plica. Changes induced by inflammation include alteration of the viscosity of the synovial fluid, caused by the elaboration of enzymes or free radicals that degrade hyaluronic acid and lubricin.[57] This breakdown of hyaluronic acid decreases smooth movement of the articular surfaces (crepitations) as a result of a decrease in the viscosity of the synovial fluid. This is important in choice of further treatment.

Infrapatellar fat pad

As mentioned previously, substance P-immunoreactive nerve fibres and type IVa FNEs are found in the fat pad,[12,18,32] demonstrating the rich nerve supply of this structure.[12,32] The heavily vascularized infrapatellar fat pad, with its alar plicae, fills the anterior part of the knee joint (Figure 4.10). It is held in place by the patellar tendon, the bilateral longitudinal retinacula and the infrapatellar synovial plica, the central structure that passes posterosuperiorly to the intercondylar roof.[58]

The close anatomical relationship to the patellar tendon and the lateral superficial oblique retinaculum make the fat pad a frequent source of pain. McConnell[31] describes 78% of her patients presenting with patellar tendonitis as having an irritation of the fat pad. Impingement of the fat

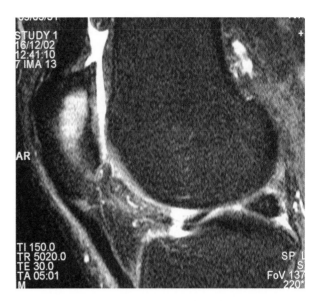

Figure 4.10 The infrapatellar fat pad fills the whole anterior part of the knee joint. It may be impinged in the patellofemoral joint, behind the patellar tendon and in the intercondylar notch (MRI, sagittal view, osteoarthritis of the patellofemoral joint)

pad is possible, especially during eccentric load in jumping or running. Also, straight leg-raising can cause pain by compression of the fat pad. In addition, chronic irritation of the synovium with joint effusion leads to swelling of the fat pad, and the risk of impingement behind the patellar tendon increases. A laterally orientated increased tension caused by a tight lateral retinaculum also may create fat pad irritation.

Understanding the biomechanical processes is necessary in order to choose the corresponding treatment. McConnell's taping technique[34] can help relieve the symptoms (see Part IV). Taping is a successful method for restoring tissue homeostasis.[59]

Subchondral bone

The subchondral bone has a rich nerve supply.[21-23] An elevated subchondral bone pressure produces pain.[16,21] The best known cause of excess pressure is the lateral patellar compression syndrome[21] (Figure 4.11). The increase

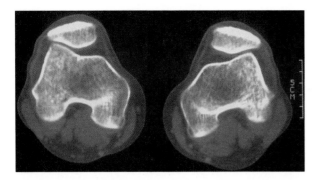

Figure 4.11   Axial CT scans showing lateral patellar tilt and displacement causing increased pressure in the lateral subchondral bone of patella and trochlea

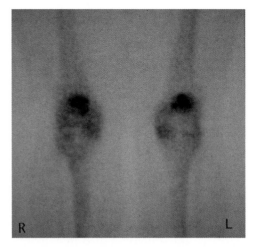

Figure 4.12   Scintiscan of a female patient with unspecific patellofemoral pain. The image shows marked increase in the activity in both patellae

of intraosseous pressure is the result of failure of the energy-absorption function of the articular cartilage caused by the decreased contact area.[21,25] Abernethy et al[26] and Minns et al[27] state that pain arises from changes in the bone caused by patellar stress patterns and loss of bone stiffness.

Waisbrod and Treiman[28] suggest that pain may originate from increasing venous engorgement in the patella in the presence of an abnormal patellofemoral rhythm and pressure. Drill holes or patellar osteotomies can decrease the subchondral pressure and improve the articular contact area in the patellofemoral joint.[30,60] Both techniques are capable of relieving pain.

Pain in the subchondral bone also can be caused by dynamic metabolic adaptations characterized by increased turnover and remodelling.[20] Dye and Chew[20] describe multiple triggers, including mechanical neurovascular and hormonal factors, that may initiate increased osseous metabolic activity. The increased activity is detectable with technetium scintigraphy (Figure 4.12). Dye and Chew[20] believe that chronic supraphysiological loading or abnormal joint mechanics combine with chronic excessive periarticular cytokine production to produce the increased remodelling in most patients. They also note that persistently increased osseous metabolic activity of periarticular bone identifies a subgroup at risk for early structural changes.[20]

In contrast to the increased pressure in the lateral patellar compression syndrome, the medial patellofemoral joint shows hypopressure of cartilage on the patellar and femoral surfaces.[21] This incongruity is also seen in dysplastic patellae. Hypopressure and disuse of the medial facet may cause malnutrition and early degenerative changes of the articular cartilage.[21] This may explain why early lesions of the cartilage in patients with lateralization of the patella are usually noted on the medial patellar facet, and why late lesions on patellar facets and osteoarthritis are more advanced in the lateral patellar facet.[21]

Retinacula

Neuropeptide-containing nerve fibres[15,17,19] and type IVa FNEs[12] are documented in the lateral and medial retinacula. Thus, the retinacula may be an important factor or trigger point in patellofemoral pain.[36] Fulkerson[38] concludes that the lateral retinaculum itself is painful, although it is difficult to distinguish retinacular pain from pain in the underlying synovium. The observations reported by Sanchis-Alfonso and colleagues[16,17] provide a neuroanatomical basis for anterior knee pain syndrome in active young patients with patellofemoral malalignment, and support the clinical observation that the lateral retinaculum may have a key role in the origin of this pain.

Recently, Sanchis-Alfonso et al[16] concluded that histological changes in the nerves of the lateral retinaculum may be an important cause of pain in patients with patellofemoral malalignment, as there is direct correlation between the severity of pain and severity of nerve injuries. Moreover, they believe that instability in patients with patellofemoral malalignment can be explained, at least in part, by the damage to nerves of the lateral retinaculum, which can be related to proprioception.

Some studies also implicate neural damage and hyperinnervation in the lateral retinaculum as a possible source of pain in patients with patellofemoral malalignment[16,17,36,61,62] (Figure 4.7). In reviewing the literature, we note that hyperinnervation is a factor implicated in the pathophysiology of pain in other orthopaedic pathologies.[63–65] The mechanisms by which this neural proliferation is produced in the lateral retinaculum, however, is currently unknown.

Sanchis-Alfonso and Roselló-Sastre[17] observed the presence of neural growth factor (NGF) and substance P in the lateral retinaculum of patients with isolated symptomatic patellofemoral malalignment. The NGF is a cytokine neurotrophin that is released during axonogenesis; inflammation stimulates neural sprouting.[2] It is involved in pain mechanisms by stimulating the release of neuroceptive mediators, such as substance P, and attracting lymph cells and mastocytes, which can potentially release more cytokines, including NGF, thus perpetuating the cycle.[17] Sanchis-Alfonso and Roselló-Sastre[17] demonstrated that nerve proliferation in patellofemoral malalignment primarily depends on nociceptive sensory substance P-positive nerves in the lateral retinaculum. Moreover, the group of patellofemoral malalignment patients with pain as their predominant symptom showed higher levels of NGF than patellofemoral

malalignment patients with instability as the main complaint.[2] This NGF is detected primarily in the vessel walls and in the large neural structures and is found as active precursors of 35 kDa, which means that the nerve fibres of these lateral retinacula must still be in a proliferative phase.[2]

Neural growth factor synthesis can be induced by ischaemia.[29,66–68] Moreover, it is observed that NGF hastens neural proliferation in vessel walls,[69,70] and it is this pattern of hyperinnervation that is seen in the lateral retinaculum of patients with painful patellofemoral malalignment.[65,70] The authors hypothesize that ischaemia may be the main problem in painful patellofemoral malalignment[2,70] as a result of a mechanism of vascular torsion secondary to patellar malalignment–medial traction over a retracted lateral retinaculum, in contrast with the lax lateral retinaculum in knees with patellar instability; periodic episodes of ischaemia are promoted and could trigger NGF release. Once NGF is present in the tissues, it leads to hyperinnervation, substance P release, pain, and attraction of mastocytes,[17,71] leading to the ischaemia–hyperinnervation–pain cycle (Table 4.2).

Biedert and Sanchis-Alfonso[2] suggested that two different pathobiological mechanisms lead to a symptomatic patellofemoral malalignment: (a) pain as the predominant symptom, with

Table 4.2 Ischaemia–hyperinnervation–pain cycle

Patellar malalignment
↓
Vascular torsion
↓
Ischaemia
↓
Increased neural growth factor synthesis
↓
Hyperinnervation, substance P release, pain, attraction of mastocytes

detectable levels of NGF that provoke hyperinnervation and stimulus of substance P release; and (b) instability as the predominant symptom, whereby there is less local NGF release, less neural proliferation and less nociceptive stimulus.

Damage to these neuroproprioceptive fibres can alter the proprioceptive innervation[16] and stability of the patella.[30] Jerosch and Prymka[61] found a reduction in knee proprioception after patellar dislocation compared with the asymptomatic contralateral knee, which can be explained by proprioceptive loss. This also may explain why elastic knee bandages can improve knee stability by increasing proprioceptive feedback from skin mechanoreceptors.

Summary

Patellofemoral pain represents a significant and complex problem. The knowledge of the underlying neurosensory principles of pain, the pathophysiology of the numerous involved structures, and the different mechanisms causing pain are mandatory to understand the characteristics and genesis of patellofemoral pain. The pathophysiological mechanisms are variable and may change. They can be present in combination, they can be cumulative, and they can interact in complex ways. These considerations are essential in understanding the basics of this complicated topic. The pathophysiology with respect to the specific involved structures and activities must be recognized to determine the path to successful treatment.

References

1. Dye SF (1996) The knee as a biologic transmission with an envelope of function: a theory. *Clin Orthop* **325**: 10–18
2. Biedert RM, Sanchis-Alfonso V (2002) Sources of anterior knee pain. *Clin Sports Med* **21**: 335–347
3. Biedert RM, Kernen V (2001) Neurosensory characteristics of the patellofemoral joint: what is the genesis of patellofemoral pain? *Sports Med Arthrosc Rev* **9**: 295–300
4. Guyton AC, Hall JE (1996) *Textbook of Medical Physiology.* Philadelphia, PA, WB Saunders
5. Zimmermann M (1979) Peripheral and central nervous mechanisms of nociception, pain, and pain therapy: facts and hypotheses. In: Bonica JJ (ed), *Advances in Pain Research and Therapy*, volume 3. New York, Raven, pp 3–32
6. Kennedy JC, Alexander IJ, Hayes KC (1982) Nerve supply of the human knee and its functional importance. *Am J Sports Med* **10**: 329–335
7. Skoglund S (1973) Joint receptors and kinesthesis. In: *Handbook of Sensory Physiology*, volume I. New York, Springer-Verlag, pp 111–136
8. Barrack RL, Lund PJ, Skinner HB (1994) Knee joint proprioception revisited. *J Sports Rehab* **3**: 18–42
9. Barrack RL, Skinner HB (1990) The sensory function of knee ligaments. In: Daniel DM, Akeson WH, O'Connor JJ (eds), *Knee Ligaments: Structure, Function, Injury, and Repair.* New York, Raven, pp 95–114
10. Fontaine C (1983) L'innervation de la routule. *Acta Orthop Belg* **49**: 425–436
11. Freeman MA, Wyke B (1967) The innervation of the knee joint. An anatomical and histological study in the cat. *J Anat* **101**: 505–532
12. Biedert RM, Stauffer E, Friederich NF (1992) Occurrence of free nerve endings in the soft tissue of the knee joint. A histologic investigation. *Am J Sports Med* **20**: 430–433
13. Johansson H, Sjolander P, Sojka P (1991) Receptors in the knee joint ligaments and their role in the biomechanics of the joint. *Crit Rev Biomed Eng* **18**: 341–368
14. Menkes CJ, Renoux M, Laoussadi S et al (1993) Substance P levels in the synovium and synovial fluid from patients with rheumatoid arthritis and osteoarthritis. *J Rheumatol* **20**: 714–717
15. Witonski D, Wagrowska-Danielewicz M (1999) Distribution of substance P nerve fibers in the knee joint in patients with anterior knee pain syndrome. A preliminary report. *Knee Surg Sports Traumatol Arthrosc* **7**: 177–183
16. Sanchis-Alfonso V, Roselló-Sastre E, Monteagudo-Castro C, Esquerdo J (1998) Quantitative analysis of nerve changes in the lateral retinaculum in patients with isolated symptomatic patellofemoral

malalignment. A preliminary study. *Am J Sports Med* **26**: 703–709

17. Sanchis-Alfonso V, Roselló-Sastre E (2000) Immunohistochemical analysis for neural markers of the lateral retinaculum in patients with isolated symptomatic patellofemoral malalignment. A neuroanatomic basis for anterior knee pain in the active young patient. *Am J Sports Med* **28**: 725–731

18. Walsh DA, Salmon M, Mapp PI et al (1993) Microvascular substance P binding to normal and inflamed rat and human synovium. *J Pharmacol Exp Ther* **267**: 951–960

19. Wojtys EM, Beaman DN, Glover RA, Janda D (1990) Innervation of the human knee joint by substance-P fibers. *Arthroscopy* **6**: 254–263

20. Dye SF, Chew MH (1993) The use of scintigraphy to detect increased osseous metabolic transmission with an envelope of function. *J Bone Joint Surg Am* **75**: 1388–1406

21. Doucette SA, Goble EM (1992) The effect of exercise on patellar tracking in lateral patellar compression syndrome. *Am J Sports Med* **20**: 434–440

22. Percy EC, Strother RT (1985) Patellalgia. *Physician Sportsmed* **13**: 43–59

23. Reimann I, Christensen SB (1977) A histological demonstration of nerves in subchondral bone. *Acta Orthop Scand* **48**: 345–352

24. Dye SF, Boll DA (1986) Radionuclide imaging of the patellofemoral joint in young adults with anterior knee pain. *Orthop Clin North Am* **17**: 249–262

25. Grana WA, Hinkley B, Hollingsworth S (1984) Arthroscopic evaluation and treatment of patellar malalignment. *Clin Orthop* **186**: 122–128

26. Abernethy PJ, Townsend PR, Rose RM, Radin EL (1978) Is chondromalacia patellae a separate clinical entity? *J Bone Joint Surg Br* **60**: 205–210

27. Minns RJ, Birnie AJ, Abernethy PJ (1979) A stress analysis of the patella, and how it relates to patellar articular cartilage lesions. *J Biomech* **12**: 699–711

28. Waisbrod H, Treiman N (1980) Intraosseous venography in patellofemoral disorders. A preliminary report. *J Bone Joint Surg Br* **62**: 454–456

29. Sanchis-Alfonso V, Roselló-Sastre E (1998) [Hyperinnervation and ischemia]. *Rev Patol Rodilla* **3**: 60–63

30. Schneider U, Graf J, Thomsen M et al (1997) Das Hypertensionssyndrom der Patella: Nomenklatur, Diagnostik, und Therapie. *Z Orthop Ihre Grenzgeb* **135**: 187–188

31. McConnell J (2002) The physical therapist's approach to patellofemoral disorders. *Clin Sports Med* **21**: 363–387

32. Krenn V, Hofmann S, Engel A (1990) First description of mechanoreceptors in the corpus adiposum infrapatellare of man. *Acta Anat (Basel)* **137**: 187–188

33. Dye SF, Stäubli HU, Biedert RM, Vaupel GL (1999) The mosaic of pathophysiology causing patellofemoral pain: therapeutic implications. *Operative Tech Sports Med* **7**: 46–54

34. McConnell J (1986) The management of chondromalacia patellae: a long-term solution. *Aust J Physiother* **32**: 215–223

35. Biedert RM (2000) A new perspective of patellofemoral pain. Where is the pain coming from? In: Symposia Handouts and Abstracts of the 67th Annual Meeting of the American Academy of Orthopaedic Surgeons, Orlando, FL, p 247

36. Fulkerson JP, Tennant R, Jaivin JS, Grunnet M (1985) Histologic evidence of retinacular nerve injury associated with patellofemoral malalignment. *Clin Orthop* **197**: 196–205

37. Kramers-de Quervain IA, Biedert R, Stüssi E (1997) Quantitative gait analysis in patients with medial patellar instability following lateral retinacular release. *Knee Surg Sports Traumatol Arthrosc* **5**: 95–101

38. Fulkerson JP (1982) Awareness of the retinaculum in evaluating patellofemoral pain. *Am J Sports Med* **10**: 147–149

39. Goldring MB (2000) The role of the chondrocyte in osteoarthritis. *Arthritis Rheum* **43**: 1916–1926

40. Cameron ML, Frondoza CG, Holland C, Hungerford DS (1999) Expression of proinflammatory IL-1 and TNF by osteoarthritic chondrocytes in altered response to mechanical stress. *Trans Orthop Res Soc* **24** (abstr): 606

41. Westacott CI, Barakat AF, Wood L et al (2000) Tumor necrosis factor alpha can contribute to focal loss of cartilage in osteoarthritis. *Osteoarthr Cartilage* **8**: 213–221

42. van den Berg WB (1999) The role of cytokines and growth factors in cartilage destruction

in osteoarthritis and rheumatoid arthritis. *Z Rheumatol* **58**: 136–141

43. Smith MD, Triantafillou S, Parker A et al (1997) Synovial membrane inflammation and cytokine production in patients with early osteoarthritis. *J Rheumatol* **24**: 365–371

44. Krenn V, Hensel F, Kim HJ et al (1999) Molecular IgV(H) analysis demonstrates highly somatic mutated B cells in synovialitis of osteoarthritis: a degenerative disease is associated with a specific, not locally generated immune response. *Lab Invest* **79**: 1377–1384

45. Ishii H, Tanaka H, Katoh K et al (2002) Characterization of infiltrating T cells and Th1/Th2-type cytokines in the synovium of patients with osteoarthritis. *Osteoarthr Cartilage* **10**: 277–281

46. Poole AR (1995) Imbalances of anabolism and catabolism of cartilage matrix components in osteoarthritis. In: Kuettner KE, Goldberg VM (eds), *Osteoarthritic Disorders*. Rosemont, IL, American Academy of Orthopaedic Surgeons, pp 247–260

47. Ushiyama T, Chano T, Inoue K, Matsusue Y (2003) Cytokine production in the infrapatellar fat pad: another source of cytokines in knee synovial fluids. *Ann Rheum Dis* **62**: 108–112

48. Moos V, Fickert S, Muller B, Weber U, Sieper J (1999) Immunohistological analysis of cytokine expression in human osteoarthritic and healthy cartilage. *J Rheumatol* **26**: 870–879

49. Moos V, Sieper J, Herzog W, Müller B (2001) Regulation of expression of cytokines and growth factors in osteoarthritic cartilage explants. *Clin Rheumatol* **20**

50. Gambardella RA (1999) Technical pitfalls of patellofemoral surgery. *Clin Sports Med* **18**: 897–903

51. Dzioba RB (1990) Diagnostic arthroscopy and longitudinal open lateral release. A four-year follow-up study to determine predictors of surgical outcome. *Am J Sports Med* **18**: 343–348

52. Dye SF, Vaupel GL, Dye CC (1998) Conscious neurosensory mapping of the internal structures of the human knee without intraarticular anesthesia. *Am J Sports Med* **26**: 773–777

53. Mori Y, Kuroki Y, Yamamoto R et al (1991) Clinical and histological study of patellar chondropathy in adolescents. *Arthroscopy* **7**: 182–197

54. Biedert RM (1999) Sensory–Motor Function of the Knee Joint. Histologic, Anatomic, and Neurophysiologic Investigations. Thesis, University of Basel, Switzerland

55. de Andrade JR, Grant C, Dixon ASTJ (1965) Joint distension and reflex muscle inhibition in the knee. *J Bone Joint Surg Am* **47**: 313–322

56. Hughston JC, Walsh WM, Puddu G (1984) *Patellar Subluxation and Dislocation. Saunders Monographs in Clinical Orthopaedics*, volume V. Philadelphia, PA, WB Saunders

57. Simon LS (1999) Viscosupplementation therapy with intra-articular hyaluronic acid. Fact or fantasy? *Rheum Dis Clin North Am* **25**: 345–357

58. Hunziker EB, Stäubli HU, Jakob RP (1992) Surgical anatomy of the knee joint. In: Jakob RP, Stäubli HU (eds), *The Knee and the Cruciate Ligaments*. Heidelberg, Springer-Verlag, pp 31–47

59. Dye SF (1999) Invited commentary on Watson CJ, Propps M, Galt W, Redding A, Dobbs D. Reliability of McConnell's classification of patellar orientation in symptomatic and asymptomatic subjects. *J Orthop Sports Phys Ther* **29**: 378–393

60. Morscher E (1978) Osteotomy of the patella in chondromalacia. Preliminary report. *Arch Orthop Trauma Surg* **92**: 139–147

61. Jerosch J, Prymka M (1996) Knee joint proprioception in patients with posttraumatic recurrent patella dislocation. *Knee Surg Sports Traumatol Arthrosc* **4**: 14–18

62. Mori Y, Fujimoto A, Okumo H, Kuroki Y (1991) Lateral retinaculum release in adolescent patellofemoral disorders: its relationship to peripheral nerve injury in the lateral retinaculum. *Bull Hosp Jt Dis Orthop Inst* **51**: 218–229

63. Coppes MH, Marani E, Thomeer RT, Groen GJ (1997) Innervation of 'painful' lumbar discs. *Spine* **22**: 2342–2349; discussion, 2349–2350

64. Freemont AJ, Peacock TE, Goupille P et al (1997) Nerve ingrowth into diseased intervertebral disc in chronic back pain. *Lancet* **350**: 178–181

65. Sanchis-Alfonso V, Roselló-Sastre E, Subias-López A (1999) Mechanisms of pain in jumper's knee. A histological and immunohistological study. *J Bone Joint Surg Br* **81** (suppl 82)

66. Abe T, Morgan DA, Gutterman DD (1997) Protective role of nerve growth factor against postischemic dysfunction of sympathetic coronary innervation. *Circulation* **95**: 213–220

67. Lee TH, Kato H, Kogure K, Itoyama Y (1996) Temporal profile of nerve growth factor-like immunoreactivity after transient focal cerebral ischemia in rats. *Brain Res* **713**: 199–210

68. Woolf CJ, Allchorne A, Safieh-Garabedian B, Poole S (1997) Cytokines, nerve growth factor, and inflammatory hyperalgesia: the contribution of tumour necrosis factor alpha. *Br J Pharmacol* **121**: 417–424

69. Isaacson LG, Crutcher KA (1995) The duration of sprouted cerebrovascular axons following intracranial infusion of nerve growth factor. *Exp Neurol* **131**: 174–179

70. Kawaja MD (1998) Sympathetic and sensory innervation of the extracerebral vasculature: roles for p75NTR neuronal expression and nerve growth factor. *J Neurosci Res* **52**: 295–306

71. Malcangio M, Garrett NE, Cruwys S, Tomlinson DR (1997) Nerve growth factor- and neurotrophin-3-induced changes in nociceptive threshold and the release of substance P from the rat isolated spinal cord. *J Neurosci* **17**: 8459–8467

Suggested reading

Biedert RM, Sanchis-Alfonso V (2002) Sources of anterior knee pain. *Clin Sports Med* **21**: 335–347

Biedert RM, Kernen V (2001) Neurosensory characteristics of the patellofemoral joint: what is the genesis of patellofemoral pain? *Sports Med Arthrosc Rev* **9**: 295–300

Dye SF, Stäubli HU, Biedert RM, Vaupel GL (1999) The mosaic of pathophysiology causing patellofemoral pain: therapeutic implications. *Op Tech Sports Med* **7**: 46–54

5 Physical Examination

Roland M. Biedert

The physical examination is the cornerstone for achieving the correct diagnosis. Routine evaluation of the patellofemoral joint must include examination of both lower extremities. Understanding of the functional anatomy and knowledge about what is normal are the basics of the physical examination.

A complete knee examination is performed on each patient to determine the cause of the patellofemoral pain or instability and to eliminate other possible causes. Physical examination consists of different parts with the patient in the standing, walking, seated and supine positions. A checklist is provided at the end of this chapter (*see* Table 5.2). The examination always has a static (passive) and a dynamic (active) part with inspection and palpation.

Standing position

The physical examination begins with the patient standing barefoot to determine weightbearing alignment, torsional deformities and foot position[1] (Figure 5.1). Foot disorders such as overpronation (Figure 5.2) cause increased internal tibial and femoral torsion with 'kneeing-in' (Figure 5.3) in the one-leg standing posi-tion. Excessive pronation affects patellofemoral mechanics and may lead to consecutive lateral subluxation of the patella. Orthotic arch support compensates for abnormal pronation.

The next step of the physical examination consists of observation of the lower extremities for varus or valgus as well as angular deformities occurring only in the tibia.[2] Tibia vara with varus deformity is often combined with external tibial torsion and internal femoral torsion. Tibia vara located in the proximal third of the tibia leads to a different appearance (grasshopper-eyes kneecaps) than varus of the entire lower extremity[2] (Figure 5.4). Obesity and atrophy are important factors overloading the patellofemoral joint; these must be evaluated. Atrophy is limited in most cases to the quadriceps and in special cases to the hip rotator and abductor muscles. Quadriceps atrophy may be measured for the purposes of documentation and follow-up comparison during rehabilitation. Atrophy of the external hip rotator muscles may cause pathological increased internal femoral torsion with secondary valgus alignment and kneeing-in. Normal hip abductor strength stabilizes the pelvis and provides a stable base for gait. Hip abductor weakness may cause sagging of the contralateral

Patellofemoral Disorders: Diagnosis and Treatment. Edited by Roland M. Biedert
© 2004 John Wiley & Sons, Ltd   ISBN: 0-470-85011-6

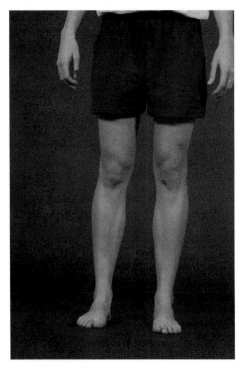

Figure 5.1   The standing position allows assessment of both lower extremities (alignment, rotation, foot position)

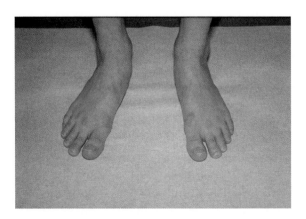

Figure 5.2   Overpronation of both feet cause increased internal rotation of the lower extremities

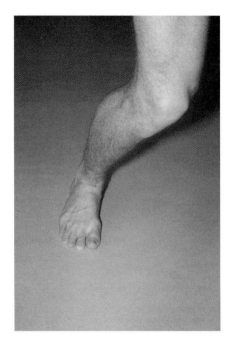

Figure 5.3   'Kneeing in' of the right leg with increased valgus alignment caused by overpronation of the foot

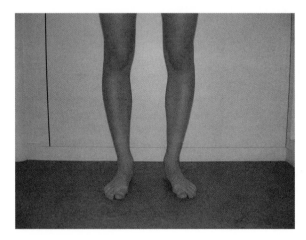

Figure 5.4   Tibiae varae with grasshopper-eyes kneecaps

pelvis, thus creating increased tension on the iliotibial band and the lateral retinacula. This should be addressed in the treatment plan, as well as a correction of leg-length discrepancies greater than 10 mm.

From the standing position, we let the patient go into knee flexion with full weightbearing. This gives information about the sensorimotor stabilizing capabilities of the patient (Figure 5.5). Kneeing-in documents muscular weakness. Weakness in the ankle joint or overpronation must be excluded.

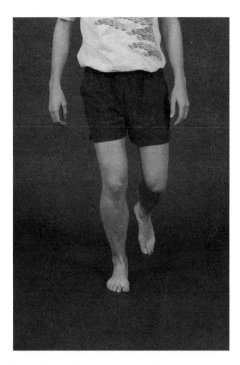

Figure 5.5 Sensorimotor control of the knee in weight-bearing flexion

By watching the patient squat and then stand, dynamic patellar tracking is evaluated. This simple movement can be painful and difficult for disabled patients. Pathological patellar tracking during the beginning of flexion is described as the 'J-sign'. It refers to the inverted J course of the patella that begins lateral to the trochlea and suddenly moves medially to enter the trochlea. The J-sign may be observed during squatting, actively or passively during open kinetic chain movements. During active motion, vastus medialis obliquus deficiency may be the pathoanatomical cause during active motion. During passive motion, bone morphology and imbalance of the patellofemoral soft tissue may be the sign of the J-sign's course.

Sideways observation may show normal alignment (full extension), hyperextension (genu recurvatum) or lack of full extension (genu flexum). Alignment has an important influence on the patella. Hyperextension decreases the osseous stabilization of the patella, whereas lack of extension increases the pressure on the patella in the trochlea.

Walking

Observation of walking on the flat floor and then up and down stairs can reveal functional deficits. Compensating mechanisms due to pain are frequent.

Seated position

Observation of the patient in the seated position (Figures 5.6, 5.7 and 5.8) with the knees flexed to 90° off the end of the table provides information regarding patellar position (alta, baja, lateralization or medialization), tibial torsion and the tubercle–sulcus angle.[1,2]

When the tibial tubercle is lateral to the mid-patella, this may indicate pathological lateralization with reference to the midtrochlea, since most patellae are centred within the trochlea at 90° of knee flexion.[1,2] This measurement has been described as the tubercle–sulcus angle or Q angle in the flexed position and is defined by referencing a point at the centre of the patella to a point at the centre of the tibial tubercle[1] (Figure 5.9).

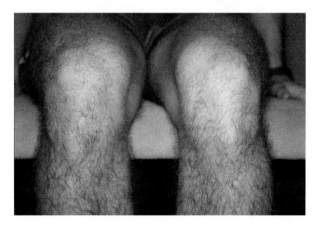

Figure 5.6 Assessment of the position of the tibial tubercle relative to the mid-patella. Minimal lateralization of the tibial tubercle in 90° of knee flexion due to increased tibial external rotation on both sides

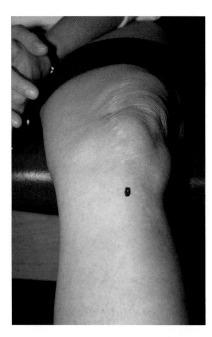

Figure 5.7 Superolateral patella subluxation. High and too lateral position of subluxed left patella following unsuccessful surgical treatment (seated, 50°, contracted)

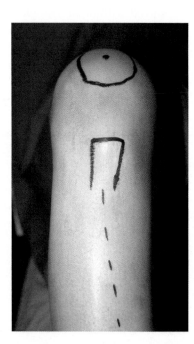

Figure 5.8 Abnormal medialization of the tibial tubercle following overcorrection to medial (- - -, axis tibia, right knee, sitting, 90°, relaxed, circle around the patella, point in the centre)

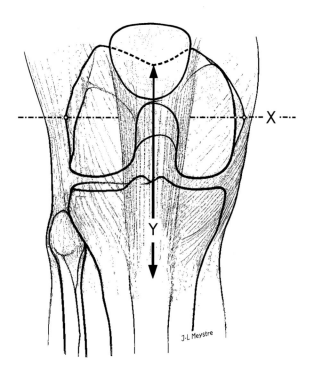

Figure 5.9 Tubercle−sulcus angle at 90° of knee flexion. The angle is delineated by a line perpendicular to the transepicondylar axis (X), and a second line (Y) passing through the centre of the tibial tubercle and the centre of the patella[1]

This is a more accurate assessment of the quadriceps angle (Q angle) than measuring in extension, because the patella is centred in the trochlea and rotational abnormalities are accounted for. A normal tubercle−sulcus angle is 0°, while greater than 10° is definitely abnormal.[1] Excessive lateralization of the tibial tubercle with respect to the midtrochlea may affect the patellar gliding mechanism and cause lateral subluxation and/or lateral patellar compression syndrome. This situation represents one of the rare and specific indications for mild medialization of the tibial tubercle with lengthening of the lateral retinaculum. The correction is made in reference to the tubercle−sulcus angle.

Still in the seated position, the patient is asked to extend the knee. The active excursion of the patella from 90° to full extension is assessed. Pain and abnormal movements like catching, locking, lateralization or medialization of the kneecap may be observed easily (Figure 5.7).

Supine position

The patient lies down on the table with both legs fully extended. Measurement of the Q angle is a standard estimate of the valgus moment acting on the patellofemoral joint. The degree of valgus at the knee may affect alignment. Abnormal patellar alignment is described as one of the extrinsic factors that can cause patellofemoral pain. An exact determination of patellar alignment or malalignment does not exist.[3] Nevertheless, a common tool to assess malalignment is the Q angle.[4] An abnormal or increased Q angle is considered a relevant pathological factor in patellofemoral disorders.[5,6] Many authors[6] use a so-called 'pathological' Q angle (measured in extension) as an indication for medial transposition of the tibial tuberosity. But the Q angle varies, depending on whether the patient's knee is in an extended or flexed position, whether the quadriceps muscle is relaxed or contracted, whether the patient is a woman or a man, and whether the position is supine or standing.[4] Clinical findings and measurements of the Q angle in extension only may be elusive in many cases.[7]

Q angle measurements

Q angle measurements are obtained clinically with subjects lying down and their knees in 0° of flexion (knees extended)[4,8] (Figure 5.10). A line is drawn from the middle of the patella to the centre of the tibial tubercle, and a second line from the middle of the patella to the centre of the anterior-superior iliac spine. The angle between these two lines, the Q angle, is measured with a goniometer.

A prospective study[9] showed that no correlation exists between the Q angle, measured in extension (0° of knee flexion), and the position of the patella in the trochlea, measured with CT imaging. Although the Q angle has some value as an estimate of the degree of the theoretical

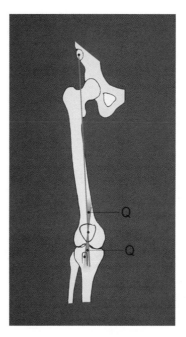

Figure 5.10   Measurement of the Q angle[8]

skeletal malalignment, we agree with Ford and Post[5] and Dandy[10] that it is an unreliable measurement and that there is no substantial proof that it correlates with patellofemoral pain.

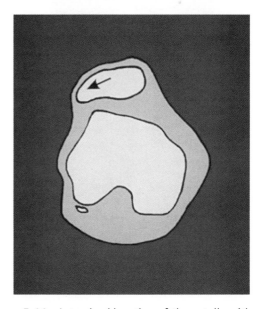

Figure 5.11   Lateral subluxation of the patella with dysplastic trochlea (axial, right knee)

Table 5.1   Factors influencing the Q angle[4,5,9,10,12]

Q angle	
Increased	Decreased
♦ High femoral anteversion ♦ Genu valgum ♦ External tibial torsion ♦ Laterally positioned tibial tuberosity ♦ Deficiencies supporting muscles ♦ Medial subluxation of the patella ♦ Defective medial trochlea	♦ Genu varum ♦ Internal tibial torsion ♦ Lateral subluxation of the patella ♦ Medialization of the tibial tuberosity over the midline of the trochlea ♦ Tight lateral retinaculum ♦ Defective lateral trochlea

There are many factors that increase or decrease the Q angle (Table 5.1) (Figures 5.11 and 5.12).

The Q angle value depends directly on the position of the patella in the trochlea (centred or not centred), e.g. a normally centred patella in combination with a laterally positioned tibial tuberosity causes a high ('pathological') Q angle value (Figure 5.13). In contrast, a laterally subluxed patella in combination with a laterally positioned tibial tuberosity shows a low ('normal') Q angle value (Figures 5.14 and 5.15). This

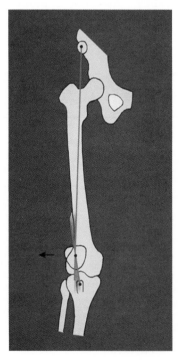

Figure 5.12   Decreased Q angle caused by lateral patellar subluxation

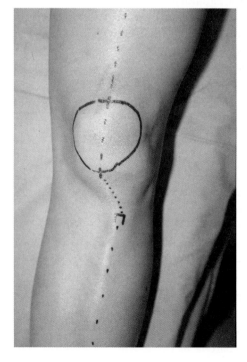

Figure 5.13   High Q angle value in a patient with documented well-centred patella (left knee)

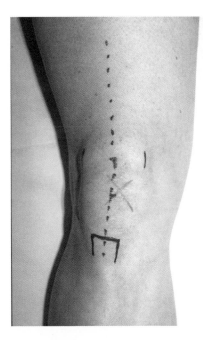

Figure 5.14 Low Q angle value in a patient with laterally subluxed patella (right knee)

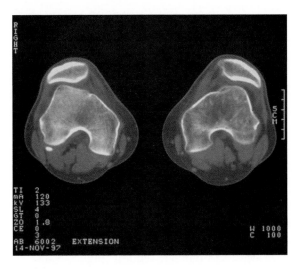

Figure 5.15 Axial CT scan documenting the lateral patella subluxation on both sides in the same patient as in Figure 5.14 (quadriceps relaxed)

explains how a normal patella position can cause 'abnormal' Q angle values, and why a pathological patella position can show 'normal' Q angle values. This leads to the conclusion that high and low Q angles have no clinical significance.[9]

Although many clinicians use Q angle measurements for clinical assessment, no universally accepted method with detailed description exists. Additionally, no exact data on what is normal, increased or abnormal are available. Measurements of the Q angle have been reported even though the range of normal values is variable and there are minimal quantifiable data supporting its diagnostic relevance.[4,9] Rillmann et al[6] and Kujala et al[11] consider an abnormal Q angle as a relevant pathological factor, even without presenting values of what exactly is 'abnormal'. Based on a literature review, different ways of measuring the Q angle exist. Messier et al[8] measured the Q angle using a goniometer, as described above. They considered Q angles in excess of 16° to be significantly associated with patellofemoral pain. Ford and Post[5] and Caylor et al[4] defined the Q angle in the same way. Q angle values of 15° or less were considered to be normal; angles greater than 20° were considered abnormal. The question of how values between 16° and 19° should be regarded remained unanswered. Papagelopoulos and Sim[12] generally considered Q angle values greater than 20° as abnormal and associated with patellofemoral pain. Caylor et al[4] measured the Q angle in two different standing positions. Finally, Guzzanti et al[7] performed the examination of the Q angle by using CT scans in 15° of flexion. They found average values of 19.4° in symptomatic patients and 20.2° in the healthy control group.

We recognize that there is an immense controversy about how to measure the Q angle and what its 'normal' values are.[9] It is dangerous to draw the conclusion that an 'abnormal' Q angle is always an aetiological factor in patellofemoral disorders and malalignment.

Effusion

Effusion may be present in patients with patellofemoral derangement (Figure 5.16). Chronic effusion is often combined with synovial thickening as the result of chronic irritation caused by

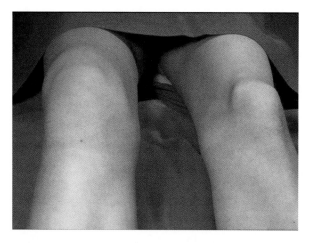

Figure 5.16 Chronic effusion with synovial thickening caused by chronic irritation in a young female patient suffering from a suprapatellar plica (right knee)

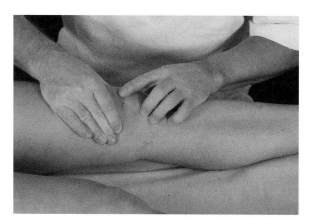

Figure 5.17 Palpation of joint effusion. Mild pressure is applied to one side, moving the liquid under the patella to the opposite side

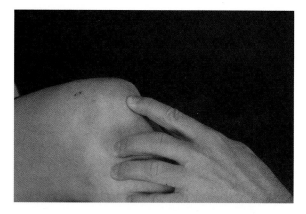

Figure 5.18 Painful palpation on the distal pole of the patella and the proximal patellar tendon in a patient with chronic proximal jumper's knee

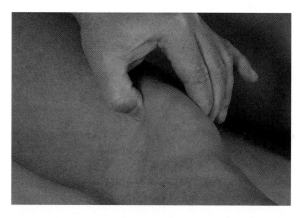

Figure 5.19 Palpation of the lateral retinaculum. Differentiation of the superficial oblique and the deep transverse retinacula is possible

plicae, articular degeneration and instability.[2,13] The seeding of the synovium with cartilaginous debris may cause chronic synovitis.[13] Effusion is evident by careful palpation (Figure 5.17). With this, the presence of minimal liquid may be also be determined.

Palpation

Systematic palpation is necessary to define the exact painful areas and the structures involved.

Palpation is a careful procedure to assess the areas of tenderness, swelling and thickening. Areas to be palpated include the insertions of the quadriceps and patellar tendon (Figure 5.18), the medial and lateral retinacula (Figure 5.19), the medial (medial shelf) (Figure 5.20) and suprapatellar plica (Figure 5.21), the patella, the fat pad, the vastus lateralis and medialis muscles and the adductor tubercle. Tenderness may represent fresh injury, inflammation, irritation, overload or neural damage.[14–17] Specific painful areas are associated with specific disorders and help to confirm the clinical diagnosis.

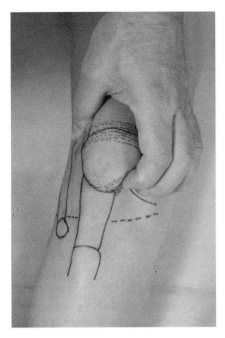

Figure 5.20 Palpation for mediopatellar plica. The knee is slightly moved in a flexed position and the fingers palpate the medial shelf more distally

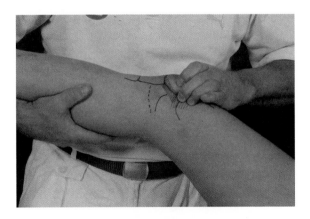

Figure 5.21 Palpation for suprapatellar plica. The leg is held in mild flexion. The patella is slightly displaced medially with fingers over the course of the plica. Passive flexion and extension movements cause pain and catching of the plica[2]

The lateral retinaculum consists of two main parts, the superficial oblique and the deep transverse retinacula (Figure 5.22). The superficial oblique retinaculum originates from the iliotibial tract, interdigitating with the longitudinally

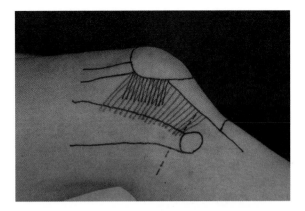

Figure 5.22 Superficial lateral retinaculum and deep oblique retinaculum (right knee)[18]

orientated fibres of the vastus lateralis and the patellar tendon.[18] The deep transverse retinaculum runs from the deep portion of the iliotibial tract directly to the lateral patella. It proceeds less far distally so that at the level of the patellar tendon, only the superficial retinaculum is present.[18]

Existing *scars* should be palpated to detect neuromas. Injecting a local anaesthetic confirms the correct diagnosis by immediate relief of pain. The same diagnostic procedure is helpful to confirm nerve entrapment syndromes, such as saphenous nerve entrapment at the adductor hiatus.

Patellar gliding mechanism

Moving the knee passively reveals information about the *gliding mechanism of the patella* in the trochlea. Stretching, impingement or compression of the peripatellar soft tissues may cause discomfort or pain. Crepitus, locking or catching may correlate with intraarticular pathology. Precise additional palpation is useful to define the area of derangement. Crepitus can also be present without complaints.[19]

Patellar mobility

To test *patellar mobility* the patient should lie supine with the quadriceps relaxed. The patella is pushed in four major directions–proximal, distal, medial and lateral (Figures 5.23 and 5.24).

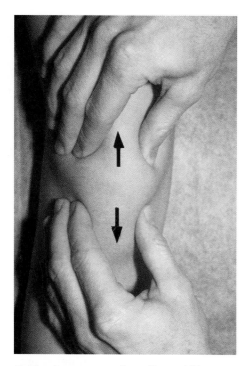

Figure 5.23 Assessment of patellar mobility: proximal–distal

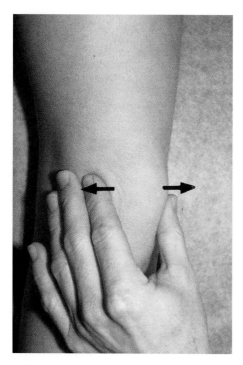

Figure 5.24 Assessment of patellar mobility: medial–lateral

Then the examiner evaluates the constraint of the different structures, the position of the patella (baja, alta, lateralized, medialized) and the rotation of the patella. Comparison with the opposite side helps to detect any pathology. Besides manual assessment of patellar mobility, instrumented measurement improves precision and documentation. To diagnose instability especially, the examiner should apply a displacing standardized force to one-half of the joint (i.e. to the patella and not also to the femur) and then measure the amount of displacement.

Patellar tests

Patellar glide test

This test indicates medial or lateral retinacular tightness. It estimates patellar translation relative to the width of the patella and with this the patellar balance. The patellar glide test is performed in extension and at 30° of flexion with the quadriceps relaxed.[1] The patella is divided into longitudinal quadrants (Figure 5.25). The

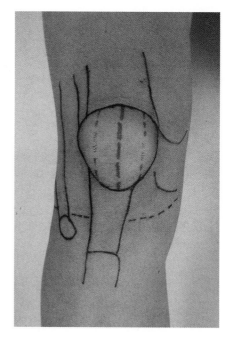

Figure 5.25 Patellar glide test: division of the patella into quadrants

patella is displaced in a medial and then a lateral direction under the guidance of the examiner's hand. Translation is recorded as quadrants of the patella and determines lateral and medial parapatellar tightness. Three quadrants of medial or lateral glide suggest incompetent restraints (lateral or medial); a glide of four quadrants (dislocatable patella) is obviously indicative of deficient restraint.[1] A medial glide of three or four quadrants suggests a hypermobile patella. One quadrant or less of medial translation is consistent with excessive lateral tightness.[1] Decreased superior patellar glide may also be present in patients with knee flexion contracture or infrapatellar contracture syndrome with thickening of the peripatellar soft tissues and infrapatellar fat pad. Patients with arthrofibrosis or 'fibrotic healers' have decreased patellar glide. The patellar glide test is more sensitive in full extension, because in extension there is less stability from the bony geometry. Examination in 30° of flexion gives patients a more secure feeling, allowing them to relax the muscles.

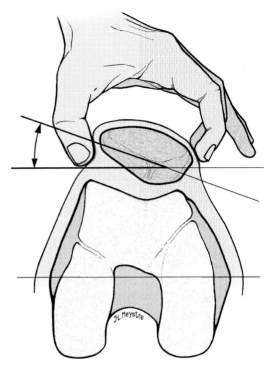

Figure 5.26 Passive patellar tilt test. The lateral edge of the patella is lifted from the lateral femoral condyle

Passive patellar tilt test

The tilt test is performed with the patient supine and relaxed (Figure 5.26). The examiner lifts the lateral edge of the patella from the lateral femoral condyle (Figure 5.27). Lateral subluxation during examination must be avoided. Excessively tight lateral restraints show a neutral or negative angle to the horizontal.[1] A high positive angle reveals deficiencies of the lateral constraints, such as over-release of the lateral retinaculum (*see* Case Study 20). Clinically, it is useful to quantify the correction of patellar tilt as less than neutral, neutral, or greater than neutral. Males' lateral restraints tend to be tighter than females' lateral restraints on the average.[1]

Patellar apprehension test

This test is carried out with the knee flexed between 20° and 30°; the patella is forced laterally by medial manual pressure[13] (Figure 5.28).

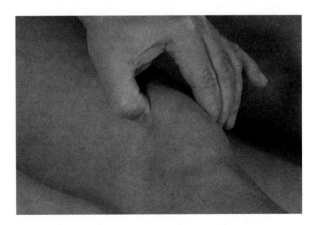

Figure 5.27 Passive patellar tilt test. Physical examination

The test is positive when the patient feels pain and/or fear of lateral subluxation of the patella and resists this manouevre[13] or when the patient instantly recognizes instability symptoms. This is suggestive of lateral patellar instability.

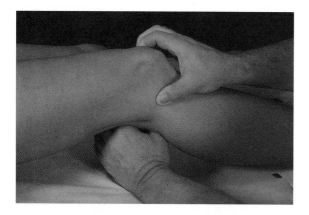

Figure 5.28 Patellar apprehension test. Medial manual pressure is applied to the patella to subluxate the patella laterally

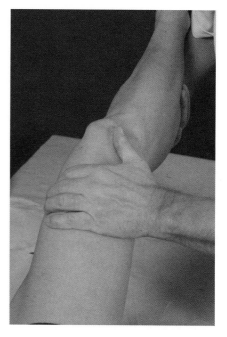

Figure 5.30 Patellar relocation test (examination for medial patellar instability)

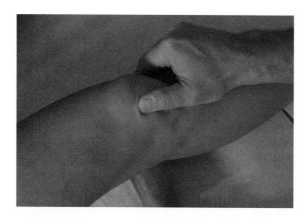

Figure 5.29 Reverse apprehension test (examination for medial patellar instability)

Special tests

Certain other tests are useful to document medial patellar instability, especially in patients with previous patellofemoral surgery and persisting complaints. The *reverse apprehension test* depicts painful medial subluxation of the patella with discomfort and fear following manual medial translation[20,21] (Figure 5.29). The *patellar relocation test* is done by manual displacement of the patella to medial and then, while holding the patella medially, flexing the knee actively or passively (Figure 5.30). Relocation of the patella into the trochlea is the painful movement and

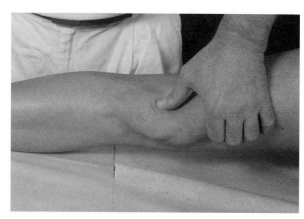

Figure 5.31 Gravity subluxation test (examination for medial patellar instability)

reproduces the patient's complaints. The *gravity subluxation test* was described by Nonweiler and DeLee[20] (Figure 5.31). The patient is placed in the lateral decubitus position, the patella is manually displaced medially toward the table and subluxed. The test is positive when the patient is unable to reduce the subluxation voluntarily.

Table 5.2 Checklist for physical examination

Standing position
- Weightbearing alignment
  Valgus, normal, varus
  Hyperextension, normal, flexion
  Position pelvis
  Leg length
  Atrophy
  Obesity
- Foot position
  Varus, valgus position calcaneus
  Pronation

Walking
- Functional deficits
- Compensations, indulgence

Seated position
- Patella position
  Alta
  Baja
  Lateralization
  Medialization
- Femoral torsion
  Internal
  External
- Tibial torsion
  Internal
  External
- Tubercle–sulcus angle
- Active knee extension

Supine position
- Extensor mechanism

- Torsion lower extremities
  Internal femoral torsion
  External tibial torsion
  Hip rotators and abductors
- Flexion movements, squatting
  Sensorimotor control
  J-sign
  In extension and flexion
  With and without contraction of
    the quadriceps
- Effusion
- Palpation
  All anatomical structures
  All scars
- Patellar mechanisms
  Gliding
  Mobility
  Glide test
  Tilt angle
- Lateral instability
  Apprehension test
- Medial instability
  Reverse apprehension test
  Patellar relocation test
  Gravity subluxation test
- Dynamic contraction
  Comparison with static situation
    (relaxed)
  Lateral pull sign

Patellar activity during gait

Thigh musculature must be performed with the quadriceps both contracted and relaxed. Both situations, *static* and *dynamic*, are important because there is a considerable period during functional activities, such as level gait, when the muscles round the patella are inactive.

During level gait, the quadriceps is active during late swing and weight acceptance only.[22-24] The medial and lateral heads of the quadriceps are normally silent while the knee is rapidly bending in preparation for the swing phase. This is a delicate time during function for maltracking of the patella to occur (*see* Case Study 17).

Lateral pull sign

Active contraction of the thigh muscles is useful to determine the vector of the extensor mechanism. The patient contracts the quadriceps with the leg in extension and the patella is observed for movement.[1] The patella should move in a straight proximal direction. When the pull is in a superolateral or lateral direction, the test is abnormal, representing a lateral overpull by the quadriceps.[1] This test is called the *lateral pull sign*.[1] Functionally, the dynamic forces are responsible for this result, especially the muscles involved. Atrophy of the vastus medialis obliquus or hypertrophy of the vastus lateralis or other lateral structures may influence the direction of the pull. Additionally, insufficient medial patellofemoral ligament and medial retinaculum or insufficient bony stabilization (e.g. trochlear dysplasia) alter the results. An abnormal *lateral pull sign* (Figure 5.32) corresponds to increased lateral translation of the patella with

subluxation. Therefore, it may explain pain and discomfort during training and strengthening in patients with active superolateral subluxation. This sign is also important in patients with pain during physical therapy and rehabilitation and should be addressed in the treatment plan.

References

1. Kolowich PA, Paulos LE, Rosenberg TD, Farnsworth S (1990) Lateral release of the patella: indications and contraindications. *Am J Sports Med* 18: 359–365
2. Hughston JC, Walsh WM, Puddu G (1984) *Patellar Subluxation and Dislocation. Saunders Monographs in Clinical Orthopaedics*, volume V. Philadelphia, PA, WB Saunders
3. Fulkerson JP, Hungerford DS (1990) *Disorders of the Patellofemoral Joint*, 2nd edn. Baltimore, MD, Williams & Wilkins
4. Caylor D, Fites R, Worrell TW (1993) The relationship between quadriceps angle and anterior knee pain syndrome. *J Orthop Sports Phys Ther* 17: 11–16
5. Ford DH, Post WR (1997) Open or arthroscopic lateral release. Indications, techniques, and rehabilitation. *Clin Sports Med* 16: 29–49
6. Rillmann P, Dutly A, Kieser C, Berbig R (1998) Modified Elmslie–Trillat procedure for instability of the patella. *Knee Surg Sports Traumatol Arthrosc* 6: 31–35
7. Guzzanti V, Gigante A, Di Lazzaro A, Fabbriciani C (1994) Patellofemoral malalignment in adolescents. Computerized tomographic assessment with or without quadriceps contraction. *Am J Sports Med* 22: 55–60
8. Messier SP, Davis SE, Curl WW et al (1991) Etiologic factors associated with patellofemoral pain in runners. *Med Sci Sports Exerc* 23: 1008–1015
9. Biedert RM, Warnke K (2001) Correlation between the Q angle and the patella position: a clinical and axial computed tomography evaluation. *Arch Orthop Trauma Surg* 121: 346–349
10. Dandy DJ (1996) Chronic patellofemoral instability. *J Bone Joint Surg Br* 78: 328–335
11. Kujala UM, Kormano M, Osterman K et al (1992) Magnetic resonance imaging analysis of patellofemoral congruity in females. *Clin J Sports Med* 2: 21–26

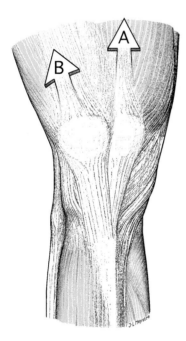

Figure 5.32 Lateral pull sign. (a) Well-centred patella, relaxed quadriceps. (b) Superolateral subluxation of the patella, external rotation of the thigh musculature under maximum contraction of the quadriceps

12. Papagelopoulos PJ, Sim FH (1997) Patellofemoral pain syndrome: diagnosis and management. *Orthopedics* **20**: 148–157; quiz, 158–159

13. Percy EC, Strother RT (1985) Patellalgia. *Physician Sportsmed* **13**: 43–59

14. Biedert RM, Kernen V (2001) Neurosensory characteristics of the patellofemoral joint: what is the genesis of patellofemoral pain? *Sports Med Arthrosc Rev* **9**: 295–300

15. Fulkerson JP, Tennant R, Jaivin JS, Grunnet M (1985) Histologic evidence of retinacular nerve injury associated with patellofemoral malalignment. *Clin Orthop* **197**: 196–205

16. Biedert RM, Vogel U, Friederich NF (1997) Chronic patellar tendonitis: a new surgical treatment. *Sports Exerc Injury* **3**: 150–154

17. Mori Y, Fujimoto A, Okumo H, Kuroki Y (1991) Lateral retinaculum release in adolescent patellofemoral disorders: its relationship to peripheral nerve injury in the lateral retinaculum. *Bull Hosp Jt Dis Orthop Inst* **51**: 218–229

18. Fulkerson JP, Gossling HR (1980) Anatomy of the knee joint lateral retinaculum. *Clin Orthop* **153**: 183–188

19. Johnson LL, van Dyk GE, Green JR III et al (1998) Clinical assessment of asymptomatic knees: comparison of men and women. *Arthroscopy* **14**: 347–359

20. Nonweiler DE, DeLee JC (1994) The diagnosis and treatment of medial subluxation of the patella after lateral retinacular release. *Am J Sports Med* **22**: 680–686

21. Miller PR, Klein RM, Teitge RA (1991) Medial dislocation of the patella. *Skeletal Radiol* **20**: 429–431

22. Kramers-de Quervain IA, Biedert R, Stüssi E (1997) Quantitative gait analysis in patients with medial patellar instability following lateral retinacular release. *Knee Surg Sports Traumatol Arthrosc* **5**: 95–101

23. Kadaba MP, Ramakrishnan HK, Wootten ME et al (1989) Repeatability of kinematic, kinetic, and electromyographic data in normal adult gait. *J Orthop Res* **7**: 849–860

24. Murray MP, Mollinger LA, Gardner GM, Sepic SB (1984) Kinematic and EMG patterns during slow, free, and fast walking. *J Orthop Res* **2**: 272–280

Suggested reading

Kolowich PA, Paulos LE, Rosenberg TD, Farnsworth S (1990) Lateral release of the patella: indications and contraindications. *Am J Sports Med* **18**: 359–365

Biedert RM, Warnke K (2001) Correlation between the Q angle and the patella position: a clinical and axial computed tomography evaluation. *Arch Orthop Trauma Surg* **121**: 346–349

6 Radiographs

Elvire Servien, Philippe Neyret, Tarik Aït Si Selmi and **Roland M. Biedert**

Radiological evaluation of the patellofemoral joint includes several planes. Two examinations are necessary for a complete evaluation of the patellofemoral joint – conventional radiology and computed tomography (CT) scans. To analyse the patellar tendon and the cartilage, magnetic resonance imaging (MRI) can be done.

The radiological evaluation comprises three standardized planes:

♦ *Monopodal anteroposterior view.* This plane is not important for the patellofemoral joint, but it is important to show femorotibial abnormalities.

♦ *Lateral view.* The patient is placed supine with the knee in 30° of flexion. The profile radiograph is strictly lateral, with the posterior borders of the two condyles superimposed. The central ray is focused along the femorotibial articular line.[1]

♦ *Axial view of the patella with the knee in 30° of flexion.* This plane is not so important but shows osseous abnormalities of the patellofemoral joint.

By definition, the analysis of an articulation includes evaluation and relation of the two anatomical structures. For the patellofemoral joint, this includes the trochlea and the patella. During the last 80 years,[2] a multitude of morphological factors of patellar instability have been documented, such as trochlear dysplasia, patella alta, patellar tilt and excessive tibial tuberosity–trochlear groove displacement. These factors of patellar instability have been identified and documented by comparing a group of patients with recurrent patellar dislocations (objective patellar instability, the term used by Dejour, is still called '*habitual dislocation*') with a normal control group. With this study,[3] the analysis of the patellar instability was possible.

Origin and formation of the patellofemoral joint

The patellofemoral joint is formed during the learning period of walking.[4] Before this learning period (under the age of 2 years), the oblique angle of the femur is zero – the femur is upright. Only when the child begins to walk does the extensor system transform into a valgus axis. Later, during adolescence, the femoral epiphysis is modified and the trochlea is transformed. Under the age of 11–12

Patellofemoral Disorders: Diagnosis and Treatment. Edited by Roland M. Biedert
© 2004 John Wiley & Sons, Ltd ISBN: 0-470-85011-6

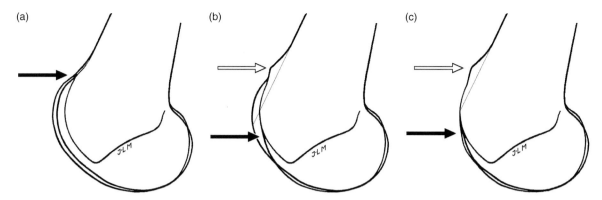

Figure 6.1   Trochlear dysplasia. (a) Type I: the crossing of both condylar outlines with the outline of the trochlear floor is proximal and symmetrical (→). (b) Type II: the crossing of the two condylar outlines with the outline of the trochlear floor is asymmetrical (→) (⇒, recentring beak). (c) Type III: the crossing of the two condylar outlines with the outline of the trochlear floor is distal and asymmetrical (→). At the crossing point, the trochlea is flat (⇒, recentring beak)

years, the trochlea is flat and symmetrical. With the strong growth during adolescence, the trochlea is deepened and the lateral femoral condyle is formed. The diagnosis of a dysplastic trochlea is difficult when the patient is under the age of 10 years.

Analysis of the trochlea

Trochlear dysplasia

The dysplastic trochlea is the most frequent abnormality found in patients presenting with habitual dislocation of the patella (objective patellar instability).[5,6] It is documented in 96% of cases, according to Dejour et al,[3] and in only 77.5% of the cases according to Verjux et al (handout for presentation at the International Patellofemoral Study Group Meeting, Lyon, France, 1998). The crossing sign is the pathognomic factor of dysplastic trochlea. The analysis is made with a lateral radiograph in 30° of knee flexion.

Crossing sign

Trochlear dysplasia is expressed by the crossing of both condylar outlines (internal and external) with the outline of the trochlear floor. Three types of trochlear dysplasia can be defined, according to the level of crossing.[1] The dysplasia is more severe with the crossing point situated more distally (Figures 6.1a, b, c, 6.2).

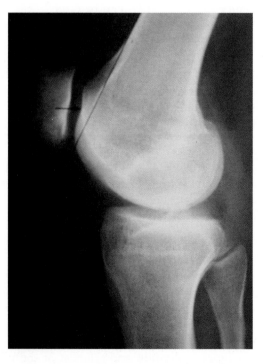

Figure 6.2   Lateral radiograph showing trochlear dysplasia with crossing sign type II, recentring beak and positive prominence of the trochlea (straight line)

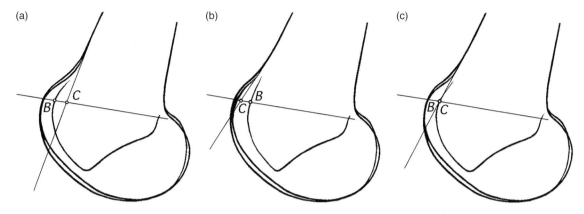

(a) (b) (c)

Figure 6.3 Prominence of the trochlea (a) Positive. (b) Negative. (c) Zero (normal)

Recentring beak

The existence of a recentring beak has been described by Dejour et al.[3] After the crossing, the line ends frequently with a recentring beak (Figure 6.1b, c). This beak appears in the criteria of classification by Tavernier and Dejour.[7]

Prominence of the trochlea

To analyse the trochlea on a true lateral radiographic view, a straight line is drawn tangential to the anterior femoral cortex along its distalmost 10 cm. The floor of the trochlea is measured at the most anterior point. According to the position of this point (anterior, posterior, or flush with the anterior cortical line), the floor of the trochlea can be positive, zero (normal) or negative, measured in millimeters. A translation of more than 3 mm is considered as pathological (positive or negative prominence). It corresponds to the distance from B to C (Figures 6.3a, b, c, 6.2).[8]

Trochlear depth

The most anterior point of the trochlear floor corresponds with the lowest depth of the trochlea. The depth is the distance from A to B. To measure this distance most consistently, a line (y) is drawn perpendicular to the tangent of the

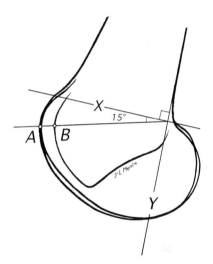

Figure 6.4 Measurement of the trochlear depth, which is the distance A–B (in mm)

posterior femoral cortex and the summit of both condylar outlines. The distance from A to B is then measured along a line (x) subtended 15° to the right angle from this tangent (Figure 6.4).

Classification

A new and more precise classification of trochlear dysplasia was described by Tavernier and Dejour.[7] It replaces the former system.[9] The new classification consists of four degrees – A, B, C and D. Besides the standard radiology, the additional evaluation requires CT scans (Figure 6.5a, b, c, d).

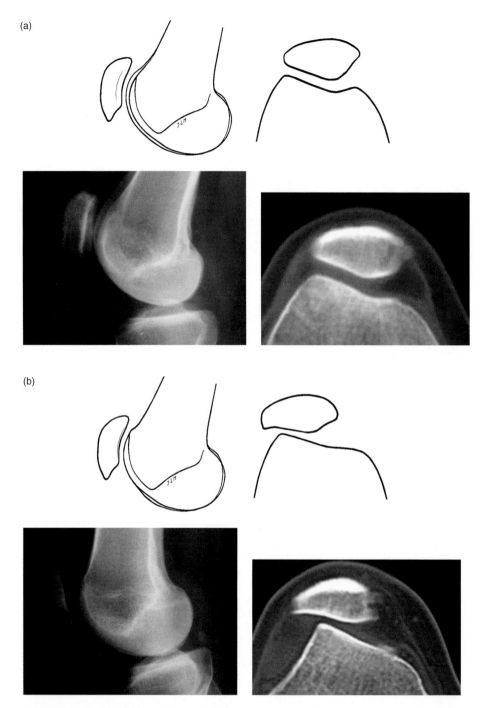

Figure 6.5   Classification of trochlear dysplasia. (a) Degree A: crossing sign with minimal trochlear depth, plus axial and sagittal CT scans. (b) Degree B: recentring beak with flat trochlea, plus axial and sagittal CT scans. (c) Degree C: hypoplasia of the medial trochlea with double contour, plus axial and sagittal CT scans. (d) Degree D: most severe trochlear dysplasia with recentring beak and double contour, plus axial and sagittal CT scans

(c)

(d)

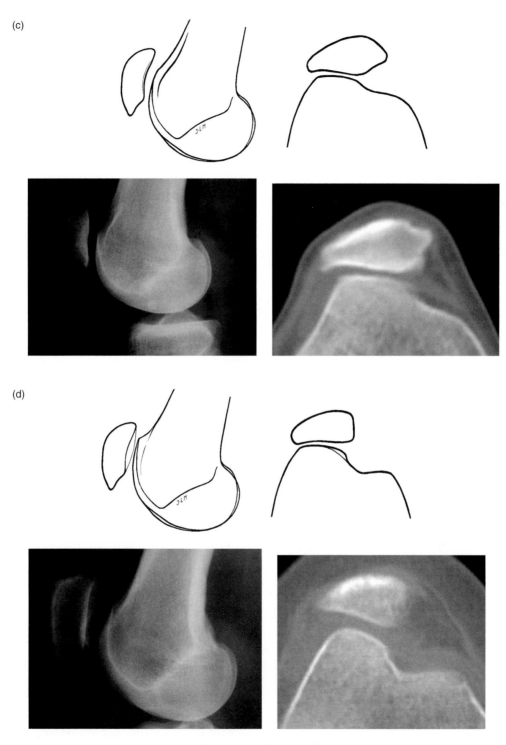

Figure 6.5   (*continued*)

The analysis with CT is performed following a first cut of reference at the level of the trochlea, where the cartilage begins. Rémy et al[10] validated the reproducibility of this new classification by analysing the two most important factors of the trochlear dysplasia – the crossing sign and the recentring beak.

Trochlear angle

The trochlear angle is measured on the axial view in 30° of knee flexion.[11] The angle is formed by a line tangential to the lateral slope of the trochlea and a line tangential to the medial slope. The angle is considered normal if it is between 135° and 145°. Other methods of measuring the trochlear angle also exist. Hughston[12] measured it in 55° of knee flexion; this 'sulcus angle' has a mean value of 118°. Merchant et al[13] measured the trochlear angle at 45° of knee flexion with mean values of 138° and a range of 126–150°. In all methods, a holding device is needed to guarantee measurements at the desired angles of flexion.

Trochlear height

The measurement of trochlear height is rarely used.[8] The *index of trochlear height* (IHT,

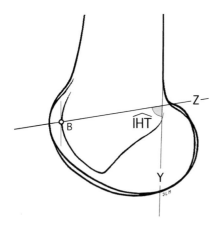

Figure 6.6 Trochlear height. Geometric reconstruction of the IHT angle for analysis of the trochlea. The angle is formed by the lines Y and Z

Figure 6.6) corresponds to an angle. This angle is defined by the crossing point of reference of two straight lines, one as the tangential line of the posterior cortex of the femur (Y) with another line (Z) from the most anterior point of the inter-condylar groove (B) to the posterior outline of the femoral condyle. The angle is formed by these two lines. This measurement helps to define and to document dysplastic trochlea type 3. We have observed that the lower the trochlear height, the greater is the dysplasia.

Analysis of the patella

Patellar height

Numerous indices are described to calculate the patellar height (Figure 6.7a–e). Four major indices are used to evaluate the patellar height *with reference to the tibia*. These include the methods described by Caton et al,[11] Insall and colleagues[14,15] and Blackburne and Peel.[16] They are all calculated on lateral radiographs in 30° of knee flexion, in a lying position. A specific index (or ratio) has been developed for each of these methods to determine the presence of a patella alta or baja:

♦ The index by Caton et al[17] (Figure 6.7a) is represented by the ratio of the distance from the lower edge of the articular surface of the patella to the anterosuperior angle of the tibial outline to the length of the articular surface of the patella.

♦ The index by Insall and colleagues[14,15] (Figure 6.7b) is represented by the ratio of the length of the patellar tendon to the longest sagittal diameter of the patella, as published by Insall and Salvati[15] in 1971. It must be noted that Insall et al,[14] 1 year later, published one series with the same index, but inverse.

♦ The index by Insall–Salvati was modified later by Grelsamer et al[18] (Figure 6.7c). It is represented by the ratio of the length of the

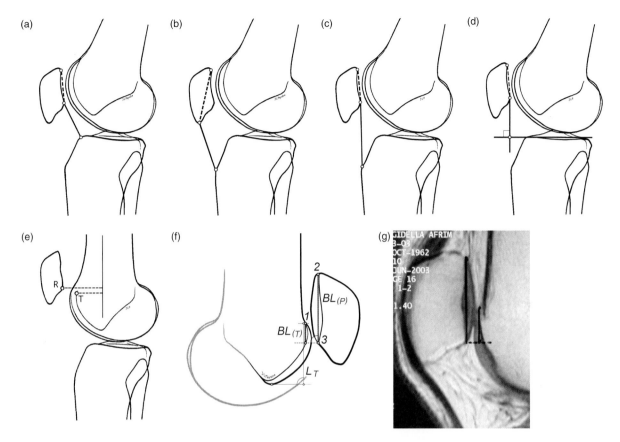

Figure 6.7 Patellar height. Measurements of patellar height according to: (a) Caton–Deschamps; (b) Insall–Salvati; (c) Insall–Salvati modified (Grelsamer); (d) Blackburne–Peel; (e) Bernageau

patellar tendon to the length of the articular surface of the patella.

♦ The index by Blackburne and Peel[16] (Figure 6.7d) is represented by the ratio of the perpendicular line of the inferior pole of the articular surface of the patella to the tangent of the tibial plateau and the length of the articular surface of the patella.

The different ratios of the methods are summarized in Table 6.1.

Other indices evaluate the patellar height *with reference to the trochlea*, but only one is used. The method by Bernageau et al[19] analyses a lateral radiograph in extension with contraction of the quadriceps muscle. The distance between the superior line of the trochlea (T) and the

Table 6.1 Indices of the patella height

Indices	Patella baja	Patella alta
Caton–Deschamps	0.6	1.2
Insall–Salvati	0.8	1.2
Insall–Salvati modified	No definition	2
Blackburne–Peel	0.5	1.0

inferior edge of the articular surface of the patella (R) is calculated. Patella alta is present if the distance is 6 mm or more; patella baja is present if the distance is 6 mm or less (Figure 6.7e). CT scans can also give information about the presence of patella alta.[3] On CT scans through the femoral condyle, where the notch has the form of a Roman arch, the patella is not visible in the case of patella alta. This sign, called the *sign of Dejour*, is even more evident, as it can be only unilateral, with a visible patella on the other side. The relation of the trochlea to the patella is especially qualitative and allows no appreciation of the amount of distalization in case of a patella alta.

A more specific and precise investigation can be needed in some cases because the index by Insall–Salvati is often inadequate. The MRI[20] is a much more precise method for measuring the length of the patellar tendon than lateral radiographs, because the insertion of the tendon at the tibial tuberosity can be measured in millimeters and is easily reproducible (Figure 6.8). The MRI reveals, for example, whether the patellar tendon is abnormally long, the aetiology of patella alta.[21] Neyret et al[21] found a mean length of the patellar tendon of 61 mm in a group of patients with an objective patellar instability, in comparison to

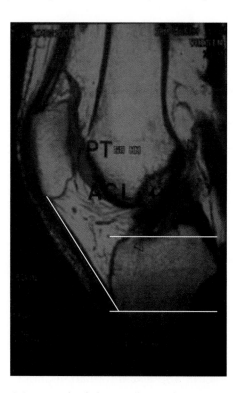

Figure 6.8 Length of the patellar tendon. Measurement on a sagittal MRI

a mean length of 53 mm in the control group. In our study[22] comprising 190 operated knees with the diagnosis of objective patellar instability, the mean length was 53.8 mm. The measurement of the patellar tendon can therefore be helpful in analysing patellofemoral pathology. Additionally, MRI allows the measurement of the most distal point of the patella, still called the 'nose' of the patella. A correlation exists between the length of the patellar tendon and the nose of the patella – the shorter the nose, the longer the patellar tendon.[22]

Biedert and Albrecht (RM Biedert and S Albrecht, in presentation at the International Patellofemoral Study Group, Naples, Florida, 2003) described the patellotrochlear index to measure patellar height on sagittal MRI (Figure 6.7f and g). The patellotrochlear index is calculated as the baseline trochlea (BL_T):baseline patella (BL_P) ratio.

In contrast to the different radiological methods, where the articular cartilage is not visible, this method documents the true articular cartilage relationship in the patellofemoral joint. Only the ratio between the articular cartilage of the patella and the trochlear cartilage is significant in determining exact patellar height and for all subsequent clinical disorders. This index considers the significant differences in the articular joint cartilage geometry and the corresponding subchondral osseous anatomy of the patella and the femoral trochlea.

The patellotrochlear index measured on sagittal MR images is a reliable and reproducible method for determining patellar height. An index between 10% and 50% may be considered as normal. Patella alta is suggested at values under 10%, patella baja over 50%. This index, in comparison to the common radiographic assessments of patellar position, has several advantages:

♦ Exact measurement of the patellotrochlear articular correlation.

♦ Osseous form variations of the patella do not affect the ratio.

- Length and shape of the trochlea are considered.

- Variations of the patellar tendon attachment areas are insignificant.

- No dependence on the position of the tibial tuberosity (Osgood–Schlatter's disease or following surgical interventions).

- Measurements obtained in 0° of knee extension are easier to obtain than measurements in 30° of flexion.

Patellar tilt

On lateral radiographs with the knee in 30° of flexion, Maldague and Malghem[23] described a classification of the patellar tilt. The morphology of the sagittal patella allows, according to three different grades, a preview of the amount of the patellar tilt on axial radiographs (Figure 6.9).

Numerous measurements can be made on the axial views.

Laurin angle

The Laurin angle[24] is measured on axial views with the knee in 20° of flexion. This angle is formed by two lines, one joining the summits of the two trochlear slopes, the other tangential to the lateral slope of the patella.[1] This angle can be positive (open laterally), null (lines parallel), or negative (open medially). A negative Laurin angle means a lateral tilt[1] (Figure 6.10a, b, c).

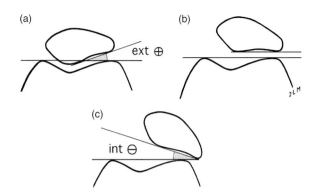

Figure 6.10 Laurin angle, measuring patellar tilt. (a) Positive; (b) null; (c) negative

Merchant angle (congruence angle)

The Merchant angle[13] is calculated on axial views with the knee flexed 45°. To measure the congruence angle, the bisector of the trochlear angle is drawn and a second line is drawn from the deepest point of the intercondylar groove to the most posterior point of the articular surface of the patella. The angle is positive if the patellar point is lateral to the bisector line (lateral subluxation) (Figure 6.11a,b).

Other studies

Julliard[25] described another radiological method. He proposed to analyse the instability of the patella on an axial patellofemoral view in 30° of knee flexion, with external rotation of the tibia to increase the lateral subluxation of the patella.

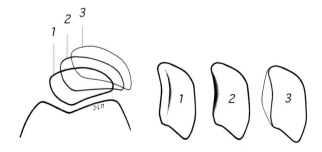

Figure 6.9 Patellar tilt. Morphology of the patella in the sagittal plane according to the amount of patellar tilt

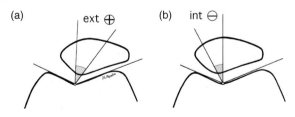

Figure 6.11 Merchant angle. Measurement of the congruence angle (according to Merchant). (a) Positive. (b) Negative

Bernageau et al[19] estimated the patellar tilt on a simple lateral radiograph in full extension with and without contraction of the quadriceps muscle.

With CT scans, the patellar tilt is measured in extension, also with and without quadriceps contraction. Therefore, two cuts are performed for each knee. For each cut, the analysis of the patellar tilt is made by calculating the angle of two lines. One line is the transverse axis of the patella; the second line connects the posterior borders of both condyles. An angle of more than 20° is considered pathological. An increase of the patellar tilt demonstrates an abnormal functional quadriceps contraction (Figure 6.12).

Nove-Josserand and Dejour[26] demonstrated the existence of the abnormal functional quadriceps contraction. Their study compared three groups, i.e. a control group, a group with habitual dislocations and a group with contralateral asymptomatic knees. In the control group, quadriceps contraction modified the patellar tilt only a little (+1.6°). On the contrary, the patellar tilt increased in the contralateral asymptomatic knees to 13° and in knees with objective patellar instability to 6°.

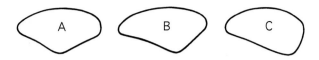

Figure 6.13   Classification of patellar morphology (types A–C)

Patellar morphology

The morphology of the patella is not well studied. A small patella is seen in habitual dislocations, especially in the 'nail patella syndrome' and the other 'small patella syndrome'.[27] Only a few objective studies identify different types of patellae. We remember the classification by Wiberg[28] with three types. Nevertheless, we should not forget that this analysis may vary with the degree of knee flexion. Type C corresponds to patellar dysplasia (Figure 6.13a, b, c). This classification is no longer used clinically.

Position of the anterior tibial tuberosity and the trochlear groove

The tibial tuberosity–trochlear groove defined by Bernageau et al[19] is the distance between the anterior tibial tuberosity and the deepest point of the trochlear groove.[29,30] The distance is calculated on CT scans by the superimposition of two perpendicular cuts to the posterior bicondylar line: one tibial cut passing through the summit of the anterior tibial tuberosity and one femoral cut passing through the deepest point of the trochlear groove where the intercondylar notch has the form of a Roman arch[2] (Figure 6.14).

The distance is measured in millimeters. It gives information about two parameters – the lateral positioning of the anterior tibial tuberosity and the external tibial torsion, which are two individually variable values.

According to the radiological protocol, the measurements can be performed with the knee in extension or flexion. The mean values of the tibial tuberosity–trochlear groove are different according to the position of the knee during the

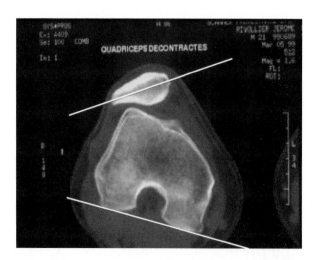

Figure 6.12   Patellar tilt: measurement of the patellar tilt with axial CT scan

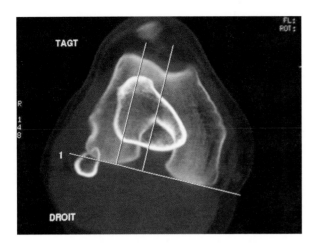

Figure 6.14 Measurement of the distance between the anterior tibial tuberosity and the trochlear groove (1, posterior bicondylar line)

examination. In a flexed knee, the mean value is 9 mm ($\pm$ 4.3 mm); in extension, the mean value is 16 mm ($\pm$ 4 mm). If the distance is over 20 mm, it is considered pathological.

The measurement of the tibial tuberosity–trochlear groove is the key for indicating a surgical procedure to move the tibial tuberosity medially and the amount of the medialization. This measurement allows objective quantification of the valgus component of the extensor mechanism of the knee, which can be estimated clinically with the Q angle or the bayonet sign.[31] However, Stäubli et al[32] argued that by this method only the shape of the subchondral bone is measured (and corrected) and not the real articular congruence of the cartilage. Therefore, they recommended MRI for documentation of the articular cartilage congruence.

The role of MRI

The MRI might play a secondary role in the analysis of the patellar tendon. Additionally, Stäubli et al[32] described the benefit of MRI to measure the thickness of the cartilage (see Chapter 2). They documented that the corresponding point of the cartilage at the floor of the trochlear

groove in most cases did not correspond to the point of the subchondral bone at the floor of the trochlear groove.

The study by Stäubli et al[32] implies that there is a significant difference between the radiologic and MRI measurements. MRI shows sometimes significant differences between the corresponding points of cartilage and bone of up to 7 mm. Although MRI allows more reproducible measurements than radiographs (length of the patellar tendon), it does not replace CT scans.

In reality, MRI of the tibial tuberosity–trochlear groove has not been studied sufficiently. New imaging methods, such as weightbearing MRI,[33] also include tibial rotation. Upcoming methods will measure the external tibial rotation and the position of the anterior tibial tuberosity.

Summary and present concepts

Present concepts

The present concepts of radiological evaluation for all patients suffering from patellofemoral problems are summarized in Table 6.2. In practice, we perform and analyse lateral radiographs obtained in 30° of knee flexion.

Lateral radiographs obtained with the knee flexed 30°

To look for a *dysplastic trochlea,* we study the level of the crossing sign or prominence of the trochlea. Both have diagnostic value and allow measurement of the depth. To determine whether the patient suffers from *patella alta,* we obtain a measurement of the patellar height with reference to the tibia, according to the method described by Caton et al.[17] If the Caton–Deschamps index is more than 1.2, the patient suffers from patella alta. Exact measurement of patellar height can only be achieved using the patellotrochlear index on MRI.

Table 6.2   Summary of radiological evaluations

	Problem knee	Contralateral knee
Standard radiographs, anteroposterior and lateral, in 30° of knee flexion	Yes	Yes
Axial radiographs in 30° of knee flexion	Yes	Yes
CT scans in extension with 15° external rotation of the feet, with and without quadriceps contraction	Yes	Yes
MRI	Prospective	No

Table 6.3   Therapeutic strategies based on pathological findings

Pathology	Treatment
Dysplastic trochlea	Trochlearplasty: deepening of the trochlear groove
Patella alta	
Normal trochlear depth	Distalization of the anterior tibial tuberosity
Decreased trochlear depth	Medialization of the anterior tibial tuberosity
Excessive tibial tuberosity–trochlear groove distance	Medialization of the anterior tibial tuberosity
Patellar tilt	Reconstruction of the vastus medialis obliquus muscle and shortening of the medial patellofemoral ligament. Lengthening of the lateral retinaculum or lateral release is performed

CT scan

If the *tibial tuberosity–trochlear groove* is more than 20 mm, then the anterior tibial tuberosity is inserted too laterally. Additionally, in cases with unilateral problems, a significant difference between the two knees can be found.

The *patellar tilt* is measured with and without quadriceps contraction. A value of more than 20° documents an imbalance in the horizontal plane between the dynamic and static medial and lateral structures.

The *morphology of the trochlea* is measured; then the examiner searches for a sign of *patella alta* (Dejour's sign). When all these values are normal, or when an isolated patella alta exists, MRI can be useful to analyse the patellar tendon and the cartilage. In some instances, MRI can be superior to CT, but comparative studies between a control group and patients with 'habitual dislocations of the patella' are necessary to determine precisely the normal values, the threshold and the pathological values.

Therapeutic strategies

The therapeutic concept and strategies depend on the documented pathology, as summarized in Table 6.3.

Postoperative analysis

Postoperative analysis includes radiological views in the anteroposterior, lateral and axial planes in 30° of flexion. The height of the patella is analysed, especially in cases of patella alta. With persisting patella alta, we look for an insufficient correction. The appearance of a patella baja is rare.

In patients with persisting pain following medialization, postoperative CT scans must be analysed to measure the tibial tuberosity–trochlear groove distance. This allows us to document a 'hypermedialization' of the anterior tibial tuberosity and to detect a medial conflict. Our aim is to have a postoperative mean tibial tuberosity–trochlear groove distance of 12 mm.

Conclusions

Measurement of the different parameters described allows precise analysis of the patellofemoral joint and determination of specific pathological factors. Additionally, the measurements furnish essential preoperative information about the patellofemoral joint. Three-dimensional reconstruction of the patellofemoral joint will give more qualitative appreciation, but no quantitative interpretations can be applied to these images up to the present time.

References

1. Galland O, Walch G, Dejour H, Carret JP (1990) An anatomical and radiological study of the femoropatellar articulation. *Surg Radiol Anat* **12**: 119–125
2. Dejour H, Walch G (1987) La pathologie fémoro-patellaire. In: *6èmes Journées Lyonnaises de Chirurgie du Genou.* University of Lyon
3. Dejour H, Walch G, Nove-Josserand L, Guier C (1994) Factors of patellar instability: an anatomic radiographic study. *Knee Surg Sports Traumatol Arthrosc* **2**: 19–26
4. Tardieu C, Dupont JY (2001) [The origin of femoral trochlear dysplasia: comparative anatomy, evolution, and growth of the patellofemoral joint]. *Rev Chir Orthop Reparatrice Appar Mot* **87**: 373–383
5. Dejour H, Walch G, Neyret P, Adeleine P (1990) [Dysplasia of the femoral trochlea]. *Rev Chir Orthop Reparatrice Appar Mot* **76**: 45–54
6. Neyret P, Dejour D, Ait Si Selmi T (2000) *Die trochleare Dysplasie. Das patellofemorale Schmerzsyndrom.* Darmstadt, Steinkopff-Verlag
7. Tavernier T, Dejour D (2001) [Knee imaging: what is the best modality?]. *J Radiol* **82**: 387–405, 407–408
8. Walch G, Dejour H (1989) [Radiology in femoro-patellar pathology]. *Acta Orthop Belg* **55**: 371–380
9. Carillon Y, Dejour D, Tavernier T, Dejour H (1997) Aspect scannographique de la trochlée fémorale en cas d'instabilité rotulienne objective. In: *XXIV Groupe d'Etude et de Travail d'Imagerie Osteo-articulatife*, University of Lyon, pp 215–225
10. Rémy F, Gougeon F, Ala Eddine T et al (2001) Reproductibilité de la nouvelle classification de la dysplasie de la trochlée fémorale selon Dejour et valeur prédictive sur la sévérité de l'instabilité fémoro-patellaire sur 47 genoux. *Rev Chir Orthop Reparatrice Appar Mot* **87**(suppl 2): 60
11. Carson WG Jr, James SL, Larson RL et al (1984) Patellofemoral disorders: physical and radiographic evaluation. Part II: radiographic examination. *Clin Orthop* **185**: 178–186
12. Hughston JC (1968) Subluxation of the patella. *J Bone Joint Surg Am* **50**: 1003–1026
13. Merchant AC, Mercer RL, Jacobsen RH, Cool CR (1974) Roentgenographic analysis of patellofemoral congruence. *J Bone Joint Surg Am* **56**: 1391–1396
14. Insall J, Goldberg V, Salvati E (1972) Recurrent dislocation and the high-riding patella. *Clin Orthop* **88**: 67–69
15. Insall J, Salvati E (1971) Patella position in the normal knee joint. *Radiology* **101**: 101–104
16. Blackburne JS, Peel TE (1977) A new method of measuring patellar height. *J Bone Joint Surg Br* **59**: 241–242
17. Caton J, Deschamps G, Chambat P et al (1982) [Patella infera. À propos of 128 cases]. *Rev Chir Orthop Reparatrice Appar Mot* **68**: 317–325
18. Grelsamer RP, Meadows S (1992) The modified Insall–Salvati ratio for assessment of patellar height. *Clin Orthop* **282**: 170–176

19. Bernageau J, Goutallier D, Debeyre J, Ferrane J (1969) Nouvelle technique d'exploration de l'articulation fémoro-patellaire. Incindinces axiales quadriceps contracté et décontracté. *Rev Chir Orthop Reparatrice Appar Mot* **61**(suppl 2): 286–290

20. Lapra C, Lecoultre B, Ait Si Selmi T, Neyret P (1997) Le tendon rotulien dans l'instabilité rotulienne: étude IRM. In: *XXIV Groupe d'Etude et de Travail d'Imagerie Osteo-articulatife*, University of Lyon pp 227–231

21. Neyret P, Robinson AH, Le Coultre B et al (2002) Patellar tendon length – the factor in patellar instability? *The Knee* **9**: 3–6

22. Servien E (2001) La luxation de rotule: étude rétrospectivede 190 cas opérés et analyse de la dysplasie fémorale-patellaire. Thesis, University of Lyon

23. Maldague B, Malghem J (1985) [Significance of the radiograph of the knee profile in the detection of patellar instability. Preliminary report]. *Rev Chir Orthop Reparatrice Appar Mot* **71** (suppl 2): 5–13

24. Laurin CA, Levesque HP, Dussault R et al (1978) The abnormal lateral patellofemoral angle: a diagnostic roentgenographic sign of recurrent patellar subluxation. *J Bone Joint Surg Am* **60**: 55–60

25. Julliard R (1989) Diagnostic radiographique de l'instabilité rotulienne. Les défilés en rotation externe. *J Chir* **3**: 169–175

26. Nove-Josserand L, Dejour D (1995) [Quadriceps dysplasia and patellar tilt in objective patellar instability]. *Rev Chir Orthop Reparatrice Appar Mot* **81**: 497–504

27. Scott JE, Taor WS (1979) The 'small patella' syndrome. *J Bone Joint Surg Br* **61**: 172–175

28. Wiberg G (1941) Roentgenographic and anatomic studies on the femoropatellar joint. *Acta Orthop Scand* **12**: 319–410

29. Goutallier D, Bernageau J (1997) Intérêt pratique de la TA-GT. Le genou traumatique et dégênératif. In: *XXIV Groupe d'Etude et de Travail d'Imagerie Osteo-articulatife*, University of Lyon, pp 259–270

30. Goutallier D, Bernageau J, Lecudonnec B (1978) [The measurement of the tibial tuberosity. Patella groove distanced technique and results (author's trans)]. *Rev Chir Orthop Reparatrice Appar Mot* **64**: 423–428

31. Trillat A, Dejour H, Couette A (1964) Diagnostic et traitement des sublaxations récidivantes de la rotule. *Rev Chir Orthop Reparatrice Appar Mot* **50**: 813–824

32. Stäubli HU, Dürrenmatt U, Porcellini B, Rauschning W (1999) Anatomy and surface geometry of the patellofemoral joint in the axial plane. *J Bone Joint Surg Br* **81**: 452–458

33. Karrholm J, Brandsson S, Freeman MA (2000) Tibiofemoral movement 4: changes of axial tibial rotation caused by forced rotation at the weight-bearing knee studied by RSA. *J Bone Joint Surg Br* **82**: 1201–1203

7 Computed Tomography Examination

Roland M. Biedert

Computed tomography (CT) examination is an excellent technique for evaluating the patellofemoral joint through the complete range of motion.[1,2] Assessment of the patellofemoral joint between full extension and less than 30° of knee flexion is of special importance.[1,3–5] Near full extension, the patella becomes more unstable because it moves more proximally and the bony stability is decreased.[1] Therefore, the axial CT examination between extension and 30° of flexion is superior to MRI or MR-arthrotomography (*see* Chapter 8). Axial CT scans reveal the most reliable documentation of the underlying pathoanatomy and secondary effects, such as a trochlear bump (primary pathology) or a subsequent patellar subluxation (resulting condition).

Axial CT scans are performed at different degrees of knee flexion and under various conditions (Table 7.1).

Technical equipment

CT examination, at our centre, was performed with Siemens Somatom Plus 4 Volume Zoom equipment (Siemens, Germany) (Figures 7.1, 7.2).

The following technical specifications were used to produce CT scans: 150 mAs, 140 kV, 1 second scanning time, slice 5.0 mm, multislice CT (four lines), sequence technique (4 × 1 axial scan) and mixed window bone–soft tissues 1500/450.

Examination techniques

The patient lies in the supine position. CT examination starts with the selection of the best CT sections. The first section runs through the centre of the patella, where the cartilage area is normally thickest (Figure 7.3). The proximal and distal halves of the patella are divided and the sections performed through the middle (Figure 7.4).

Table 7.1 Axial CT evaluation on both sides

In extension:
  Quadriceps relaxed
  Quadriceps contracted
  With or without manual pressure on the patella from medial and/or lateral (stress CT)
In 30° of knee flexion
In 60° of knee flexion

Patellofemoral Disorders: Diagnosis and Treatment. Edited by Roland M. Biedert
© 2004 John Wiley & Sons, Ltd ISBN: 0-470-85011-6

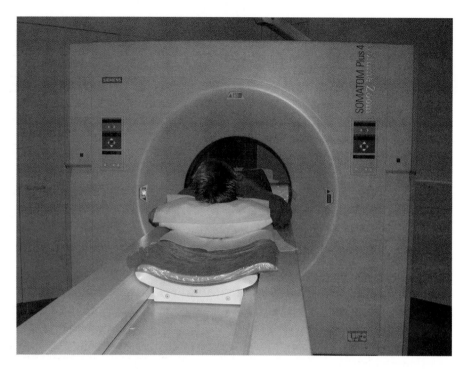

Figure 7.1   Siemens Somatom equipment (Plus 4 Volume Zoom), Siemens, Germany

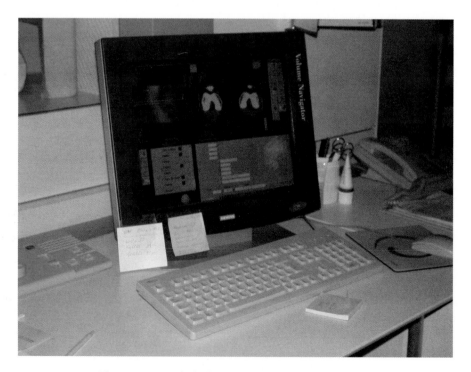

Figure 7.2   Technical equipment (Siemens Somatom)

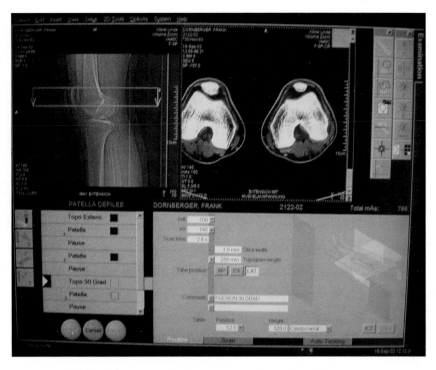

Figure 7.3   Identification of the correct axial CT sections

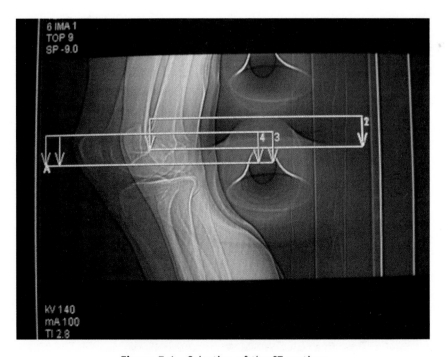

Figure 7.4   Selection of the CT sections

Axial CT scans are then performed under the desired conditions, always on both sides at the same time.

Examination in extension, with and without quadriceps contraction

Examination, quadriceps relaxed

The first examination is performed with the quadriceps muscle relaxed (Figure 7.5). This documents the static situation. The knees are free from skin fixation.[1,3,6,7] The leg is fixed with a foam coil or roll to prevent excessive external foot rotation.[6] The correct selection of the CT sections is controlled in the first three images (Figures 7.6, 7.7 and 7.8). The best views of the patellofemoral joint are necessary for measurement of the tomogram parameters.

Extension, quadriceps contracted

Second, examination with maximal isometric voluntary contraction of the quadriceps

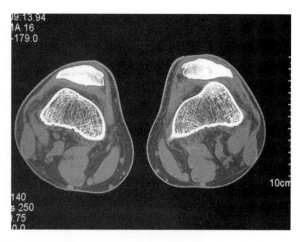

Figure 7.6   Axial CT image in extension. Proximal section: severe patellar subluxation, on the left more than on the right side

muscle is performed, the feet held in dorsal extension[1,5,8] (Figure 7.9). This documents the dynamic evaluation.

With quadriceps contraction, the patella moves in most cases to proximal and lies on the upper

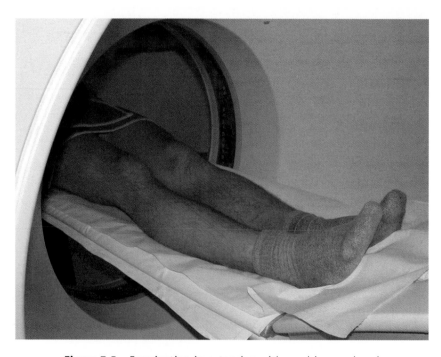

Figure 7.5   Examination in extension with quadriceps relaxed

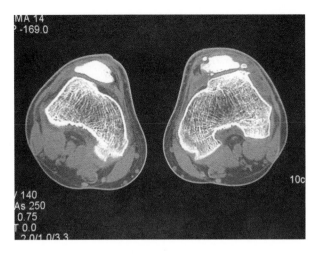

Figure 7.7 Axial CT image in extension. Middle section: central bump of the trochlea with multifragmented patella

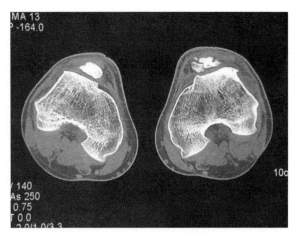

Figure 7.8 Axial CT image in extension. Distal section: the distal contact area of the patella lies more medially

end of the trochlea.[1,6] Various pathological positions of the patella can occur under contraction (subluxation, dislocation, lateralization, medialization) as the result of a complex balance between the different structures involved. Examination with full quadriceps contraction may document pathological situations that would have been missed under quadriceps-relaxed conditions (Figures 7.10, 7.11 and 7.12).

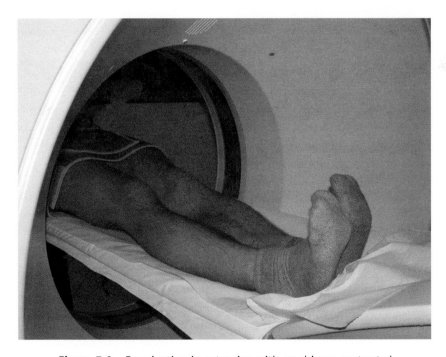

Figure 7.9 Examination in extension with quadriceps contracted

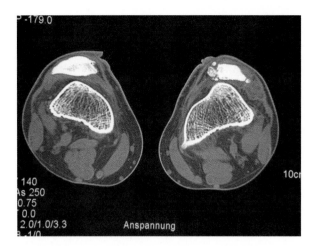

Figure 7.10 Axial CT image in extension with quadriceps contracted. Proximal section: quadriceps contraction causes almost complete lateral patellar dislocation (same patient as in Figure 7.6)

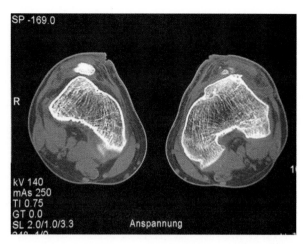

Figure 7.12 Axial CT image in extension with quadriceps contracted. Distal section: the patella moved to proximal and only bone fragments are visible; severe trochlear dysplasia with central bump on the left side

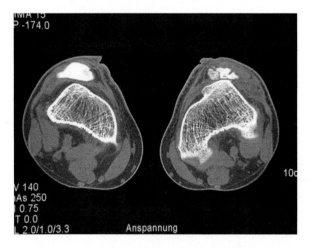

Figure 7.11 Axial CT image in extension with quadriceps contracted. Middle section: severe subluxation of the multifragmented patella; sclerosis and patellofemoral joint space narrowing document the osteoarthritis; excessive central bump

Examination in extension with manual pressure (stress CT)

If patellar instability (primary or secondary) or excessive laxity is suspected, manual pressure from the medial and/or lateral side may help to document the most pathological position of the

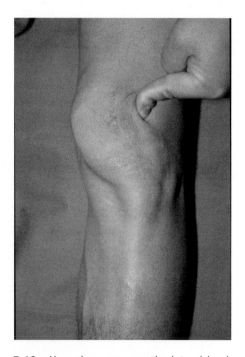

Figure 7.13 Manual pressure on the lateral border of the patella to document secondary medial instability (left knee) (incision after lateral retinaculum release)

patella.[9,10] Force is applied to the medial and the lateral aspect of the patella by the patient's finger (Figures 7.13, 7.14, 7.15, 7.16). This represents a

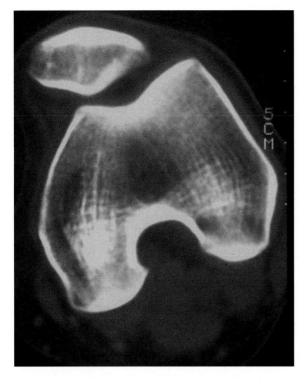

Figure 7.14 Documentation of secondary medial patellar instability

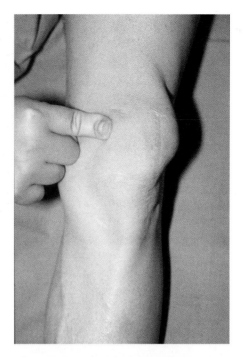

Figure 7.15 Manual pressure on the medial border of the patella to document lateral patellar instability

most valuable, reliable, and simple technique to document the different forms of patellar instability that might be overlooked by performing only standard CT examination.[9,10]

Examination in 30° of knee flexion

The next step of examination is performed with the knees flexed to 30°. A stiff radiograph-transparent roll is placed under the knee. The angle is controlled while the examiner measures with a goniometer (Figure 7.17). In this position, the patella lies more distally in the trochlear groove and the osseous stabilization is improved. Routinely, quadriceps contraction is not necessary because the effect, if any, is minimal.[9] With this examination, differences between the patella position in 30° of flexion (Figure 7.18), in extension with relaxed quadriceps (Figure 7.19) and extension with quadriceps contraction (Figure 7.20) are obvious.

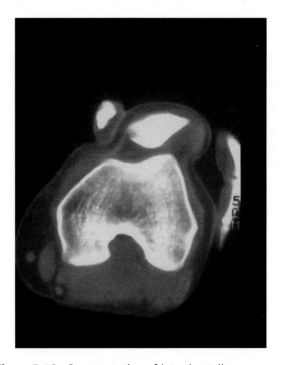

Figure 7.16 Documentation of lateral patellar instability using manual pressure (fingers on the medial facet)

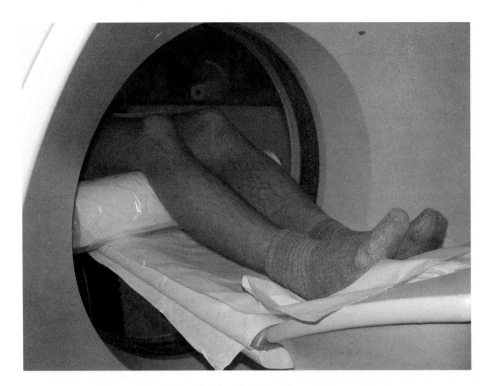

Figure 7.17   Examination in 30° of knee flexion, relaxed

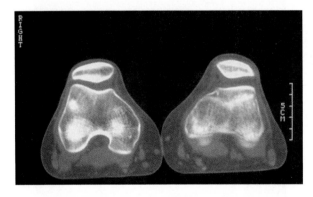

Figure 7.18   Almost normal position of the patella in the dysplastic trochlea (axial views, 30°)

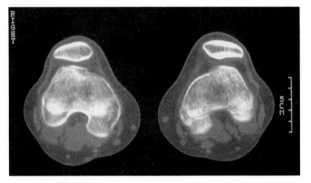

Figure 7.19   Lateral patellar subluxation with trochlear dysplasia. Same female patient as in Figure 7.18 (axial views, extension, relaxed)

Examination in 60° of knee flexion

The last step of examination is performed with the knees flexed to 60°. Two rolls are placed under the knees and the angle is controlled (Figure 7.21). Normally the patella is well-centred at this angle of knee flexion.[1] This examination

documents the situation more in flexion (walking up and down the stairs) and includes the normal and physiological corrections and adaptations of the femoral and tibial torsion. The examination in 60° of knee flexion may simulate the normal patellar position (Figure 7.22) in cases with

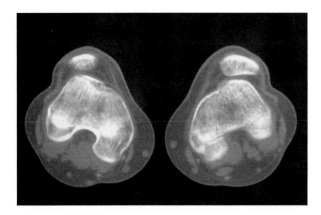

Figure 7.20 Severe lateral patellar subluxation in the same patient as in Figures 7.18 and 7.19 (axial views, extension, contracted)

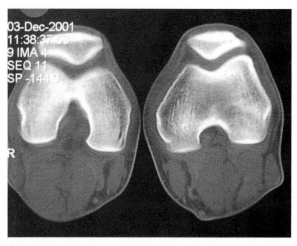

Figure 7.22 Well-centred patellae on both sides in 60° of flexion. Correct osseous stabilization (axial views, relaxed)

severe trochlea dysplasia and patellar subluxation in extension (Figure 7.23). Examination at 60° of knee flexion may also be helpful to document pathological patella position following surgery, i.e. medial subluxation of the patella following over-correction (*see* Case Study 19). Additional examination with quadriceps contraction is not necessary.

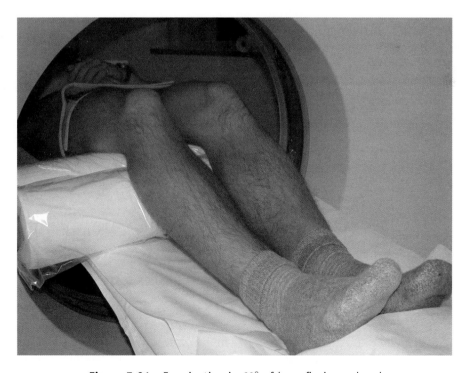

Figure 7.21 Examination in 60° of knee flexion, relaxed

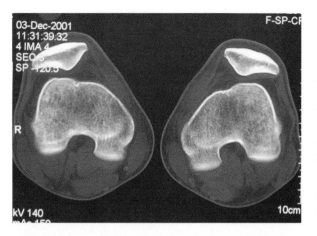

Figure 7.23 Lateral patellar subluxation with dysplastic trochlea in the same patient as in Figure 7.22 (axial views, extension, relaxed)

Clinical implications

The CT examination is extremely helpful in evaluating the patellofemoral joint through the whole range of motion. In most cases, it documents the underlying pathology, the causal pathoanatomy and the influence of voluntary muscle contraction. It helps to plan the necessary treatment and to evaluate the efficacy of surgical treatments. What can we see on the CT images? How can we measure and document what we see? What conclusions can we draw? We need to look at specific attributes within several different CT sections: with the knee in extension and the quadriceps relaxed, in extension with the quadriceps contracted, and in flexion at both 30° and 60°.

In extension, quadriceps relaxed

♦ The spontaneous position of the patella in the trochlea (proximal, distal, lateral, medial).

♦ The condition of the patellofemoral joint (degenerative changes, joint space narrowing).

♦ The shape of the patella and trochlea (dysplastic, flat lateral condyle, small medial trochlea, central bump).

♦ The balancing of the patella in the trochlea comparing the most proximal and distal sections (subluxation, tilt, joint space narrowing).

Note that in the case of patella alta, the patella is positioned proximal to the trochlea, sometimes even on the distal femoral shaft. The patellar articular surface lies tangentially to the distal femur rather than being firmly apposed to it.[1] In such cases, sections through the patellofemoral joint are not through the height of the Roman arch of the condyle but much more proximal on the femur (*see* Case Study 8).

In extension, quadriceps contracted

♦ The patellar movement to proximal (lateral, well-centred, medial).[1]

♦ The changed position of the patella in the trochlea (subluxation, dislocation, tilt).

Quadriceps contraction substitutes for the tension of the quadriceps muscle during load bearing[3] and more closely simulates dynamic conditions.[1,5,8] The patella may move more toward proximal–lateral in a subluxation position, which indicates impairment of patellar balancing during contraction and explains why some patients suffer more pain when performing a strengthening programme. However, in some cases, contraction leads to dynamic repositioning of a subluxed patella into the trochlear groove or even to mild medialization.

In 30° and 60° of flexion

♦ Patellar movement to distal (lateral, well-centred, distal)

♦ Changed position of the patella in the trochlea (subluxation, tilt)

The osseous stabilization of the patella in the trochlea is normally improved in these positions. In many cases, we find almost normal conditions at more than 30° of flexion. This underlines the fact that most pathologies occur between 0° and

30° of knee flexion. But it is still important to know the shape of the trochlea and the position of the patella in the trochlear groove in higher knee-flexion positions; they may have therapeutic consequences.

Summary

The CT examination documents patellofemoral balancing through the clinically most important range of motion (0–60°) and under different conditions (relaxed, contracted, applied stress). A close relationship exists between clinical findings and the data of the CT examination. The decision to perform a CT examination in favour of MRI or MR-arthrotomography should be carefully considered and must have therapeutic consequences, but in specific cases only CT examination reveals the true pathoanatomy.[1–3,6]

References

1. Biedert RM, Gruhl C (1997) Axial computed tomography of the patellofemoral joint with and without quadriceps contraction. *Arch Orthop Trauma Surg* **116**: 77–82
2. Fulkerson JP, Schutzer SF, Ramsby GR, Bernstein RA (1987) Computerized tomography of the patellofemoral joint before and after lateral release or realignment. *Arthroscopy* **3**: 19–24
3. Sasaki T, Yagi T (1986) Subluxation of the patella. Investigation by computed tomography. *Int Orthop* **10**: 115–120
4. Schutzer SF, Ramsby GR, Fulkerson JP (1986) Computed tomographic classification of patellofemoral pain patients. *Orthop Clin North Am* **17**: 235–248
5. Delgado-Martins H (1979) A study of the position of the patella using computed tomography. *J Bone Joint Surg Br* **61-B**: 443–444
6. Guzzanti V, Gigante A, Di Lazzaro A, Fabbriciani C (1994) Patellofemoral malalignment in adolescents. Computed tomographic assessment with or without quadriceps contraction. *Am J Sports Med* **22**: 55–60
7. Martinez S, Korobkin M, Fondren FB, Hedlund LW, Goldner JL (1983) Diagnosis of patellofemoral malalignment by computed tomography. *J Comput Assist Tomogr* **7**: 1050–1053
8. Pinar H, Akseki D, Karaoglan O, Genc I (1994) Kinematic and dynamic axial computed tomography of the patellofemoral joint in patients with anterior knee pain. *Knee Surg Sports Traumatol Arthrosc* **2**: 170–173
9. Biedert RM, Friederich NF (1994) Failed lateral retinacular release: clinical outcome. *J Sports Traumatol* **16**: 162–173
10. Teitge RA, Faerber WW, Des Madryl P, Matelic TM (1996) Stress radiographs of the patellofemoral joint. *J Bone Joint Surg Am* **78**: 193–203

Suggested reading

Biedert RM, Gruhl C (1997) Axial computed tomography of the patellofemoral joint with and without quadriceps contraction. *Arch Orthop Trauma Surg* **116**: 77–82

Guzzanti V, Gigante A, Di Lazzaro A, Fabbriciani C (1994) Patellofemoral malalignment in adolescents. Computed tomographic assessment with or without quadriceps contraction. *Am J Sports Med* **22**: 55–60

Teitge RA, Faerber WW, Des Madryl P, Matelic TM (1996) Stress radiographs of the patellofemoral joint. *J Bone Joint Surg Am* **78**: 193–203

Comparison of Radiographs, MRI and CT

Roland M. Biedert

The pathology of patellofemoral disorders is multifactorial. Therefore, different examinations can be useful to get more insight into the causal aetiology. Radiographs, MRIs and CT scans are most frequently used to evaluate the patellofemoral joint. Bone scintigraphy[1] or ultrasound investigations need specific indications. Precise knowledge of the radiological anatomy leads to better understanding of the underlying pathology.

Different methods of investigation help to identify the real pathoanatomy. The chosen method must determine the pathognomonic features of the problem, therefore, the best methods must be selected to answer the questions about the individually different pathology. The patient's history and physical examination help the examiner to decide which method of evaluation is necessary. The results of these examinations should be helpful in making the decision for a specific therapy.

Advantages of frequently used methods are described in this chapter, with reference to clinical and therapeutic implications.

Conventional radiology

Standard radiographs are the first method of evaluation for a patient presenting with patellofemoral disorders after the history has been obtained and the patient's lower extremities have been physically examined.[2,3] Radiographs include one lateral view with the knee in 30° of flexion, an anteroposterior view, and an axial view of the patella in 30° of flexion. The specific techniques are described in Chapter 6. Each of these three views can reveal specific pathologies. Some pathologies manifest at first sight; some must be calculated. The most frequent pathologies found with conventional radiographs are summarized in Table 8.1.

Every patient presenting with a patellofemoral problem should undergo a radiological evaluation in three planes – anteroposterior, lateral at 30° of knee flexion, and axial at 30° of flexion.

Magnetic resonance imaging

The MRI, a noninvasive modality, has significant advantages compared with conventional

Patellofemoral Disorders: Diagnosis and Treatment. Edited by Roland M. Biedert
© 2004 John Wiley & Sons, Ltd   ISBN: 0-470-85011-6

Table 8.1 Frequent pathologies documented with conventional radiology

Plane	Pathology
Axial, 30°	Patellar tilt
	Subluxation
	Dislocation
	Patella multipartita* (Figure 8.1)
	Osseous fragments
	Degenerative joint disease
	Fractures
Lateral, 30°	Patella alta or baja
	Degenerative joint disease (Figure 8.2)
	Trochlear dysplasia (Figure 8.3)
	Patella multipartita*
	Osseous fragments
	Patellar tilt
	Fractures
Anteroposterior, 0°	Subluxation
	Patella multipartita*
	Osseous fragments
	Fractures (Figure 8.4)

*Patella is congenitally divided into two or more pieces.

radiographs or CT scans (Table 8.2). Soft tissues, ligaments, cartilage and bone can be represented in multiple planes and in thin slices. The true articular surfaces of the patellar and trochlear cartilage can be evaluated and the congruence of the joint can be assessed.[4,5] Gadolinium-enhanced MR-arthrotomography, using intraarticular injection of gadopentate dimeglumine and physiological saline, are helpful to appraise the true articulating surfaces.[6] Additionally, the subchondral bone and marrow can be evaluated. Intravenous gadolinium contrast (Gd–DTPA) MRI has been used to enhance the different areas.[7]

Static and *dynamic* MRI must be distinguished.[8] *Static* MRI allows visualization of the articular cartilage congruence, bone and soft-tissue structures under static conditions. Static MRI lacks views of muscle contraction, movement and loading.[8] *Dynamic* MRI offers a new perspective for dynamic study of the patellofemoral

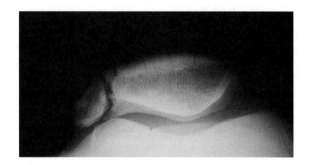

Figure 8.1   Patella multipartita (right knee, axial view)

Table 8.2   Advantages of MRI versus CT (axial views)

	MRI	CT
Soft tissues, ligaments	Visible (partial or complete tears, inflammation)	Not visible
Cartilage	Documentation of the true articular cartilage congruence; softening, fissuring, erosions and defects are visible	Only osseous contours and space between patella and trochlea are visible
Subchondral bone	Oedema, fluid, bone bruise	Not visible
Technique	No radiation	Radiation

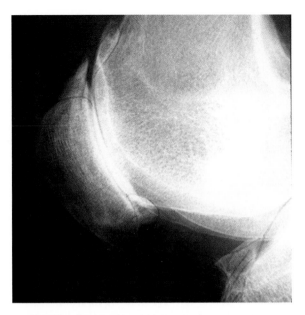

Figure 8.2 Degenerative disease of the patellofemoral joint (lateral view)

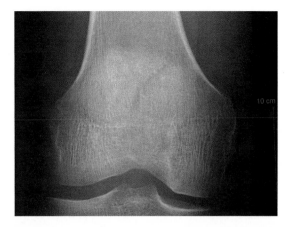

Figure 8.4 Longitudinal fracture of the patella (anteroposterior view, right side)

joint. Brossmann et al[9] documented patellar tracking during active and passive extension with motion-triggered cineMRI.[8] Bellelli and Nardis[10] used open MRI for dynamic knee examination between 0° and 120° of flexion. Shellock et al[11] compared unloaded with loaded dynamic MRI and revealed abnormalities in some patients with symptomatic patellofemoral joints. Dynamic MRI is still an experimental investigative tool that needs additional examination and a correct cost–effectiveness analysis. Eventually, it may replace diagnostic arthroscopy.[8]

Cartilage

Axial and sagittal images depict the articular cartilage, enhanced or unenhanced. Homogenous signal intensity demonstrates normal anatomy. On axial views, cartilage attenuation or erosions can be demonstrated (Figures 8.5, 8.6, and 8.7). Intraarticular liquid (joint effusion, haemarthrosis) or MR arthrotomography give improved contrast to document cartilage softening, swelling, fissuring or blistering.[7]

Inhomogeneity associated with irregular cartilage surface and thinning of the cartilage represent different grades of chondromalacia. Increased subchondral signal intensity represents local oedema or imbibed fluid; low signal intensity may represent subchondral sclerosis (Figure 8.8).

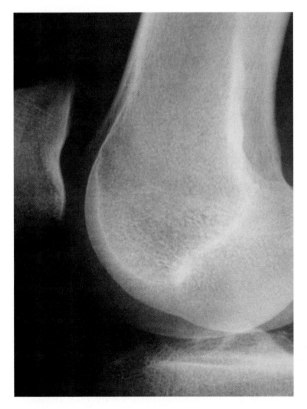

Figure 8.3 Asymmetrical crossing of the intercondylar groove and the two condyles (lateral view)

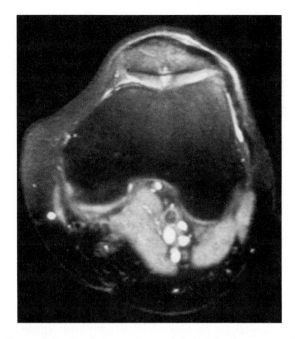

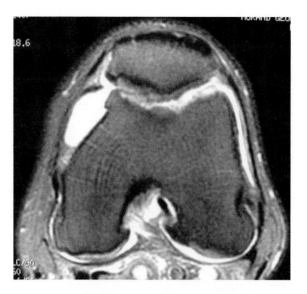

Figure 8.7   Severe cartilage destruction of the patellofemoral joint with osteoarthritis (left knee, axial view, T2-weighted)

Figure 8.5   Cartilage erosion and defect in the centre of the patella with high signal intensity changes subchondrally (left knee, axial view, T2-weighted)

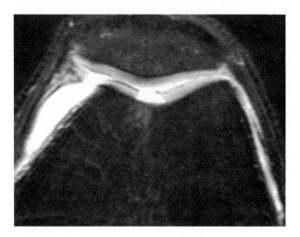

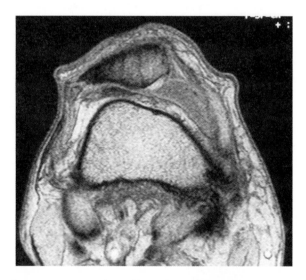

Figure 8.6   Cartilage defect in the centre of the trochlea. The lesion is filled with intraarticular fluid. Partially detached chondral flaps on both sides with fissuring to the deep articular cartilage layer may occur (left knee, T2-weighted, axial view)

Figure 8.8   Lateral patellar subluxation with subchondral sclerosis and advanced chondromalacia (right knee, axial view, T1-weighted)

Subchondral bone

Other changes of the signal intensity in the subchondral bone can be identified with MRI fol-

lowing patellar dislocation (Figure 8.9), showing, for example, a bone bruise. This lesion is confined by definition to the medullary bone.[12] On MRI, the bone bruise appears as a poorly defined area of decreased signal intensity on

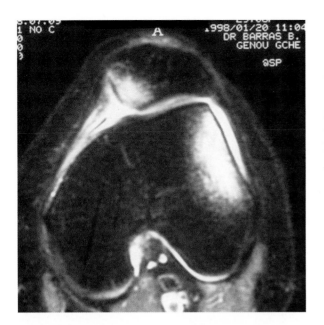

Figure 8.9 Bone bruises in the medial facet of the patella and the lateral femoral condyle following patellar dislocation with dysplastic trochlea (left knee, T2-weighted, axial view)

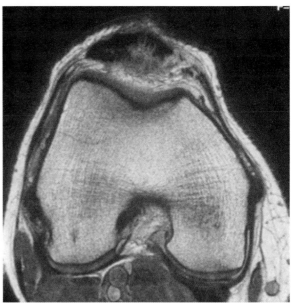

Figure 8.10 Hyperintense, subchondral imbibed-fluid signal intensity due to chronic inflammation of the distal part of the patella and the proximal patellar tendon (jumper's knee) (right knee, T1-weighted, axial view)

T1-weighted images that irregularly increase in signal intensity on T2-weighted sequences. Bone bruises are considered to be related to trauma.[13] Bone bruises pose a potential risk of chondrolysis because of microfracture of the subchondral bone. Therefore, partial weightbearing must be recommended.[14]

The subchondral signal intensity can also be changed by chronic inflammation of the attached tendon with destruction of the normal bone (Figure 8.10).

The fast spin-echo STIR (short inversion time, inversion recovery) sequence has been described as superior to the fat-suppressed fast spin-echo T2-weighted sequence for depiction of the lesions or marrow oedema.[15]

Ligaments

Partial or complete ruptures of different ligaments around the patellofemoral joint can be documented following acute trauma. Lateral patellar

dislocation is accompanied by tears of the medial retinaculum, the vastus medialis obliquus muscle and the medial patellofemoral ligament[16,17] (Figure 8.11). On the lateral opposite side, a lax retinaculum or vastus lateralis tendon is present. MRI helps in these cases to evaluate the severity of the injury, to identify the damaged structures involved and to define the precise area of the injury.[18] This evaluation also helps to determine the therapeutic approach.[18]

Chronic inflammation of a tendon, with or without partial tears, can also be seen with MRI[18,19] (Figure 8.12). The best-known disease is jumper's knee, representing patellar tendonitis.[19–21] Grade and severity of patellar tendinitis are identified by MRI.[7,19,22] Chronic tears, necrosis and inflammation lead to intratendinous foci and increased signal intensity[19] (Figures 8.13 and 8.14). In grades II and III, pain is felt after, during or before activity.

In grade IV, a severe partial tear, pain is always present.[19,21] The results of MRI evaluation determine the necessary type of treatment.[19] By

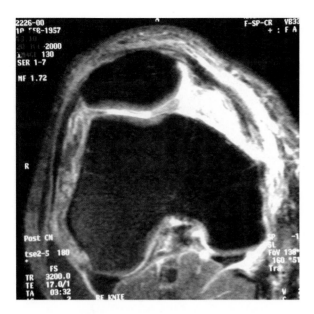

Figure 8.11 Lateral subluxation of the patella following lateral patellar dislocation. MRI shows partial tear of the medial retinaculum and rupture of the medial patellofemoral ligament close to the adductor tubercle. Joint effusion serves as a intraarticular contrast medium (right knee, T2-weighted, axial view)

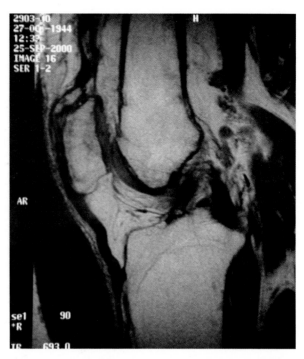

Figure 8.12 Partial chronic rupture of the quadriceps tendon close to the attachment at the upper pole of the patella with splayed tendon fibres. The tear site with the scar tissue demonstrates high signal intensity (T1-weighted, sagittal view)

excising the involved tendon and distal part of the patella, the defect can be closed with augmentation using a quadriceps bone–tendon graft.[19]

Suprapatellar and mediopatellar plicae

The plicae, both the suprapatellar and mediopatellar, are potential causes of patellofemoral pain when they are thickened, scarred or inflamed.[16] MRI is an excellent examination to document plicae in axial views (Figures 8.15 and 8.16).

Contraindications to MRI

MRI, which exposes the patient to a magnetic field,[6] has several contraindications. These include cardiac pacemakers, some types of cardiac prosthetic valves, intraorbital metallic foreign bodies, cochlear implants, metallic cerebral aneurysm clips, dorsal column stimulators and bone-growth stimulators.[8] Metallic orthopaedic hardware (joint prosthesis, plates, screws, staplers) may limit MRI. Patients suffering from claustrophobia are candidates only for open MRI. MR arthrotomography requires an intraarticular injection of a contrast medium and absolutely sterile conditions.[6]

Computed tomography

Different authors[23–27] stress the importance of using CT scans when examining the patellofemoral joint. The CT evaluation of the patellofemoral joint has specific advantages compared to conventional radiographs or MRI. But CT scans cannot replace normal radiographs, e.g. the true lateral

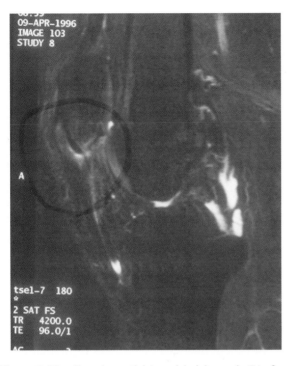

Figure 8.13 Chronic partial tear (circle), grade IV of the proximal patellar tendon in chronic jumper's knee (T2-weighted, sagittal view)

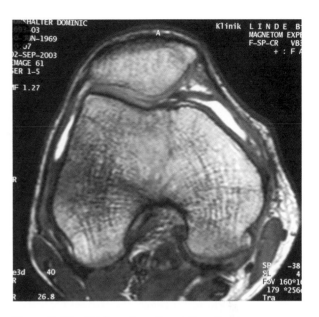

Figure 8.15 Thickened mediopatellar plica in a young female with patellofemoral pain. Normal cartilage and congruence of the patellofemoral joint (right knee, T2-weighted, axial view)

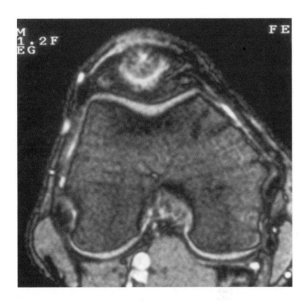

Figure 8.14 Chronic partial tear of the patellar tendon with thickening and increased signal intensity by fluid and scar tissue (right knee, T2-weighted, axial view)

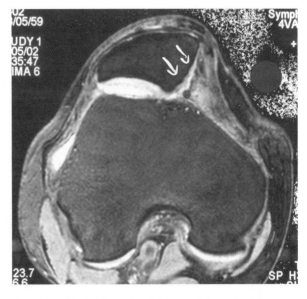

Figure 8.16 Thickened and inflamed plica ($\rightarrow$) in a female patient with chronic lateral patellar subluxation. Note the dysplastic patellofemoral joint with a flat lateral condyle and type C patellar morphology (right knee, T2-weighted, axial view)

Table 8.3   Advantages (→) of CT versus radiographs

	CT	Radiographs
Axial views	In all angles → assessment of the whole range of motion	Between 30° and 90° of knee flexion
Quadriceps contraction	With and without	Normally without
Planes	Two or three dimensions	Two dimensions

views. The CT scans are additional examinations to define questions exactly and to plan the necessary treatment. They also cannot replace MRI or MR arthrotomography regarding the real articular congruence of the joint, the cartilage, soft tissues or subchondral bone. But arthro-CT scans are helpful in determining articular congruence in patients with contraindications to MRI. In Table 8.3, the advantages of the CT scan are summarized in comparison to radiographs.

CT scans provide six important advantages in comparison to MRI:

♦ Evaluation is possible in all different angles between full extension and maximum knee flexion.

♦ Evaluation is possible with and without contraction of the quadriceps muscle.

♦ Comparison of both sides.

♦ Assessment and documentation of medial and/or lateral patellar instability.

♦ Evaluation of the rotation of the whole lower extremity is possible.

Table 8.4   Advantages (→) of CT versus MRI (axial views)

	CT	MRI
Side	→ Comparison of both sides	Only one side
Quadriceps contraction	With and without; → static and dynamic evaluation	Normally without contraction
Angle	In all angles 0°, 30° and 60° of knee flexion; → assessment of the whole range of motion	Normally in extension
Instability	Stress CT scans; → documentation possible using an applied force (medial and/or lateral)	No force can be applied
Assessment of limb alignment in the horizontal plane	Femoral antetorsion, torsion of the bicondylar axis, internal or external tibial torsion; → evaluation of the rotation of the lower extremity	No assessment of the femoral or tibial torsion is possible
Magnetic field	→ No disturbance of metallic hardware	Several contraindications

♦ No contraindications for a magnetic field (Table 8.4).

Evaluation in different angles

Kujala et al[28,29] demonstrated that evaluation of the first 30° of knee flexion gives the most important diagnostic information about the underlying pathology (Figures 8.17 and 8.18). This corresponds to Goodfellow's biomechanical studies demonstrating that the most susceptible position for patella dysfunction is at the beginning of knee flexion, under 30°.[30]

In addition, serial imaging over a range of flexion between 0° and 30° is helpful to see

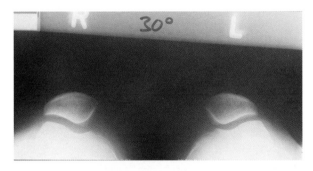

Figure 8.17 Well-centred and balanced patellae in a young female patient (axial radiographs in 30° of flexion)

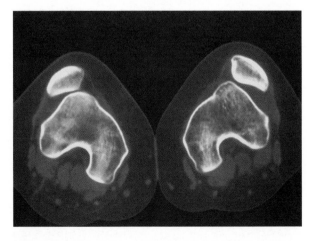

Figure 8.18 Same female patient (as in Figure 8.17) with complete patellar dislocations (CT scans, axial views, with quadriceps contracted)

deeper into the complex patellofemoral balancing mechanism.[24,31] This evaluation of the first 30° of knee flexion with CT is a major difference and advantage over standard axial radiographs, which cannot be performed under 30°.[24]

Quadriceps muscle contracted

The second important difference between CT, MRI and standard radiographs is the possibility of performing CT scans with and without the quadriceps contracted. An examination in extension with quadriceps muscle contraction is needed to obtain a more comprehensive picture of the patellofemoral relationship.[24,30,32] Muscle contraction might partially substitute for the normal tension of the quadriceps muscle during load bearing, which comes closer to a more dynamic evaluation.

We have shown that, in 30° of knee flexion, no significant difference of the patellar position exists with or without quadriceps contraction.[24] This means that axial CT scans in 30° of flexion with quadriceps contracted give no further information about the dynamic influence of muscle contraction, because the patella normally has an osseous stabilization and centralization in this position.

Different effects of quadriceps muscle contraction in extension are known. Kujala et al[29] reported that the lateral patellar tilt can decrease with contraction and that the patella may move either laterally or medially. Sasaki and Yagi[25] found an increased tilt component of up to 8.8°. They also reported that the lateral shift of the patella increased significantly in knees with subluxation compared to normal knees.

We have demonstrated that the patella can move laterally or medially or stay well-centred with quadriceps contraction.[24] The direction of the displacement depends on the underlying pathology. Near full extension, the lateral condyle gives less support to the patella. In this position, the integrity of the soft-tissue structures (medial and lateral retinacula, medial

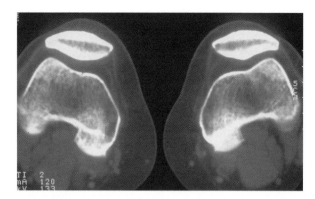

Figure 8.19   Nearly normal position of the patella in a female patient (axial CT, extension, quadriceps relaxed)[24]

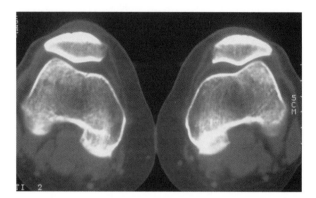

Figure 8.20   Same patient as Figure 8.19, presenting lateral patellar subluxation and lateral hypercompression with full activation of the quadriceps muscle (axial CT, extension, quadriceps contracted)[24]

patellofemoral ligament, vastus medialis and lateralis muscles) determine the position of the patella. With full muscle contraction, the force vector of the quadriceps muscle determines the position of the patella. A force vector directed to lateral subluxates the patella to lateral, especially in combination with tight lateral retinacula and weak medial structures. This explains why non-specific muscle training may worsen the situation in patients suffering from patellofemoral pain (Figures 8.19 and 8.20). Dynamic lateralization of the patella can be caused by an insufficiency of the medial patellofemoral ligament. Medialization with full quadriceps contraction can be

caused after excessive release of the lateral structures (retinacula and tendon of the vastus lateralis muscle).[33,34] The best indices for measuring the effect of maximal quadriceps muscle contraction at 0° of knee flexion and its documentation are the lateral patellar displacement and the patellar tilt.[24,26,35]

A special situation is present in patients with patella alta.[24] The patellar articular surface lies tangentially to the distal femur, rather than being firmly apposed to it. In addition, the patella has, in full extension or hyperextension, the lowest passive osseous stabilization with a contact surface of under 12%.[24,36] The influence of the muscle contraction becomes even more important in this unstable osseous situation. Patella alta is therefore often related to a functional imbalance of the extensor mechanism and is thus a critical risk factor for patellofemoral disorders (Figures 8.21, 8.22, 8.23).

In conclusion, axial CT scans in 0° of knee flexion with and without contraction of the

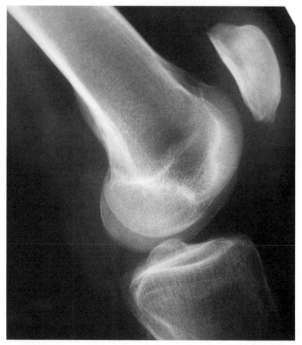

Figure 8.21   Patella alta (lateral radiograph in 30° of flexion)

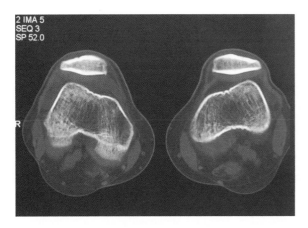

Figure 8.22 Patella alta: patella positioned proximal in the trochlea (axial view, extension, quadriceps relaxed)

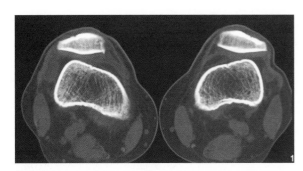

Figure 8.23 Increased lateral subluxation of the proximally positioned patella (axial view, extension, quadriceps contracted)

Table 8.5 Influence of quadriceps muscle contraction on the patellar position

Constant abnormality	
Relaxed	Contracted
Patellar subluxation	Patellar subluxation
	♦ Unchanged
	♦ Increased (Figures 8.24 and 8.25)
	♦ Decreased (Figures 8.26 and 8.27)
Inconstant abnormality	
Relaxed	Contracted
Patella centred	Patellar subluxation
	♦ Lateral (Figures 8.28 and 8.29)
	♦ Medial (Figures 8.30 and 8.31)

quadriceps muscle can demonstrate an abnormal patellofemoral relationship that might be overlooked using only cuts from different levels of the patellofemoral joint.[24] The static (not contracted) and dynamic (contracted) position of the patella must be compared, especially in full extension. With this, different types of biomechanical deficiencies of the patellofemoral joint must be distinguished: *constant abnormality* of the patellar position in the femoral groove and *inconstant abnormality*, caused and present only with full contraction of the quadriceps[24] (Table 8.5).

The comparison of static and dynamic aspects allow clear identification of the type of patellofemoral incongruence, knowledge of which is mandatory for the selection of treatment.

Comparison of both sides

Another major advantage of CT in comparison to MRI is the possibility of evaluating both knees at the same time with one single investigation. This is especially important in cases where prior surgery has been performed. The nonoperated side serves as a marker of the given normal or abnormal patellofemoral congruence in each patient (Figures 8.32 and 8.33).

Comparison of the two sides gives important information about the present pathology and helps to determine the type and amount of therapy necessary. This bilateral comparison can be performed between 0° and 60° of knee flexion, with and without quadriceps contraction.

Assessment of instability

Instability can be described objectively as abnormal stability with excessive limits of motion in

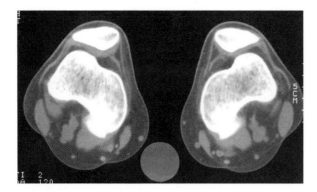

Figure 8.24   Constant abnormality. Lateral patellar subluxation (axial view, extension, relaxed)

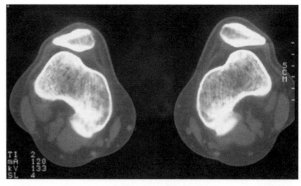

Figure 8.25   Constant abnormality. Increased dynamic patellar subluxation (axial view, extension, contracted)

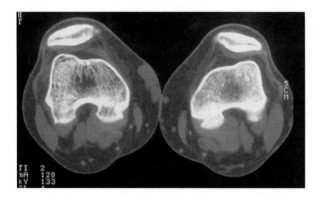

Figure 8.26   Constant abnormality. Lateral patellar subluxation (axial view, extension, relaxed)

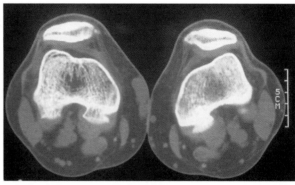

Figure 8.27   Constant abnormality. Decreased patellar subluxation (axial view, extension, contracted)

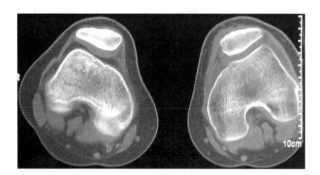

Figure 8.28   Inconstant abnormality. Well-centred patella (axial view, extension, relaxed)

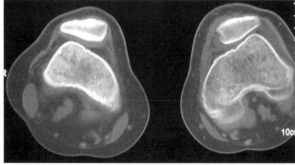

Figure 8.29   Inconstant abnormality. Dynamic lateral subluxation (axial view, extension, contracted)

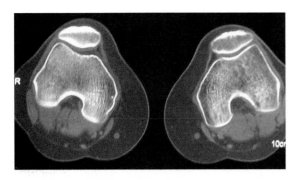

Figure 8.30 Inconstant abnormality. Well-centred patella (axial view, extension, relaxed)

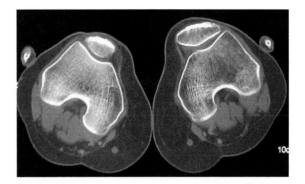

Figure 8.31 Inconstant abnormality. Dynamic medial subluxation, left side (axial view, extension, contracted)

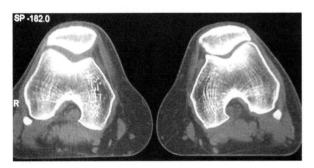

Figure 8.32 Normal congruence of the nonoperated side (right knee). Operated side (left knee) with degenerative changes (axial views, extension, relaxed)

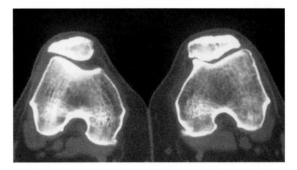

Figure 8.33 Abnormal congruence of the nonoperated side (right) with patellar subluxation to lateral. The operated left side presents medial subluxation of the patella, with osteoarthritis of the medial patellofemoral joint following over-correction with medialization of the tibial tuberosity (axial views, extension, relaxed)

the three translational planes and about the three rotational axes.[37] Regarding the patellofemoral joint, objective instability must be distinguished from subjectively perceived functional instability, e.g. caused by pain or quadriceps weakness. This differentiation is not always easy. Instability can exist with normal radiographs. Standard radiographs may show potential for instability (i.e. risk factors) but not ultimate displacement.[38] CT evaluation with axial views can be useful to document stability or instability of the important passive structures (capsule, retinacula, ligaments).

Instability results from a lack of adequate restraint or too much of a displacing force.[38] Muscles are not primary joint stabilizers and are therefore not the topic of this type of CT evaluation. Adequate restraint of the patellofemoral joint comes from ligaments (lateral retinacula,

medial patellofemoral ligament, medial and lateral patellomeniscal ligaments) and the bone geometry (trochlear depth, width and length). Patellar instability has numerous aetiological factors (Table 8.6). It can be caused by trochlear dysplasia, e.g. shallow femoral groove. Femoral dysplasia is a common cause for recurrent patellar dislocation.

Injured ligaments following patellar dislocation can cause instability by insufficient healing. This instability and the amount of displacement can be measured with a force applied to the patella from either the lateral, medial or both sides, depending on the suspected pathology. Stress CT scans are so far the most sensitive examinations available for documenting pathological displacement and

Table 8.6   Aetiological factors of patellar instability

Subjective instability
   Pain
   Muscular weakness
Objective instability
   Primary
   ◆ Lateral
     Tight lateral structures
     Muscular imbalance
     Increased femoral antetorsion
     Increased foot pronation
   ◆ Lateral and/or medial
     Trochlear dysplasia
     Patella alta
   Secondary
   ◆ Lateral
     Following traumatic injury
   ◆ Lateral and medial
     Over-release
   ◆ Medial
     Lateral retinacular release
     Excessive medialization of the tibial
       tuberosity

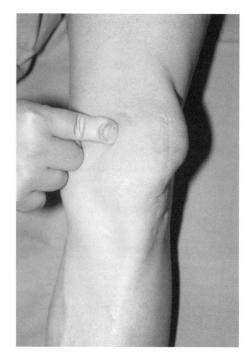

Figure 8.34   Finger pressure from medial leading to lateral patellar subluxation in a male patient following excessive lateral release (left knee)

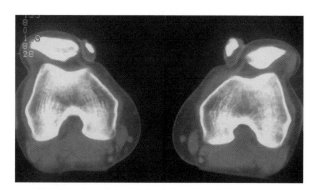

Figure 8.35   Documentation of lateral patellar instability on both sides. Note the fingers on both medial sides of the patella to apply the force (axial views, extension, relaxed)

instability.[38] Comparison of the normal side (if available) with the abnormal side using stress examinations is more important than the absolute amount of displacement.

Stress CT scans can be performed with applied finger pressure (Figures 8.34, 8.35, 8.36, and 8.37).

The possibility of documenting patellar instability is of great importance[33,38] and CT scans allow quantification of instability. Documentation of secondary instability following lateral retinaculum release helps us to understand the persisting postoperative problems and to determine the necessary treatments.[33,38,39]

Assessment of limb alignment

Normal limb alignment means 12–13° of femoral antetorsion and external torsion of the tibia of about 23° (less in males than females) in the horizontal plane.[2,3,38]

To analyse the alignment of the lower extremity by using CT scans, the patient lies supine with a plantar support under the foot; the foot is held

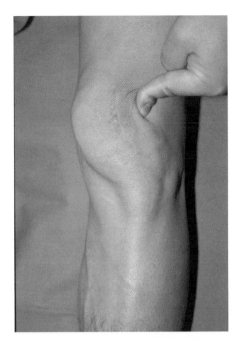

Figure 8.36 Finger pressure from lateral leading to medial patellar subluxation (left knee)

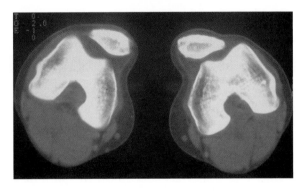

Figure 8.37 Documentation of the medial instability on both sides in the same patient (axial views, extension, relaxed)

in 15° of external rotation.[3] Several sections with the quadriceps relaxed can be performed, depending on the suggested pathological aetiological factor.

Femoral antetorsion

This is the angle formed by the intersection of a line joining the centre of the femoral head and femoral neck at the top of the trochanteric fossa (x) with a line tangential to the posterior aspects of the femoral condyles (y)[3] (Figure 8.38). Increased (pathological) femoral antetorsion causes increased internal rotation of the distal femur[38] (Figure 8.39).

If the knee rotates inward, a side force vector is produced that subluxates the patella laterally. Additionally, higher strain on the medial patellofemoral ligament and increased compression force on the lateral patellar facet occur (Figures 8.40 and 8.41).

Exact analysis of the pathological femoral antetorsion has an important clinical implication and determines the necessary treatment. Teitge

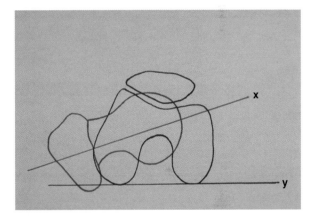

Figure 8.38 Measurement of femoral antetorsion (right knee)

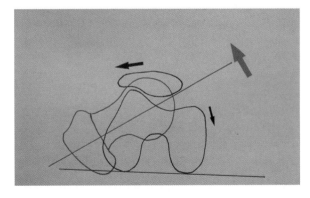

Figure 8.39 Increased femoral antetorsion with lateral patellar subluxation (right knee)

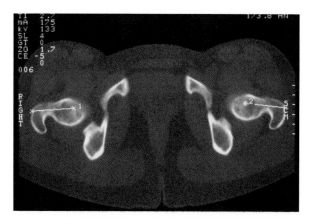

Figure 8.40   Section through the femoral neck and head at the top of the trochanteric fossa (27 year-old female)

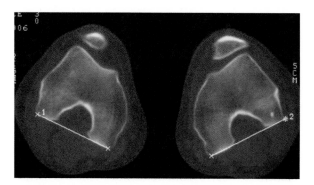

Figure 8.41   Tangential line to the posterior aspects of the femoral condyles in the same patient. The measurement of the angle documents increased femoral antetorsion

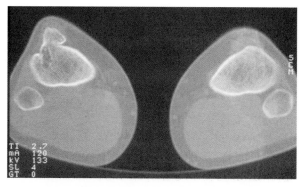

Figure 8.42   Documentation and comparison of the exact position of the tibial tuberosity following medialization on the right side (24 year-old female)

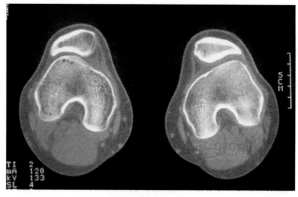

Figure 8.43   Persistent lateral patellar subluxation in spite of medialization of the tibial tuberosity on the right side (same patient as Figure 8.42)

(RA Teitge, handout, 1999) reported that intertrochanteric rotational femoral osteotomies lead to a major reduction in pain, crepitation, giving-way and weakness. His treated patients included some with arthrosis, some with pain only, some with instability, and most with some combination of all three (*see* Case Study 12).

Tibial tuberosity

CT scan sections that pass through the tibial tuberosity document the exact position of the tibial tuberosities, so that both sides can be compared. These sections are especially important

after surgical medialization of the tuberosity (Figure 8.42). They also document the position of the patella in the trochlear groove after medialization of the tuberosity (Figure 8.43). They document the effect of other previous surgery and help to define the type of correction, a re-Elmslie procedure in cases of over-correction.

External tibial torsion

Exact documentation of the complete tibial torsion is possible by scanning various sections on different levels. External tibial torsion is formed by the line tangential to the posterior aspect of the plateau (head of the tibia) (Figure 8.44) and the line

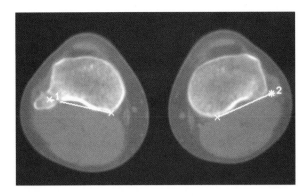

Figure 8.44 Tangential line to the posterior aspects of the proximal tibial head

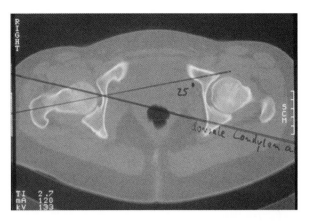

Figure 8.47 Section through the femoral neck and head

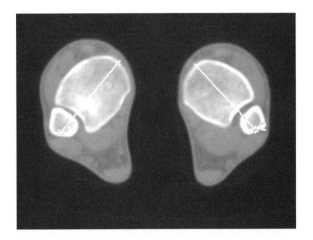

Figure 8.45 Section through the bimalleolar axis

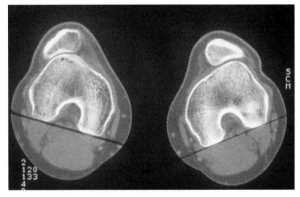

Figure 8.48 Axis of the femoral condyles, using tangential lines to the posterior aspects

midtibial shaft (Figure 8.46). The torsion has an indirect influence on patellofemoral function.[2] Tibial torsion also can be calculated in reference to femoral torsion, using sections through the femoral neck and condyle (Figures 8.47 and 8.48).

Conclusion and summary

Understanding of radiological, MRI and CT analyses of the patellofemoral joint, with the corresponding advantages of each technique, leads to better understanding of the present pathology and the necessary treatment. Anatomical factors can be distinguished and every problem can be treated precisely. A brief physical examination at the beginning helps to determine which individual

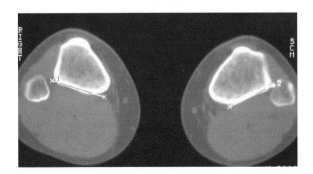

Figure 8.46 Tangential line to the posterior border of the mid-tibial shaft

through the bimalleolar axis (Figure 8.45).[3] In addition, we can determine the torsion of the

investigation is necessary to guarantee the best additional information. Dynamic evaluation is of special interest to take into account all the functional aspects as fully as possible.

Static, dynamic and kinematic three-dimensional analyses of CT and MRI, through the whole range of motion, comparing both sides, loaded and unloaded, will increase the fundamental knowledge and understanding of patellofemoral joint pathology in future.

References

1. Dye SF, Chew MH (1993) The use of scintigraphy to detect increased osseous metabolic transmission with an envelope of function. *J Bone Joint Surg Am* **75**: 1388–1406

2. Galland O, Walch G, Dejour H, Carret JP (1990) An anatomical and radiological study of the femoropatellar articulation. *Surg Radiol Anat* **12**: 119–125

3. Dejour H, Walch G, Nove-Josserand L, Guier C (1994) Factors of patellar instability: an anatomic radiographic study. *Knee Surg Sports Traumatol Arthrosc* **2**: 19–26

4. Stäubli HU, Durrenmatt U, Rauschning W (1997) Zur Frage der Kongruenz von Gelenkknorpeloberflächen und subchondralem Knochen des Femoropatellargelenks in der axialen Ebene. *Arthroskopie* **10**: 66–71

5. Bosshard C, Stäubli HU, Rauschning W (1997) Konturinkongruenz von Gelenkknorpeloberflächen und subchondralem Knochen des Femoropatellargelenks in der sagittalen Ebene. *Arthroskopie* **10**: 72–76

6. Stäubli HU, Dürrenmatt U, Porcellini B, Rauschning W (1999) Anatomy and surface geometry of the patellofemoral joint in the axial plane. *J Bone Joint Surg Br* **81**: 452–458

7. Stoller DW (1993) *Magnetic Resonance Imaging in Orthopaedics and Sports Medicine.* Philadelphia, PA, JB Lippincott

8. Witonski D (2002) Dynamic magnetic resonance imaging. *Clin Sports Med* **21**: 403–415

9. Brossmann J, Muhle C, Schroder C et al (1993) Patellar tracking patterns during active and passive knee extension: evaluation with motion-triggered cine MR imaging. *Radiology* **187**: 205–212

10. Bellelli A, Nardis P (1997) [Dynamic magnetic resonance of the knee. Considerations on techniques and anatomy with a magnetic resonance system with open magnet]. *Radiol Med (Torino)* **93**: 199–205

11. Shellock FG, Mink JH, Deutsch AL et al (1993) Patellofemoral joint: identification of abnormalities with active-movement, 'unloaded' versus 'loaded' kinematic MR imaging techniques. *Radiology* **188**: 575–578

12. Deutsch AL, Mink JH, Shellock FG (1990) Magnetic resonance imaging of injuries to bone and articular cartilage. Emphasis on radiographically occult abnormalities. *Orthop Rev* **19**: 66–75

13. Dienst M, Blauth M (2000) Bone bruise of the calcaneus. A case report. *Clin Orthop* **378**: 202–205

14. Johnson DL, Bealle DP, Brand JC Jr et al (2000) The effect of a geographic lateral bone bruise on knee inflammation after acute anterior cruciate ligament rupture. *Am J Sports Med* **28**: 152–155

15. Lazzarini KM, Troiano RN, Smith RC (1997) Can running cause the appearance of marrow edema on MR images of the foot and ankle? *Radiology* **202**: 540–542

16. Hughston JC, Walsh WM, Puddu G (1984) *Patellar Subluxation and Dislocation. Saunders Monographs in Clinical Orthopaedics*, volume V. Philadelphia, PA, WB Saunders

17. Sallay PI, Poggi J, Speer KP, Garrett WE (1996) Acute dislocation of the patella. A correlative pathoanatomic study. *Am J Sports Med* **24**: 52–60

18. King J (2000) Patellar dislocation and lesions of the patella tendon. *Br J Sports Med* **34**: 467–470

19. Biedert RM, Vogel U, Friederich NF (1997) Chronic patellar tendonitis: a new surgical treatment. *Sports Exerc Injury* **3**: 150–154

20. Eifert-Mangine M, Brewster C, Wong M et al (1992) Patellar tendinitis in the recreational athlete. *Orthopedics* **15**: 1359–1367

21. Blazina ME, Kerlan RK, Jobe FW et al (1973) Jumper's knee. *Orthop Clin North Am* **4**: 665–678

22. el-Khoury GY, Wira RL, Berbaum KS et al (1992) MR imaging of patellar tendinitis. *Radiology* **184**: 849–854

23. Martinez S, Korobkin M, Fondren FB et al (1983) Diagnosis of patellofemoral malalignment by

computed tomography. *J Comput Assist Tomogr* 7: 1050–1053

24. Biedert RM, Gruhl C (1997) Axial computed tomography of the patellofemoral joint with and without quadriceps contraction. *Arch Orthop Trauma Surg* **116**: 77–82

25. Sasaki T, Yagi T (1986) Subluxation of the patella. Investigation by computerized tomography. *Int Orthop* **10**: 115–120

26. Schutzer SF, Ramsby GR, Fulkerson JP (1986) Computed tomographic classification of patellofemoral pain patients. *Orthop Clin North Am* **17**: 235–248

27. Delgado-Martins H (1979) A study of the position of the patella using computerised tomography. *J Bone Joint Surg Br* **61-B**: 443–444

28. Kujala UM, Osterman K, Kormano M et al (1989) Patellar motion analyzed by magnetic resonance imaging. *Acta Orthop Scand* **60**: 13–16

29. Kujala UM, Kormano M, Osterman K et al (1992) Magnetic resonance imaging analysis of patellofemoral congruity in females. *Clin J Sports Med* **2**: 21–26

30. Goodfellow J, Hungerford DS, Woods C (1976) Patello-femoral joint mechanics and pathology. 2. Chondromalacia patellae. *J Bone Joint Surg Br* **58**: 291–299

31. Pinar H, Akseki D, Karaoglan O, Genc I (1994) Kinematic and dynamic axial computed tomography of the patellofemoral joint in patients with anterior knee pain. *Knee Surg Sports Traumatol Arthrosc* **2**: 170–173

32. Caylor D, Fites R, Worrell TW (1993) The relationship between quadriceps angle and anterior knee pain syndrome. *J Orthop Sports Phys Ther* **17**: 11–16

33. Biedert RM, Friederich NF (1994) Failed lateral retinacular release: clinical outcome. *J Sports Traumatol* **16**: 162–173

34. Hughston JC, Deese M (1988) Medial subluxation of the patella as a complication of lateral retinacular release. *Am J Sports Med* **16**: 383–388

35. Laurin CA, Levesque HP, Dussault R et al (1978) The abnormal lateral patellofemoral angle: a diagnostic roentgenographic sign of recurrent patellar subluxation. *J Bone Joint Surg Am* **60**: 55–60

36. Hille E, Schulitz KP, Henrichs C, Schneider T (1985) Pressure and contract-surface measurements within the femoropatellar joint and their variations following lateral release. *Arch Orthop Trauma Surg* **104**: 275–282

37. Jakob RP, Stäubli HU (1990) *The Knee and the Cruciate Ligaments.* Berlin and Heidelberg, Springer-Verlag

38. Teitge RA, Faerber WW, Des Madryl P, Matelic TM (1996) Stress radiographs of the patellofemoral joint. *J Bone Joint Surg Am* **78**: 193–203

39. Kramers-de Quervain IA, Biedert R, Stüssi E (1997) Quantitative gait analysis in patients with medial patellar instability following lateral retinacular release. *Knee Surg Sports Traumatol Arthrosc* **5**: 95–101

Suggested reading

Biedert RM, Gruhl C (1997) Axial computed tomography of the patellofemoral joint with and without quadriceps contraction. *Arch Orthop Trauma Surg* **116**: 77–82

Kramers-de Quervain IA, Biedert R, Stüssi E (1997) Quantitative gait analysis in patients with medial patellar instability following lateral retinacular release. *Knee Surg Sports Traumatol Arthrosc* **5**: 95–101

Galland O, Walch G, Dejour H, Carret JP (1990) An anatomical and radiological study of the femoropatellar articulation. *Surg Radiol Anat* **12**: 119–125

Dejour H, Walch G, Nove-Josserand L, Guier C (1994) Factors of patellar instability: an anatomic radiographic study. *Knee Surg Sports Traumatol Arthrosc* **2**: 19–26

Biedert RM, Vogel U, Friederich NF (1997) Chronic patellar tendonitis: a new surgical treatment. *Sports Exerc Injury* **3**: 150–154

Sallay PI, Poggi J, Speer KP, Garrett WE (1996) Acute dislocation of the patella. A correlative pathoanatomic study. *Am J Sports Med* **24**: 52–60

9 Nonoperative Treatment

Roland M. Biedert and **Vroni Kernen**

The key to successful treatment of patellofemoral disorders is to decrease the symptoms and maximize the individual patient's function.[1] The goals of nonoperative treatment described by the European League Against Rheumatism (EULAR)[2] and the American College of Rheumatology (ACR)[3] are to control pain, to minimize disability and to educate the patient about the disorder and its therapy.[4] Correct identification of the source of patellofemoral pain is essential to determine the methods of treatment.[5] Treatment should be tailored to the individual patient, taking into account factors such as age, co-morbidity and expectations for the future. Treatment may be surgical or nonoperative. In this chapter, nonoperative treatment is described.

Optimal nonoperative treatment of patellofemoral pain requires a combination of nonpharmacological and pharmacological treatment modalities. The components of both modalities are outlined in Table 9.1.

Nonpharmacological modalities

Nonpharmacological modalities offer additional benefit over and above the use of analgesics. Nonsurgical treatment includes exercise

Table 9.1 Proposals for nonoperative treatment modalities of patellofemoral disorders

Nonpharmacological treatment

Patient education
Physical therapy
Orthoses and insoles
Sleeves and braces
Walking aids
Weight reduction (if overweight)

Pharmacological treatment

Oral
Paracetamol-acetaminophen
Nonsteroidal antiinflammatory drugs (NSAIDs)
Selective cyclooxygenase-2 (COX-2) inhibitors
Other pure analgesics
Symptomatic slow-acting drugs for osteoarthritis (SYSADOA)
Vitamins A, C and E
Intraarticular
Glucocorticoids
Viscosupplementation

Patellofemoral Disorders: Diagnosis and Treatment. Edited by Roland M. Biedert
© 2004 John Wiley & Sons, Ltd ISBN: 0-470-85011-6

programmes, physical therapy, appliances, lifestyle changes and education.

Education

Patient education is an integral part of the treatment plan.[2,4] Physicians and physical therapists should explain to the patient the nature of his/her disorder, its prognosis, the requirement of investigations and what that involves, and determine with each patient the rationale and practicalities of the specific treatment plan.[2] Patients who understand their disorder communicate better than those without information and understanding about their problem. Discussions and clear explanations (such as radiographs, MRI or CT scans) improve patients' understanding and show benefits of the acceptance of the disease.

Physical therapy

There is evidence that the different modalities of physical therapy reduce complaints and improve knee functions.[6-12] Physical therapy plays a key role in the nonsurgical treatment of patellofemoral disorders. The different approaches are summarized in Part IV.

Orthoses and insoles

Orthoses are used to correct biomechanical abnormalities and to provide pain relief in weight-bearing joints.[13] Pain is often experienced during gait by shock wave transmission as the heel strikes the ground. In addition, abnormal force distribution resulting from pathological skeletal alignment, such as overpronation, can occur (Figure 9.1). The aims of lower limb orthotic interventions are to improve attenuation properties through shock absorption and ameliorate force distribution through skeletal alignment correction (Figures 9.2 and 9.3). Individual manufacture (in special cases according to the results of foot prints or force plate measurements) is

mandatory for a successful outcome (Figure 9.4). Although studies analysing the effects of orthotic interventions are of poor quality, clinical experience demonstrates a positive outcome as a result of appropriate insoles.[13]

Sleeves and braces

Orthotic devices for the patellofemoral joint consist in most cases of neoprene sleeves or elastic braces. They may have two different positive effects: (a) improvement of patellar stability in cases with subluxation or dislocation, increasing

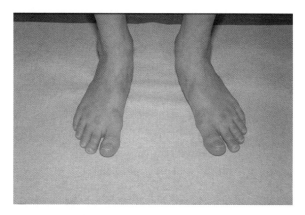

Figure 9.1 Patient with bilateral over-pronation and consecutive increased internal rotation of both lower extremities

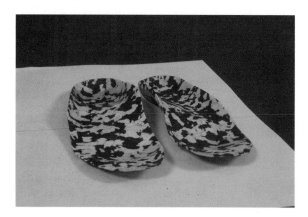

Figure 9.2 Individually adapted insoles for correction of foot position and shock absorption

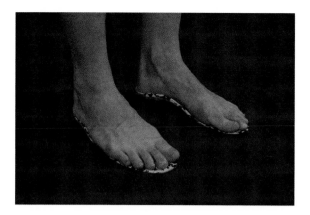

Figure 9.3 Correction of over-pronation using insoles

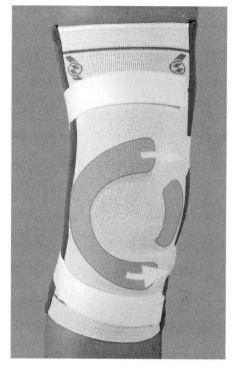

Figure 9.5 Sleeve with C-shaped thickening to resist laterally directed forces in patellar subluxation or dislocation

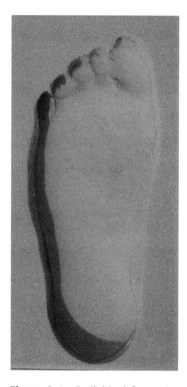

Figure 9.4 Individual foot print

compression. The outcome using orthotic devices is questionable. Only well-prepared trials will show whether or not they are beneficial.

Walking aids

Sticks (canes) or crutches can help to relieve stress on painful patellofemoral joints.[13] They are used after fresh injuries (patellar dislocations) or in cases with acute inflammation, swelling and effusion. Reducing the pain, they help to improve joint function and mobility.

Weight reduction

Avoidance of obesity is important in terms of primary and secondary prevention. There are only a few clinical trials on the effect of weight loss on knee pain.[17,18] One observational study

the function of the joint and decreasing pain (Figure 9.5); and (b) improvement of giving-way or weakness, as the sleeves or braces operate through skin proprioception, with improvement in the joint position sense.[14-16] Contrary to the positive effects, sleeves or braces that are too tight may increase pain in cases with plicae or fat pad

showed impressive reduction in prevalence of knee pain after weight loss.[17-19] A larger study reported significant improvements in pain and function in subjects with knee osteoarthritis who were able to lose more than 15% of initial body weight.[17,20]

There is good evidence that education and physical therapy reduce pain and that exercise regimens also improve function.[2] The impact of other changes, such as appropriate footwear (orthoses and insoles), seems positive but still remains to be elucidated.[17]

Pharmacological treatment

Pharmacological agents should be considered as additions to nonpharmacological measures, such as those described above, which are the cornerstone in treatment of patellofemoral disorders and should be maintained throughout the treatment period. Drug therapy for pain relief is most effective when combined with non-pharmacological strategies.[3,21] Analgesics, in general, offer additional benefit when used in addition to nonpharmacological regimens.[2] In choosing the pharmacological intervention, side-effects and interactions must be considered.[22]

Paracetamol (acetaminophen)

The European League Against Rheumatism[2] and the American College of Rheumatology[3] state that paracetamol-acetaminophen is the oral analgesic to try first, based on its overall costs, efficacy and toxicity profile.[22] Paracetamol-acetaminophen is commonly used, if success-ful, as long-term self-medication for the treat-ment of mild to moderate pain.[2,3] There are no drug interactions or common contraindications to the use of paracetamol-acetaminophen, and there is also evidence that it may be taken safely without severe side-effects over a long term.[23] Acetaminophen has a superior overall safety pro-file compared with nonsteroidal antiinflammatory drugs (NSAIDs).[24]

Nonsteroidal antiinflammatory drugs

NSAIDs, both oral and topical, should be con-sidered in patients unresponsive to paracetamol-acetaminophen.[2,22,23] They are used as the sec-ond step in the pharmacological treatment.[22] The use of NSAIDs should only be decided upon after evaluation of risk factors (gastrointestinal and renal toxicity).[22] NSAIDs may be considered in patients with effusion and a low-grade inflamma-tory component.[2]

Selective cyclooxygenase-2 (COX-2) inhibitors

NSAIDs exert their clinical effects by way of inhi-bition of prostaglandin synthesis by the cyclooxy-genase (COX) enzyme.[25] COX exists in two isoforms – a constitutively expressed COX-1 subserves physiological functions in the gut and kidney, and an inducible COX-2 is upregulated at sites of inflammation. Unlike conventional NSAIDs, which inhibit both isoforms, selective inhibitors of COX-2 have clinical antiinflam-matory efficacy with minor side-effects on the gastrointenstinal system.[25] The newer COX-2-specific inhibitors, celecoxib and rofecoxib, are comparable in efficacy with various NSAIDs.[22] The COX-2 inhibitors should be used when NSAIDs are indicated for patients who are at increased risk for serious upper gastrointesti-nal complications.[23] COX-2 inhibitors have an advantageous safety profile in comparison with nonselective NSAIDs, especially for the treat-ment of high-risk patients.[23] A further advan-tage of the COX-2-specific inhibitors is that nei-ther has a clinically significant effect on platelet aggregation or bleeding time at pharmacologi-cal doses.[3,23] This is a consideration, especially in pre- and postoperative care of patients for whom nonselective NSAIDs have been discounted. However, specific COX-2 inhibitors can cause renal toxicity.[23,26] Caution must be exercised in patients with hypertension or mild-to-moderate renal insufficiency,[23] therefore they should not be used in patients with congestive heart failure or severe renal insufficiency. In addition, celecoxib is contraindicated in patients with allergic reaction to a sulphonamide.[23]

Other pure analgesics

Tramadol

This synthetic opioid agonist is a centrally acting oral analgesic.[3,22] It is useful for the treatment of moderate to severe pain in patients who have contraindications to COX-2-specific inhibitors and nonselective NSAIDs, including impaired renal function.[3] Side-effects are common and include nausea, constipation and drowsiness.[22]

Opioids

Patients who do not respond to one of the described drug therapies and who continue to have severe pain may be considered for opioid therapy.[3,21] Opioid analgesics, such as codeine, propoxyphene or oxycodone, should be avoided for long-term use, but short-term use may be helpful for the treatment of acute exacerbations of pain.[4] The combination of codeine plus acetaminophen was shown to provide significantly better analgesia than acetaminophen alone.[3] However, side-effects such as nausea, vomiting, dizziness or constipation are frequent.

Symptomatic slow-acting drugs for osteoarthritis (SYSADOA)

There is evidence that symptomatic slow-acting drugs for osteoarthritis, such as glucosamine sulphate and chondroitin sulphate, may possess structural modification properties.[2,22] They are considered to have beneficial effects on cartilage,[27] but so far, studies have not been convincing.[22] Nevertheless, the decrease of the patients' pain, as reported in these studies, is remarkable.[22,27,28]

Vitamins A, C and E

These vitamins have been identified as having a potential for antioxidant activity in the process associated with osteoarthritis.[27,29] There are at least four possible pathways in which these nutrients can influence osteoarthritis: protection against oxidative damage; modulation of the inflammatory response; cellular differentiation; and biological actions related to bone and collagen synthesis.[29] Consuming sufficient amounts of vitamin C may slow down the progression of osteoarthritis.[27] However, no solid data from randomized controlled studies have been published so far.[27]

Glucocorticoids

Intraarticular injection of a depot (long-acting) glucocorticoid is indicated for acute exacerbation of knee pain, especially if accompanied by effusion.[2,22] Intraarticular steroids may provide marked symptomatic relief.[22] The evidence for predictors of response remains unclear.[2] In concern about the negative effect of glucocorticoids on cartilage, it is wise to give an intraarticular injection no more than every 3–4 months.[22]

Viscosupplementation

Hyaluronic acid is a linear polysaccharide. It consists of N-acetyl glucosamine and glucuronic acid.[30,31] Hyaluronic acid is found in synovial fluid, skin, cartilage and other extracellular matrices.[30] Synoviocytes, fibroblasts and chondrocytes all synthesize hyaluronic acid. The synovial lining cells (a layer one to two cells thick) produce a highly viscous lubricating fluid, which consists of different substances, such as hyaluronic acid and lubricin, in an ultrafiltrate of plasma.[30] These coat the surface of the hyaline cartilage, providing lubrication during joint movements. The highly viscous nature of the synovial fluid is important for normal joint function, providing a nearly frictionless surface for joint movement. Hyaluronic acid has a protective function and a trophic function. In addition, it has antiinflammatory and analgesic characteristics.[31] Intraarticular injection of hyaluronic acid has been referred to as 'viscosupplementation', a process whereby exogenous hyaluronic acid (or similar high molecular weight substances) provides a replacement for the lubrication that has been lost in patients with degenerative joint disease.[30]

In osteoarthritis, damage to the articular cartilage leads to a local tissue response and to mechanical changes resulting in joint function failure. Episodes of inflammation additionally affect the integrity of the individual components of the joint. The changes induced by the inflammation include stretching of the joint capsule by episodes of effusion and alteration of the viscosity of the synovial fluid, caused by the proliferation of enzymes or free radicals that degrade both hyaluronic acid and lubricin.[30] This breakdown of hyaluronic acid, which leads to a decrease in the viscosity of the synovial fluid, culminates in the loss of smooth movement of the articular surfaces.[30] This loss of lubrication may change the viscoelastic properties of the synovial fluid and may lead to further joint destruction.

Intraarticular injection of hyaluronic acid may be used in patients for whom nonpharmacological and simple analgesic therapy have failed.[22,30] The efficacy is comparable with that of NSAIDs and there is no risk of gastropathy or other consequences of systemic inhibition of prostaglandin synthesis.[22] Pain relief is less rapid than with intraarticular injection of glucocorticoids, but the duration of the pain relief may be much longer; in some patients, relief for 6 months or more has been observed.[22,32]

A special effect has been postulated. Since intraarticular injected hyaluronic acid derivates stay on average only 10–20 hours in the synovial fluid, and yet their effect continues over several months, modulation of the activity of different cells in the development and progression of the osteoarthritis (synoviocytes, chondrocytes, inflammatory cells), probably by direct effect on their specific receptors, is a result of the injected hyaluronic acid.[31] The receptors play a specific role in the migration, adhesion and activation of inflammatory cells, as well as maturation and differentiation of the chondrocytes for synthesis of the cartilage matrix.[31] A sustained increase in the production of hyaluronic acid by the chondrocytes through viscosupplementation has been shown.[31]

Intraarticular injection of hyaluronic acid (viscosupplementation) contributes at least to three important elements for the homoeostasis of the degenerative joint: (a) restoration of the elastic and viscous characteristics of the synovial fluid by stimulation of the proliferation of the chondrocytes, the synthesis of proteoglycan and the normalization of synthesis of hyaluronic acid by synoviocytes; (b) an antiinflammatory effect; and (c) a antinociceptive effect.[31] A decrease in patient complaints was shown in several studies and a delay of disease progression seems possible.[31]

References

1. Arendt EA, Fithian DC, Cohen E (2002) Current concepts of lateral patellar dislocation. *Clin Sports Med* 21: 499–519
2. Pendleton A, Arden N, Dougados M et al (2000) European League Against Rheumatism (EULAR) recommendations for the management of knee osteoarthritis: report of a task force of the Standing Committee for International Clinical Studies Including Therapeutic Trials (ESCISIT). *Ann Rheum Dis* 59: 936–944
3. American College of Rheumatology Subcommittee on Osteoarthritis Guidelines (2000) Recommendations for the medical management of osteoarthritis of the hip and knee. *Arthritis Rheum* 43: 1905–1915
4. Hochberg MC, Altman RD, Brandt KD et al (1995) Guidelines for the medical management of osteoarthritis. Part I. Osteoarthritis of the hip. *Arthritis Rheum* 38: 1535–1540

5. Insall J (1982) Current Concepts Review: patellar pain. *J Bone Joint Surg Am* **64**: 147–152

6. Timm KE (1998) Randomized controlled trial of Protonics on patellar pain, position, and function. *Med Sci Sports Exerc* **30**: 665–670

7. Rowlands BW, Brantingham JW (1999) The efficacy of patella mobilization in patients suffering from patellofemoral pain syndrome. *J Neuromusculoskel Syst* **7**: 142–149

8. Suter E, McMorland G, Herzog W, Bray R (2000) Conservative lower back treatment reduces inhibition in knee-extensor muscles: a randomized controlled trial. *J Manip Physiol Ther* **23**: 76–80

9. Antich TJ, Randall CC, Westbrook RA et al (1986) Physical therapy treatment of knee extensor mechanism disorders: comparison of four treatment modalities. *J Orthop Sports Phys Ther* **8**: 255–259

10. Jensen R, Gothesen O, Liseth K, Baerheim A (1999) Acupuncture treatment of patellofemoral pain syndrome. *J Alt Compl Med* **5**: 521–527

11. Cesarelli M, Bifulco P, Bracale M (2000) Study of the control strategy of the quadriceps muscles in anterior knee pain. *IEEE Trans Rehabil Eng* **8**: 330–341

12. Harrison EL, Sheppard MS, McQuarrie AM (1999) A randomized controlled trial of physical therapy treatment programs in patellofemoral pain syndrome. *Physiother Canada Spring*: 93–100

13. Hurley M, Walsh N (2001) Physical, functional and other nonpharmacological interventions for osteoarthritis. *Best Pract Res Clin Rheumatol* **15**: 569–581

14. Biedert RM (1999) Sensory–Motor Function of the Knee Joint. Histologic, Anatomic, and Neurophysiologic Investigations. Thesis, University of Basel, Switzerland

15. Barrack RL, Lund PJ, Skinner HB (1994) Knee joint proprioception revisited. *J Sports Rehab* **3**: 18–42

16. Jerosch J, Prymka M (1996) Knee joint proprioception in patients with posttraumatic recurrent patella dislocation. *Knee Surg Sports Traumatol Arthrosc* **4**: 14–18

17. O'Reilly S, Doherty M (2001) Lifestyle changes in the management of osteoarthritis. *Best Pract Res Clin Rheumatol* **15**: 559–568

18. McGoey BV, Deitel M, Saplys RJ, Kliman ME (1990) Effect of weight loss on musculoskeletal pain in the morbidly obese. *J Bone Joint Surg Br* **72**: 322–323

19. Balint G, Szebenyi B (1997) Non-pharmacological therapies in osteoarthritis. *Baillières Clin Rheumatol* **11**: 795–815

20. Huang MH, Chen CH, Chen TW (2000) The effects of weight reduction on the rehabilitation of patients with knee osteoarthritis and obesity. *Arthritis Care Res* **13**: 398–405

21. American Geriatrics Society Panel on Chronic Pain in Older Persons (1998) The management of chronic pain in older persons. Clinical practice guidelines. *J Am Geriatric Soc* **46**: 635–651

22. Bijlsma JW (2002) Analgesia and the patient with osteoarthritis. *Am J Ther* **9**: 189–197

23. Hochberg MC, Dougados M (2001) Pharmacological therapy of osteoarthritis. *Best Pract Res Clin Rheumatol* **15**: 583–593

24. Abramson SB (2002) Et tu, acetaminophen? *Arthritis Rheum* **46**: 2831–2835

25. Golden BD, Abramson SB (1999) Selective cyclooxygenase-2 inhibitors. *Rheum Dis Clin N Am* **25**: 359–378

26. Whelton A (2001) Renal aspects of treatment with conventional nonsteroidal antiinflammatory drugs versus cyclooxygenase-2-specific inhibitors. *Am J Med* **110**(suppl 3A): 33–42

27. Hauselmann HJ (2001) Nutripharmaceuticals for osteoarthritis. *Best Pract Res Clin Rheumatol* **15**: 595–607

28. McAlindon TE, LaValley MP, Gulin JP, Felson DT (2000) Glucosamine and chondroitin for treatment of osteoarthritis: a systematic quality assessment and meta-analysis. *J Am Med Assoc* **283**: 1469–1475

29. Sowers MF, Lachance L (1999) Vitamins and arthritis. The roles of vitamin A, C, D and E. *Rheum Dis Clin North Am* **25**: 315–332

30. Simon LS (1999) Viscosupplementation therapy with intra-articular hyaluronic acid. Fact or fantasy? *Rheum Dis Clin North Am* **25**: 345–357

31. Pandolfi S, Exer P, Schwarz HA (2002) [Viscosupplementation in arthrosis]. *Ther Umsch* **59**: 545–549

32. Brandt KD (2000) The role of analgesics in the management of osteoarthritis pain. *Am J Ther* **7**: 75–90

Suggested reading

Pendleton A, Arden N, Dougados M et al (2000) European League Against Rheumatism (EULAR) recommendations for the management of knee osteoarthritis: report of a task force of the Standing Committee for International Clinical Studies Including Therapeutic Trials (ESCISIT). *Ann Rheum Dis* **59**: 936–944

Simon LS (1999) Viscosupplementation therapy with intra-articular hyaluronic acid. Fact or fantasy? *Rheum Dis Clin North Am* **25**: 345–357

10 Patellofemoral Joint Replacement

Alan C. Merchant

Patellofemoral arthroplasty, or patellofemoral joint replacement, has been used to treat severely disabled patients who have isolated end-stage arthrosis or failed surgeries of the patellofemoral joint. Many patients in this group are too young to be considered for total knee arthroplasty. Older patients with isolated patellofemoral arthrosis benefit from replacement of only those joint surfaces that are damaged.

For over two decades various authors[1–9] have reported on different designs of patellofemoral prostheses. The good or excellent results ranged from a low of 45%[7] to a high of 96%.[6] A careful review of all these studies showed that implant design and patient selection are the two most important factors for success. The three studies using the design first reported by Lubinus[3,7,8] had the worst results. The five papers about the design reported by Blazina et al[1,2,4,6,9] averaged the best results. Of the two designs, the Blazina et al[2] design is the more anatomical with a deeper trochlear groove.

Many so-called 'failures' in these different series were caused by subsequent deterioration of the femorotibial joints, requiring revision to a total knee arthroplasty. However, the majority of patients who need patellofemoral replacement are too young to be considered for total knee arthroplasty initially. Therefore, many years ago, the current author designed a patellofemoral prosthesis whose patellar component would also articulate exactly with an existing femoral component of a total knee system. Thus, if revision to a total knee arthroplasty should be needed in the future, only the trochlear component would need to be removed and replaced with the femoral component of that system. Leaving the well-fixed patellar component intact would eliminate the unacceptably high complication rate of 33% encountered in patellar revision reported by Berry and Rand.[10] No other patellofemoral prosthesis had this modular capability.

Design and surgical considerations

Patients disabled by isolated patellofemoral arthritis and failed patellofemoral surgeries tend to be much younger than patients considered to be good candidates for total knee arthroplasty. Their relative youth demands a prosthetic design that will provide maximum longevity and survivorship. The patellar component of a total knee

Patellofemoral Disorders: Diagnosis and Treatment. Edited by Roland M. Biedert
© 2004 John Wiley & Sons, Ltd   ISBN: 0-470-85011-6

system with the longest follow-up (20 years), the best survivorship (99%) and the lowest complication rate (0.9%)[11] has been the low-contact-stress rotating patella, first described by Buechel and Pappas in 1989[12] [this low-contact-stress (LCS®) mobile bearing knee system is manufactured by DePuy Orthopedics Inc., Warsaw, IN, USA].

I modified the polyethylene bearing of this rotating patella for use as a patellofemoral implant. The trochlear component (Figure 10.1) was designed to articulate exactly with that patellar component. This new combination for patellofemoral arthroplasty takes advantage of the design features that have led to such excellent survivorship and freedom from complications. These design features are: (a) an anatomical trochlear groove that is deeper than most other knee implants, reducing the risk of patellar dislocation; (b) components with broad and congruent area contact loading, as opposed to point or line contact loading, reducing the wear rate; and (c) the self-aligning feature of the rotating patellar bearing that reduces stress on the bone–implant interface, reducing the risk of loosening.

When used in a patellofemoral prosthesis, this polyethylene rotating patellar bearing slides off the metallic trochlear component to articulate with the remaining normal femoral cartilage during full flexion. Therefore, the shape and

contour of this bearing have been redesigned. The superior–inferior dimension of the rotating bearing has been increased so that the bearing will remain in contact with the metal trochlear implant longer during acute knee flexion. The sharp, angular superior and inferior edges of the standard LCS® rotating bearing have been rounded off or contoured to avoid gouging the femoral articular cartilage during acute flexion (Figure 10.2). Because the polyethylene patellar bearing articulates with normal cartilage in full flexion, all patients are warned repeatedly to avoid weight bearing when the knee is flexed more than 90°, i.e. to avoid full squatting. Half squats are acceptable and certainly full flexion of the unweighted knee is acceptable.

However, the most important design feature of this new patellofemoral prosthesis is its modularity that eliminates the need for patellar revision, with its high complication rate, if a total knee arthroplasty should be needed in the future (Figure 10.3). Furthermore, the modified rotating polyethylene bearing can be snapped off from its base plate and exchanged for a new one if wear is found. If a size change is planned, a customized bearing can be ordered.

The trochlear component is implanted by inlaying it flush with the remaining normal

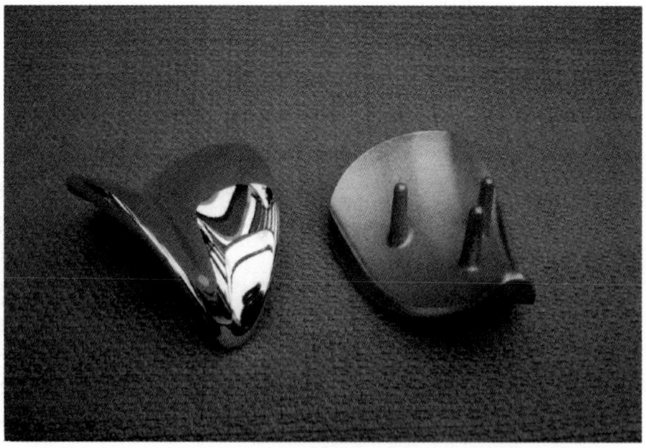

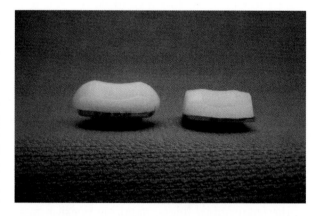

Figure 10.1 Trochlear components of the modular patellofemoral prosthesis showing the articular surface (left) and the reverse with the three fixation pins (right)

Figure 10.2 The modified rotating patella bearing (left) compared to the standard patella (right). Both are shown in a side view from the medial aspect and are different sizes

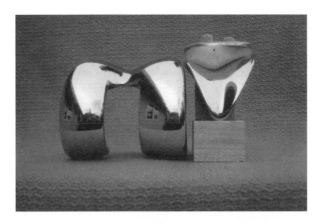

Figure 10.3 A femoral component (left) and the modular patellofemoral joint prosthesis (right) from the same system demonstrating the modularity of the three components

joint surfaces after preparing the osseous bed with small osteotomies, a routing guide and a motorized burr. It is impacted into position and secured by its three small fixation pins and bone cement. Because very little bone is removed during implantation, conversion to a total knee femoral component, if necessary at a later date, will not be complicated.

The patellar component is implanted in the usual manner, using a porous-coated, press-fit technique or cement, at the surgeon's preference.

Indications

Patellofemoral replacement is a salvage procedure, and patient selection is the single most important decision the surgeon must make to assure a successful result. There are four major indications for patellofemoral arthroplasty, and *all four must be present* to qualify a patient for this operation:

1. The surgeon must prove that the source of pain is from patellofemoral arthrosis or chondrosis. All other causes for anterior knee pain, such as tendinitis, neuromata, reflex sympathetic dystrophy and others, must be ruled out or treated first. The patellar and trochlear damage must be severe chondromalacia (grade III or IV) or true osteoarthrosis. Objective evidence from arthroscopic observation or radiographic joint narrowing, sclerosis and perhaps osteophytes must be present.

2. The amount of pain must limit the patient's ability to perform normal activities of daily living. The goal of patellofemoral arthroplasty is to return the patient to normal daily activities, not competitive sports.

3. The candidate must agree to low-demand activities after surgery. Frequently, these patients are relatively young; they tend to overuse the knee once it is pain-free. They must understand the dangers of running, jumping and full squatting. Moderate recreational activities are allowable, such as hiking, golf, moderate cycling with the seat adjusted to avoid flexion beyond 90°, and perhaps doubles tennis without tournaments.

4. All other treatment alternatives must have either been tried and failed or they are contraindicated. For instance, a comparatively simple lateral release has been shown to give satisfactory or very satisfactory long-lasting relief for 59% patients who have isolated patellofemoral arthrosis.[13] However, if the surgeon is considering anterior or anteromedial tibial tubercle transfer, Pidoriano et al[14] have shown that the presence of proximal patellar articular lesions is a contraindication to these procedures. In patients who are too young to consider total knee arthroplasty, who have both patellofemoral and medial or lateral compartment arthrosis, patellofemoral replacement can be combined with a tibial osteotomy.

Contraindications

The usual contraindications for any joint replacement surgery also apply to patellofemoral arthroplasty: infection, reflex sympathetic dystrophy, inflammatory arthritis and psychogenic pain. Patella infera is a relative contraindication. It must be corrected to normal before the patello-femoral replacement. If the surgeon has experience with the techniques to correct patella infera and understands the importance of proper extensor mechanism rehabilitation, both the correction and patellofemoral replacement can be performed at the same surgery and the postoperative course modified appropriately.

Results

The first consecutive eight patients who met the indications for this new patellofemoral replacement have been followed for an average of 4.3 years (3.0–4.75 years). None were lost to follow-up. All were female. The median age at surgery was 47.5 years (range, 26–81 years). During hospitalization, the patients followed a standard total-knee-arthroplasty protocol with full weight-bearing as tolerated. After discharge, the patients were given a home exercise programme to regain knee flexion and quadriceps strength. Formal physical therapy was used only if progress lagged. Understandably, they recovered more rapidly than total-knee-arthroplasty patients. Because this modular patellofemoral arthroplasty is a salvage procedure, I used the Activities of Daily Living (ADL) Scale published by Irrgang et al[15] and validated by Marx et al[16] as the outcome instrument. ADL scores of 85–100% were considered excellent, 70–84% good and 55–69% fair.

At the latest follow-up, seven patients (88%) were rated excellent (4) or good (3) and all were happy with their result. One patient continues to have unexplained anterior pain and has a fair result. The median ADL score for the group was 85%, and the mean score was 81%. There have been no major complications from the procedure itself, and there have been no implant loosenings or failures.

With these encouraging results and the realization that no one surgeon will perform a large number of these patellofemoral replacements, I

started a multi-surgeon prospective study using the same ADL Scale for assessment. Thus far, an additional nine cases (seven females, two males) with a median age of 41 years (30–55 years) are showing a similar trend at 1 year. The average preoperative ADL score for the group was 40%, rising to 82% 1 year after surgery.

Combining the two groups, 16 out of 17 patients (94%) had good or excellent results and one had a fair outcome.

Illustrative case reports

Case One demonstrates the use of this patello-femoral replacement for severe disability in a young patient who had failed to get relief from all other options, comprising six operations in the previous 4 years. She was a 26 year-old woman with a 2-year history of chronic left anterior knee pain who then had an impact injury to the front of her knee. Arthroscopic surgery shortly after that injury revealed a grade IV lesion of the femoral trochlear cartilage. During the next 4 years she had a total of five more unsuccessful operations, including two anteromedializations of the tibial tubercle to treat this severe and painful patellofemoral chondrosis. She was unable to work, even at a sedentary occupation. Her pre-operative axial view radiographs[17,18] demonstrated excellent congruence of the patellofemoral joint, but there was more than 50% loss of the joint space compared to the opposite side. She improved significantly after her modular patellofemoral replacement. Because the severity of her patella infera had not been recognized at the time of her patellofemoral arthroplasty, she required a 1.0 cm Z-plastic patellar tendon lengthening 23 months later. This changed her good result to an excellent one. At 3 years follow-up she was working full-time and enjoys recreational activities, such as golf, bicycling, hiking and other noncontact sports, without signs of implant loosening or wear.

Case Two, illustrated in Figures 10.4, 10.5 and 10.6, is more typical of patients who are

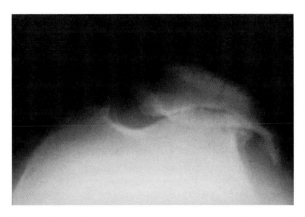

Figure 10.4 The pre-operative axial view radiograph of the right knee of Case Two. Diagnosis: chronic subluxation of the patella with secondary patellofemoral osteoarthrosis

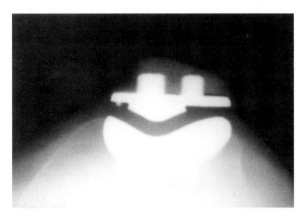

Figure 10.5 The postoperative axial view radiograph of the right knee of Case Two

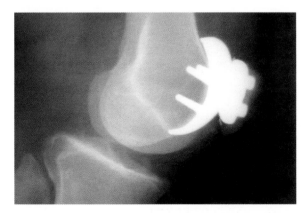

Figure 10.6 The postoperative lateral view radiograph of the right knee of Case Two

candidates for this procedure. This patient had a chronic subluxation of both patellae all her life that finally culminated in disabling isolated patellofemoral arthrosis. She was a 41 year-old office worker who had been involved in sports since childhood. For as long as she could remember, she had experienced anterior knee pain. A solitary dislocation of the right patella occurred at age 14, and at 30 she was treated with a lateral release and patellar exostectomy. Modular patellofemoral replacements were performed on both knees a few months apart. The results were excellent.

Conclusions

The modular patellofemoral replacement presented here has produced early results that are equal to or better than those of previous designs.[1-9] This design incorporates features that should provide maximum longevity with the added advantage of modularity, allowing revision to a total knee arthroplasty if necessary in the future, while avoiding patellar revision with its unacceptably high complication rate.

This modular patellofemoral arthroplasty offers a more conservative alternative compared to total knee arthroplasty, both for the younger patient for whom total knee arthroplasty is inappropriate as well as for the older patient who has no disease in the medial or lateral compartments. Laskin and van Steijn[19] and Mont et al[20] have advocated total knee arthroplasty for older patients who have only isolated patellofemoral arthrosis. It makes no sense to perform a major operation to destroy normal medial and lateral compartments if a less destructive operation, such as patellofemoral arthroplasty, will provide equally good results.

References

1. Arcerio R, Toomey H (1988) Patellofemoral arthroplasty: a three to nine year follow-up study. *Clin Orthop* **236**: 60–71

2. Blazina ME, Fox JM, Del Pizzo W et al (1979) Patellofemoral replacement. *Clin Orthop* **144**: 98–102

3. Lubinus HH (1979) Patella glide bearing replacement. *Orthopaedics* **2**: 119–127

4. Cartier P, Sanouiller JL, Grelsamer R (1990) Patellofemoral arthroplasty. 2–12 year follow-up study. *J Arthroplasty* **5**: 49–55

5. Argenson JN, Guillaume JM, Aubaniac JM (1995) Is there a place for patellofemoral arthroplasty? *Clin Orthop* **321**: 162–167

6. Krajca-Radcliffe JB, Coker TP (1996) Patellofemoral arthroplasty. A 2–18 year follow-up study. *Clin Orthop* **330**: 143–151

7. Tauro B, Ackroyd CE, Newman JH, Shah NA (2001) The Lubinus patellofemoral arthroplasty. A 5–10 year prospective study. *J Bone Joint Surg Br* **83**: 696–701

8. Smith AM, Peckett WR, Butler-Manuel PA et al (2002) Treatment of patellofemoral arthritis using the Lubinus patellofemoral arthroplasty: a retrospective review. *The Knee* **9**: 27–30

9. de Winter WE, Feith R, van Loon CJ (2001) The Richards type II patellofemoral arthroplasty: 26 cases followed for 1–20 years. *Acta Orthop Scand* **72**: 487–490

10. Berry DJ, Rand JA (1993) Isolated patellar component revision of total knee arthroplasty. *Clin Orthop* **286**: 110–115

11. Buechel FF Sr, Buechel FF Jr, Pappas MJ, D'Alessio J (2001) Twenty-year evaluation of meniscal bearing and rotating platform knee replacements. *Clin Orthop* **388**: 41–50

12. Buechel FF, Rosa RA, Pappas MJ (1989) A metal-backed, rotating-bearing patellar prosthesis to lower contact stress. An 11 year clinical study. *Clin Orthop* **248**: 34–49

13. Aderinto J, Cobb AG (2002) Lateral release for patellofemoral arthritis. *Arthroscopy* **18**: 399–403

14. Pidoriano AJ, Weinstein RN, Buuck DA, Fulkerson JP (1997) Correlation of patellar articular lesions with results from anteromedial tibial tubercle transfer. *Am J Sports Med* **25**: 533–537

15. Irrgang JJ, Snyder-Mackler L, Wainner RS et al (1998) Development of a patient-reported measure of function of the knee. *J Bone Joint Surg Am* **80**: 1132–1145

16. Marx RG, Jones EC, Allen AA et al (2001) Reliability, validity, and responsiveness of four knee outcome scales for athletic patients. *J Bone Joint Surg Am* **83**: 1459–1469

17. Merchant AC (2001) Patellofemoral imaging. *Clin Orthop* **389**: 15–21

18. Merchant AC, Mercer RL, Jacobsen RH, Cool CR (1974) Roentgenographic analysis of patellofemoral congruence. *J Bone Joint Surg Am* **56**: 1391–1396

19. Laskin RS, van Steijn M (1999) Total knee replacement for patients with patellofemoral arthritis. *Clin Orthop* **367**: 89–95

20. Mont MA, Haas S, Mullick T, Hungerford DS (2002) Total knee arthroplasty for patellofemoral arthritis. *J Bone Joint Surg Am* **84**: 1977–1981

PART III

Case Studies

CASE STUDY 1

Unspecific patellofemoral pain

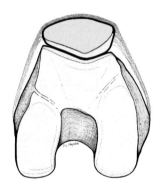

♦ What do we mean by 'unspecific'?

♦ Where is the pain coming from?

♦ What should be our treatment plan?

♦ Do we need special investigations?

Table CS1 Patellofemoral joint examination			
Diagnostic clues	Findings	Diagnostic clues	Findings
Pain	Unspecific, in flexion	Patellar gliding mechanism	Normal
Tenderness	Diffuse, unspecific	Patellar apprehension	Negative
Effusion	Sometimes	Q angle	'Normal'
Swelling	Sometimes	Catching	Sometimes
Patellar position, relaxed, 0°	Centred	Locking	None
Patellar position, contracted, 0°	Centred	Range of motion	Normal
Patellar position, 30°	Centred	Radiographs	Normal
Patellar mobility	Normal	Other	None

Patellofemoral Disorders: Diagnosis and Treatment. Edited by Roland M. Biedert
© 2004 John Wiley & Sons, Ltd   ISBN: 0-470-85011-6

History

A 31 year-old female suffered from pain and swelling in the patellofemoral joint. Pain was increased during and after sports activities, such as skiing. She felt no instability; range of motion was unlimited. The clinical examination revealed no specific findings.

Comments

Unspecific patellofemoral pain during and after sport activities is one of the classic problems, especially in the young female. 'Unspecific' means that both location and genesis of pain are not obvious upon initial physical examination.

The patient's history does not help very much to answer questions. Various pathologies (e.g. patellar instability) can be excluded. In consequence, we must try to find the sources of this unspecific pain, as described in Chapter 4 – Pathogenesis of patellofemoral pain. The relation to an anatomical structure or a pathological process can be difficult, but it is the diagnostic and therapeutic key to resolve such problems.

Course of action

Physical examination

The physical examination is the initial and the most important step to achieving the correct diagnosis. The patient must be in a position of comfort and show the painful area. Gently feel the anatomical structures, starting the examination on the pain-free side. Examine precisely the anatomical structures involved.

In the present case we found a normal-looking patellofemoral joint with full active and passive range of motion. No effusion or swelling was found. There existed an unspecific and diffuse tenderness in the whole patellofemoral joint. The patella was well-centred in a relaxed position in 0° of extension, with quadriceps muscle activation, and in 30° of knee flexion. The Q angle and tubercle–sulcus angle showed normal values. Pain was caused in the one-leg position with increased loaded flexion. The axis of the foot and the lower extremity were normal. The only pathological finding was difficulty in stabilizing the knee joint and in stabilizing the whole lower extremity during motion in the single-leg standing position. This revealed a deficit of the sensorimotor capabilities and control of dynamic stabilization.[1]

Axial CT evaluation

The anteroposterior and lateral radiographs were normal. In 0° extension with relaxed quadriceps muscle, the patella was well-centred on the axial CT scans (Figure CS1.1). The sulcus angle was normal; no tilt could be found. With full quadriceps contraction in 0° extension, the patella stayed well-centred in the trochlea, as well as in 30° of flexion (Figure CS1.2).

The distances between the medial and lateral patellofemoral facets were equal and normal. We could therefore suggest that no important defect of the articular cartilage is present. Definitive proof can be achieved by performing an MRI.

The CT evaluation was absolutely normal in this patient. This excluded many pathologies and confirmed the findings of the physical examination. A mechanical problem did not exist and

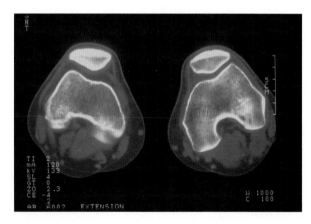

Figure CS1.1 Normal figuration of patella and trochlea. The patella is well-centred (extension, relaxed)

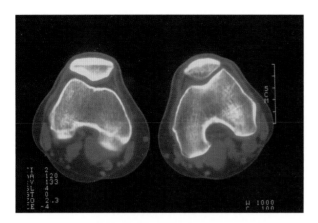

Figure CS1.2 Dynamic activation of the quadriceps muscle keeps the patella well-centred (extension, contracted)

therefore no need for a so-called 'realignment' was given.

Plan

Patients with unspecific patellofemoral pain and with normal radiographs, CT evaluation and physical examination, are in a domain of nonoperative treatment. Any surgical procedure must be strictly avoided because we have found no obvious structural pathology that has to be corrected. Surgery would probably impair the situation and create a secondary problem.

In this patient, sensorimotor training under control of the physical therapist was the key to resolving the problem.[2] Improvement of the dynamic stabilization of the patellofemoral joint during sport activities was the deciding positive step (Figures CS1.3 and CS1.4). Training in the closed kinetic chain improved the stabilization of the whole lower extremity.

Summary

Unspecific patellofemoral pain is a frequent problem, especially in females. We need a detailed physical examination to decide what kind of

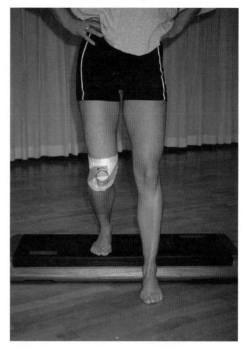

Figure CS1.3 Sensorimotor training to improve the stabilization of the knee joint. Taping of the patellofemoral joint can improve the training capabilities at the beginning

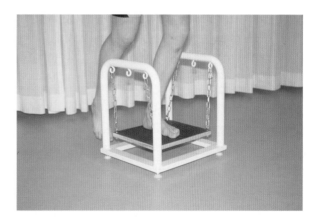

Figure CS1.4 Sensorimotor training with unstable conditions

additional investigations are necessary. Radiographs and CT evaluation help to exclude any dysplastic or mechanical pathologies. An MRI could also be performed to identify small

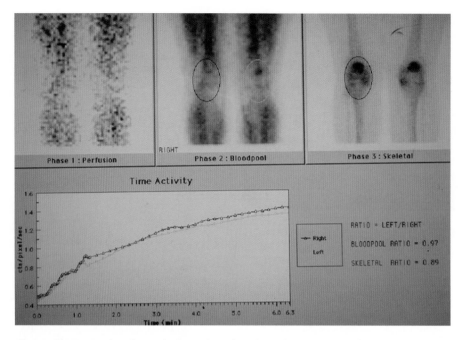

Figure CS1.5   Technetium scintiscan in a female patient. Increased uptake with time

cartilage lesions or bone bruises.[3,4] Unspecific patellofemoral pain can also be caused by increased osseous metabolic activity. The patellofemoral joint is one of several regions of dynamic metabolic adaptations characterized by increased turnover and remodelling.[5] Such dynamic osseous events can be detected by using scintigraphy with technetium imaging[3,4] (Figures CS1.5 and CS1.6).

Mechanical, neurovascular and hormonal factors may trigger increased osseous metabolic activity. Supraphysiological loading or abnormal joint mechanics (pathological kinematics, i.e. ACL insufficiency) can produce increased, painful remodelling. Unphysiological loading, such as overweight, muscular weakness or insufficient sensorimotor control, create various forms of unspecific pain in the patellofemoral joint. Successful treatment for this unspecific pain must be combined with homeostasis of the involved structures. The treatment is specific and clear only when underlying mechanical pathologies can be identified, e.g. in ACL insufficiency.

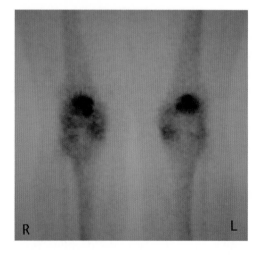

Figure CS1.6   Anterior technetium scintiscan showing increased activity in the patellofemoral joint. Overweight female patient

References

1. Biedert RM (1999) Sensory–Motor Function of the Knee Joint. Histologic, Anatomic, and Neurophysiologic Investigations. Thesis, University of Basel, Switzerland

2. Barrack RL, Skinner HB (1990) The sensory function of knee ligaments. In: Daniel DM, Akeson WH, O'Connor JJ (eds), *Knee Ligaments: Structure, Function, Injury, and Repair*. New York, Raven, pp 95–114

3. Dye SF (1996) The knee as a biologic transmission with an envelope of function: a theory. *Clin Orthop* **325**: 10–18

4. Dye SF, Chew MH (1993) The use of scintigraphy to detect increased osseous metabolic transmission with an envelope of function. *J Bone Joint Surg Am* **75**: 1388–1406

5. Dye SF, Stäubli HU, Biedert RM, Vaupel GL (1999) The mosaic of pathophysiology causing patellofemoral pain: therapeutic implications. *Operative Tech Sports Med* **7**: 46–54

Suggested reading

Dye SF (1996) The knee as a biologic transmission with an envelope of function: a theory. *Clin Orthop* **325**: 10–18

Dye SF, Chew MH (1993) The use of scintigraphy to detect increased osseous metabolic transmission with an envelope of function. *J Bone Joint Surg Am* **75**: 1388–1406

CASE STUDY 2
Specific patellofemoral pain

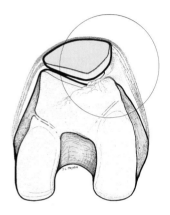

♦ What do we mean by 'specific'?

♦ What causes the pain?

♦ Which examinations are necessary?

Table CS2 Patellofemoral joint examination

Diagnostic clues	Findings	Diagnostic clues	Findings
Pain	Medial, soft tissues	Patellar gliding mechanism	With catching
Tenderness	Medial and suprapatellar plica	Patellar apprehension	Negative
Effusion	Sometimes	Q angle	Normal value
Swelling	Sometimes	Catching	Transient, painful
Patellar position, relaxed, 0°	Normal	Locking	Following longer flexion
Patellar position, contracted, 0°	Normal	Range of motion	Limited flexion
Patellar position, 30°	Normal	Radiographs	Normal
Patellar mobility	Normal	Other	Cinema (car, airplane) sign

Patellofemoral Disorders: Diagnosis and Treatment. Edited by Roland M. Biedert
© 2004 John Wiley & Sons, Ltd ISBN: 0-470-85011-6

History

A 20 year-old female presented herself with chronic pain of the patellofemoral joint when going up or down stairs and while sitting with the knee flexed, particularly when keeping the knee flexed for a long time (e.g. the length of a movie). She felt the pain like a tight bandage around the patella, with the feeling of having 'something too much' in her knee joint. Catching and locking occurred under the same conditions. She reported her first symptoms during adolescence. The pain could be relieved by extension after some minutes.

Comments

This pain in flexed position, in most cases bilateral, beginning in young age, is the classic complaint of a plica syndrome. Different parts of the synovial plica are distinguished: suprapatellar, mediopatellar and infrapatellar (Figure CS2.1). Some parts of the plica may be impinged during knee flexion (Figure CS2.2). The plica is one of the soft tissue structures with a high nerve supply.[1] Repetitive impingement causes fibrotic inflammation and thickening of the plica (Figure CS2.3). The loss of elasticity of a fibrotic plica is felt by the patient, especially in flexion, as a 'tight pain' like a bandage in or around the patellofemoral joint (Figures CS2.4 and CS2.5).

Course of action

Physical examination

In most cases, a light effusion and swelling are found after effort. The painful plica can be best palpated on the medial side (proximal–vertical, distal–horizontal) during flexion and extension movements.[2] The examining fingers feel a painful snapping and the patient confirms that 'this is the pain' (Figure CS2.6). The rest of the examination of the knee joint is normal.

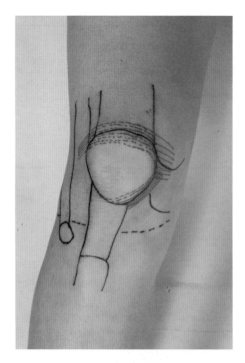

Figure CS2.1   The different parts of the synovial plica: suprapatellar, running under the quadriceps tendon from proximal–lateral to proximal–medial in the suprapatellar pouch; mediopatellar, from the suprapatellar plica on the medial side into the infrapatellar part; and infrapatellar, from the mediopatellar plica into the Hoffa fat pad

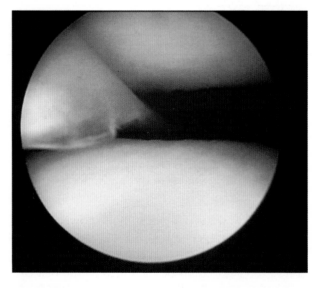

Figure CS2.2   Arthroscopic view showing impingement of a synovial mediopatellar plica (left) between the patella (top) and the femoral condyle (bottom)

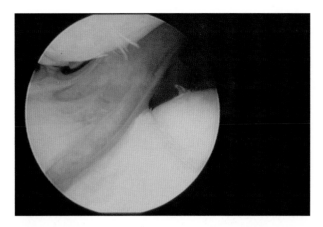

Figure CS2.3 Fibrotic mediopatellar plica (left) between the patella (top) and the femoral condyle (bottom)

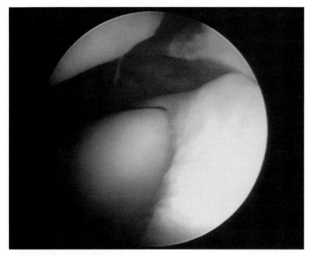

Figure CS2.4 Arthroscopic view showing friction of a mediopatellar plica (right) on the medial femoral condyle (bottom). Patella is on top

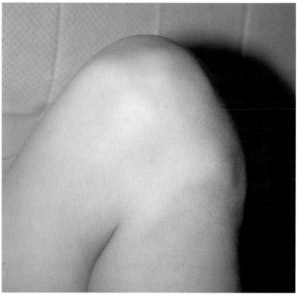

Figure CS2.5 Maximal pain during flexion caused by impingement and tension of a fibrotic plica

Axial CT evaluation

In this patient, the CT evaluation showed correct centring and balancing of the patella in the trochlea in extension and 30° of flexion. The thickened plica could be identified in the medial patellofemoral joint line (Figure CS2.7). CT evaluation was needed to exclude any pathological mechanical causes.

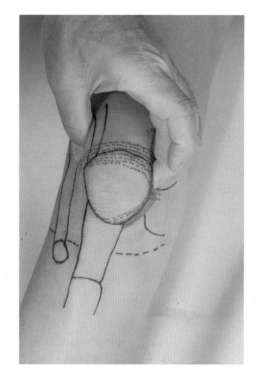

Figure CS2.6 Palpation of the painful suprapatellar plica

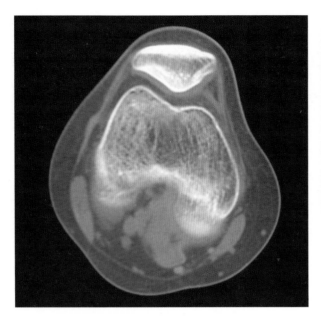

Figure CS2.7   Mediopatellar plica

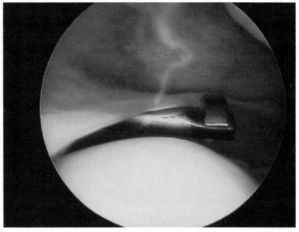

Figure CS2.9   Arthroscopic resection of a horizontal mediopatellar plica (left knee, medial condyle on bottom)

Plan

The inflamed, thickened plica can be an unequivocal cause of specific patellofemoral pain.[2,3] If the diagnosis is clear, arthroscopic resection of the plica can resolve the problem (Figures CS2.8 and

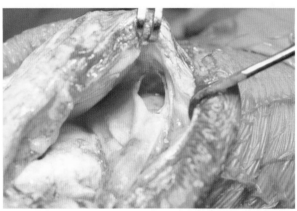

Figure CS2.10   Fibrotic plica in the suprapatellar pouch (left knee)

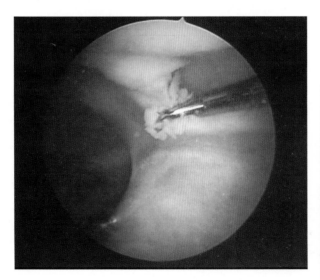

Figure CS2.8   Arthroscopic resection of a suprapatellar plica (right knee, patella on top)

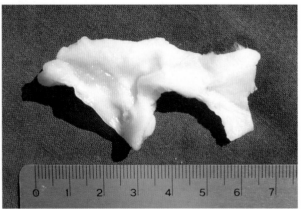

Figure CS2.11   Excised fibrotic plica

CS2.9). The plica can also be resected in combination with an open procedure (Figures CS2.10 and CS2.11).

Postoperative care and rehabilitation

Goals

♦ To decrease postoperative swelling and haemarthrosis.

♦ To increase activation of the muscle groups and strengthen.

♦ To regain full range of motion.

Timeline

♦ Hospital	1–2 days	
♦ Mobilization	1st day	
♦ Weightbearing	Partial	20 kg for 2 weeks
	Complete	Depends on swelling and muscle activation
♦ Sports	Bicycle, swimming	After 2 weeks
	Everything	Depends on final results

Specific patellofemoral pain is present when the underlying pathology is clear. The plica syndrome is a typical problem in this sense. Combinations with other pathologies, e.g. dysplastic trochlea, are possible and must be considered in the treatment plan.

References

1. Biedert RM, Stauffer E, Friederich NF (1992) Occurrence of free nerve endings in the soft tissue of the knee joint. A histologic investigation. *Am J Sports Med* 20: 430–433
2. Hughston JC, Walsh WM, Puddu G (1984) *Patellar Subluxation and Dislocation. Saunders Monographs in Clinical Orthopaedics*, volume V. Philadelphia, PA, WB Saunders
3. Biedert R, Friederich N (1996) [Femoropatellar pain syndrome: which operation is still sensible?]. *Ther Umsch* 53: 775–779

Suggested reading

Hughston JC, Walsh WM, Puddu G (1984) *Patellar Subluxation and Dislocation. Saunders Monographs in Clinical Orthopaedics*, volume V. Philadelphia, PA, WB Saunders

CASE STUDY 3

Lateral patellar hypercompression, tilt and mild lateral subluxation

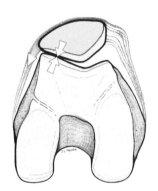

♦ What do we mean by 'hypercompression'?

♦ How can we document hypercompression?

♦ What should be our treatment plan?

Table CS3 Patellofemoral joint examination

Diagnostic clues	Findings	Diagnostic clues	Findings
Pain	Lateral patellofemoral joint in loaded flexion	Patellar gliding mechanism	Lateral tight
Tenderness	Lateral retinacula, capsule	Patellar apprehension	Negative
Effusion	None		
Swelling	Moderate lateral	Q angle	Normal value
Patellar position, relaxed, 0°	Centred	Catching	Lateral
Patellar position, contracted, 0°	Moderate lateral tilt	Locking	None
Patellar position, 30°	Moderate lateral tilt	Range of motion	Flexion decreased
Patellar mobility	Decreased	Radiographs	Normal

Patellofemoral Disorders: Diagnosis and Treatment. Edited by Roland M. Biedert
© 2004 John Wiley & Sons, Ltd ISBN: 0-470-85011-6

History

A 29 year-old male suffered from pain, swelling and catching on the lateral side of the patella during loaded flexion. Maximum flexion was decreased by pain. No effusion and no signs of instability were reported. The physical examination revealed no patellar instability, but the examination did reveal decreased mobility in the lateral patellofemoral joint with tight lateral structures.

Comments

Increased pain in the patellofemoral joint during loaded flexion represents a classic complaint in many active athletes, especially those participating in sports activities, such as volleyball, squash, tennis or skiing, that are performed in loaded flexion with rotation. In such situations, the patella has increased pressure in the trochlea. Tight lateral structures (retinacula, capsule, iliotibial tract, vastus lateralis muscle) decrease the mobility of the patella, accentuated on the lateral side, therefore creating lateral hypercompression in the patellofemoral joint.

Course of action

Physical examination

In the present case we found a painful and very tight lateral retinaculum (superficial and oblique) in combination with a sore lateral patellofemoral joint line. The contracted lateral retinaculum created the lateral patellar tilt and decreased the normal mobility of the patella (under one to two quadrants, both to medial and lateral).[1] In such cases, moderate swelling in the involved structures can be found. The patella glides very tightly on the lateral trochlea, with mild subluxation during flexion (Figure CS3.1). Catching can be noted on the lateral side.

Axial CT evaluation

In 0° extension with relaxed quadriceps muscle, the patella lays laterally and a mild tilt can be

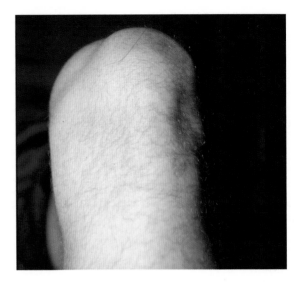

Figure CS3.1 Lateral subluxation and tilt of the patella caused by tight lateral structures (left knee, 30°, relaxed)

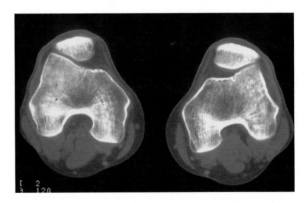

Figure CS3.2 Lateral hypercompression on both sides with tilt (extension, relaxed)

noted (Figure CS3.2). The lateral patellofemoral joint space is narrow; medially it is open. Narrowing of the bones (patella and lateral trochlea) demonstrates hypercompression with thinned cartilage on both sides. Contraction of the quadriceps muscle causes additional lateral subluxation of the patella (Figure CS3.3).

Plan

Patients with severe lateral hypercompression are in most cases not good candidates for conserva-

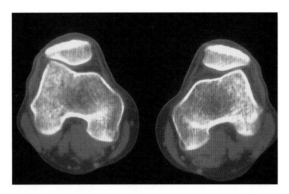

Figure CS3.3 Dynamic lateral subluxation of the patella with tilt and hypercompression (extension, contracted)

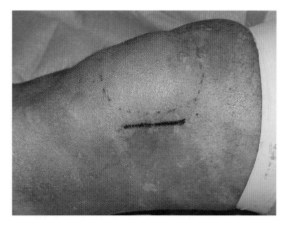

Figure CS3.4 Skin incision, 4 cm long (left knee)

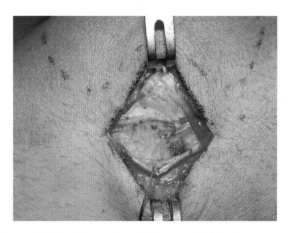

Figure CS3.5 Separation of the superficial retinaculum (hold with sutures) from the deep part (left knee)

tive treatment and physical therapy. Hypercompression leads to an important use of the cartilage and with this to consecutively more lateralization of the patella. This may lead to an elevated subchondral bone pressure,[2–4] with increased turnover and remodelling creating pain. Hypercompression can also increase venous engorgement in the patella and cause pain.[5]

Surgery must decrease the hypercompression. As mentioned in the comments, the lateral retinacula are too tight and short. These are the anatomical structures on which we must focus. Lateral retinacular release is a frequently practised operative procedure in such cases, but secondary complications, such as instability with medial patellar subluxation, are well known and described by several authors.[6–9] Therefore, lengthening of the lateral retinaculum is the therapy to choose.[10]

Through a short parapatellar lateral incision (maximum 5 cm), the superficial retinaculum is localized (Figure CS3.4). About 1 cm from the border of the patella it is longitudinally incised and carefully separated from the oblique part of the retinaculum (Figure CS3.5) in the posterior direction. Then the oblique part is cut, together with the synovial membrane; the patellofemoral joint is opened (Figure CS3.6). Intraarticular inspection is now possible. The superficial and oblique parts are readapted in about 80° of knee flexion with lengthening of the retinacula at the same time (Figures CS3.7 and CS3.8). The amount of lengthening can be checked by the present new mobility of the patella, which must be one to two quadrants to both the medial and lateral sides (Figure CS3.9). This procedure decreases the compression forces and normalizes the patellofemoral gliding mechanism.

Postoperative care and rehabilitation

Goals

♦ Protection of lengthening.

♦ Normalization of patellar balancing in the trochlea.

♦ Strengthening of the weak muscle groups.

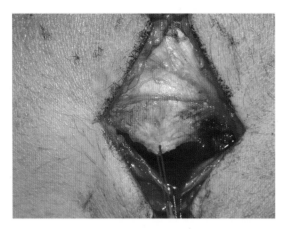

Figure CS3.6   The oblique part (top) and the superficial retinaculum (bottom) are separated and the joint opened posteriorly (left knee)

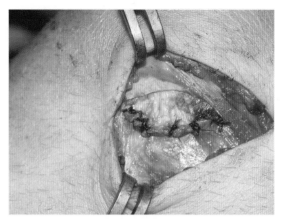

Figure CS3.7   Sutures of the adapted and lengthened retinacula: oblique (top) and superficial (bottom)

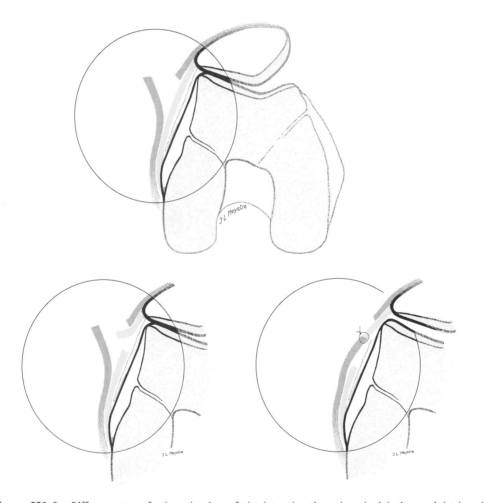

Figure CS3.8   Different steps for lengthening of the lateral retinaculum (axial views, right knee)

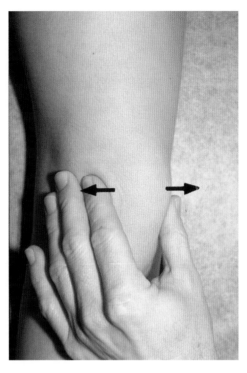

Figure CS3.9 Clinical examination of the new patellar mobility to medial and lateral after reconstruction

Timeline

- ♦ Hospital   2–4 days
- ♦ Mobilization   1st or 2nd day
- ♦ Weightbearing   Partial   20 kg for 2 weeks
  - Complete   Depends on pain and swelling
- ♦ Sports   Bicycle   After 2 weeks
  - Everything   Depends on final result after 6 weeks

Continuous passive motion is started as soon as possible. The amount of flexion is increased every day. Lengthening of the shortened structures is needed on the lateral side by smooth manual therapy. Accordingly, strengthening of the weakened muscles on the medial side starts immediately.

Summary

This case describes a clear pathology with lateral patellar hypercompression caused by tight lateral retinacula. The pathoanatomy is obvious and the necessary treatment unequivocal. Lengthening of the lateral retinacular structures has major advantages compared to lateral retinacular release.[1,7–9,11–14]

The advantages of lateral retinacular lengthening in comparison to release are:

- ♦ Avoidance of secondary medial patellar instability with subluxations or dislocations.

- ♦ Avoidance of overrelease of the lateral structures, including unintended section of the vastus lateralis tendon.

- ♦ Possibility of meticulous adaptation of length and tension of the retinacula in extension and flexion.

- ♦ Protection of nerves and vessels (lateral superior and inferior genicular arteries).

- ♦ Exact haemostasis.

References

1. Kolowich PA, Paulos LE, Rosenberg TD, Farnsworth S (1990) Lateral release of the patella: indications and contraindications. *Am J Sports Med* **18**: 359–365
2. Biedert RM, Kernen V (2001) Neurosensory characteristics of the patellofemoral joint: what is the genesis of patellofemoral pain? *Sports Med Arthrosc Rev* **9**: 295–300
3. Biedert RM (2000) A new perspective of patellofemoral pain. Where is the pain coming from? In: Symposia Handouts and Abstracts of the 67th Annual Meeting of the American Academy of Orthopaedic Surgeons, Orlando, FL, p 247
4. Biedert RM, Sanchis-Alfonso V (2002) Sources of anterior knee pain. *Clin Sports Med* **21**: 335–347

5. Waisbrod H, Treiman N (1980) Intra-osseous venography in patellofemoral disorders. A preliminary report. *J Bone Joint Surg Br* **62**: 454–456

6. Biedert RM, Gruhl C (1997) Axial computed tomography of the patellofemoral joint with and without quadriceps contraction. *Arch Orthop Trauma Surg* **116**: 77–82

7. Kramers-de Quervain IA, Biedert R, Stüssi E (1997) Quantitative gait analysis in patients with medial patellar instability following lateral retinacular release. *Knee Surg Sports Traumatol Arthrosc* **5**: 95–101

8. Biedert RM, Friederich NF (1994) Failed lateral retinacular release: clinical outcome. *J Sports Traumatol* **16**: 162–173

9. Hughston JC, Deese M (1988) Medial subluxation of the patella as a complication of lateral retinacular release. *Am J Sports Med* **16**: 383–388

10. Biedert RM (2000) Is there an indication for lateral release and how I do it. In: Proceedings of the International Patellofemoral Study Group, Garmisch-Partenkirchen, Germany

11. Teitge RA, Faerber WW, Des Madryl P, Matelic TM (1996) Stress radiographs of the patellofemoral joint. *J Bone Joint Surg Am* **78**: 193–203

12. Larson RL, Cabaud HE, Slocum DB et al (1978) The patellar compression syndrome: surgical treatment by lateral retinacular release. *Clin Orthop* **134**: 158–167

13. Nonweiler DE, DeLee JC (1994) The diagnosis and treatment of medial subluxation of the patella after lateral retinacular release. *Am J Sports Med* **22**: 680–686

14. Henry JH, Goletz TH, Williamson B (1986) Lateral retinacular release in patellofemoral subluxation. Indications, results, and comparison to open patellofemoral reconstruction. *Am J Sports Med* **14**: 121–129

Suggested reading

Biedert RM, Gruhl C (1997) Axial computed tomography of the patellofemoral joint with and without quadriceps contraction. *Arch Orthop Trauma Surg* **116**: 77–82

Biedert RM, Friederich NF (1994) Failed lateral retinacular release: clinical outcome. *J Sports Traumatol* **16**: 162–173

Biedert RM, Sanchis-Alfonso V (2002) Sources of anterior knee pain. *Clin Sports Med* **21**: 335–347

Teitge RA, Faerber WW, Des Madryl P, Matelic TM (1996) Stress radiographs of the patellofemoral joint. *J Bone Joint Surg Am* **78**: 193–203

CASE STUDY 4

Dynamic lateral patellar subluxation

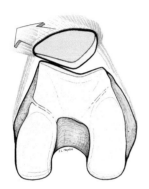

◆ What do we mean by 'dynamic'?

◆ What causes the lateralization?

◆ What is our treatment plan?

Table CS4 Patellofemoral joint examination			
Diagnostic clues	Findings	Diagnostic clues	Findings
Pain	Lateral, dynamic	Patellar apprehension	Moderate positive to lateral
Tenderness	Lateral soft tissues	Q angle	Normal value
Effusion	None	Catching	Negative
Swelling	Sometimes lateral	Locking	Negative
Patellar position, relaxed, 0°	Normal	Range of motion	Normal
Patellar position, contracted, 0°	Lateralization		
Patellar position, 30°	Normal	Radiographs	Normal
Patellar gliding mechanism	Moderate lateralization near extension	Other	Increased pain with physical therapy/ strengthening

Patellofemoral Disorders: Diagnosis and Treatment. Edited by Roland M. Biedert
© 2004 John Wiley & Sons, Ltd ISBN: 0-470-85011-6

History

A 32 year-old female suffered from patellofemoral pain going up and down stairs. At another clinic, she had been sent to physical therapy for a strengthening program to improve muscular weakness of the vastus medialis muscle (the diagnosis given there). But instead of an improvement, all strengthening exercises impaired the situation and the training was very painful and had to be stopped. Not even simple exercises like quadriceps setting or straight leg raising could be performed without pain. On the contrary, they worsened the whole problem.

Comments

We hear descriptions of this classic situation more and more from patients. Strengthening exercises exacerbate the pain at the patellofemoral joint. The local pathology is further impaired. Exercises for contracting the quadriceps are contraindicated for achieving relief of pain. Patients feel better without physical therapy, although they do not feel good.[1-4]

Course of action

Physical examination

With this problem, the lateral soft tissues (lateral retinaculum, capsule) are painful on palpation. The mobility of the patella is normal to the medial side but increased to lateral, with moderate signs of a positive apprehension test. Lateral subluxation is documented with contraction of the quadriceps muscle. The patient can repeat this dynamic lateralization by voluntary contraction. In the relaxed situation, the patella is well balanced in the trochlea. Movements near extension (0–25°) in the one-leg standing position provoke pain and crepitus.

These patients presenting dynamic patellar subluxation perform their training or the physical therapy in a biomechanically impaired situation, with chronic subluxation and relocation near extension, and therefore provoke more pain.

CT evaluation

In 0° of extension and relaxation, the patient's patella was well centred (Figure CS4.1). With contraction of the quadriceps muscle, the patella displaced laterally without a severe tilt (Figure CS4.2). Narrowing of the lateral patellofemoral joint documents the loss of articular cartilage and chronic overuse.

The patient's patella was well-centred in 30° of knee flexion by the bony configuration of the

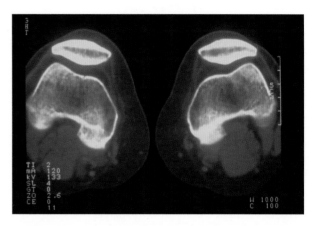

Figure CS4.1 Well-centred patella on both sides (axial views, extension, relaxed)

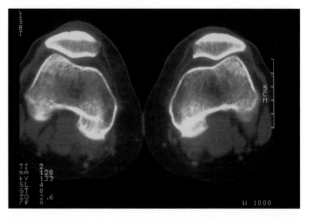

Figure CS4.2 Lateralization of both patellae without tilt (axial views, extension, contracted)

trochlea. The sulcus angle and the lateral trochlea were normal.

Plan

The most important therapeutic step is to improve centralization of the patella. Painful lateralization must be avoided because pain decreases the muscular control and stabilization. The physical therapist must find painless exercises for the strengthening programme. Medialization of the patella using a tape, as described by McConnell,[5,6] can be helpful, especially at the beginning (Figure CS4.3). Specific training of the vastus medialis obliquus is necessary to avoid a lateralization. Adjustment of the force vector of the whole extensor apparatus must be achieved with this training. Prolonged physical therapy and training are necessary to establish dynamic centralization of the patella.

Dynamic lateralization of the patella is a complaint that can be successfully treated by conservative therapy in most patients. Surgical correction is only necessary when overstretching of the medial patellofemoral ligament is documented. Frequently this is coupled with hypertrophy and shortening of the lateral soft tissue structures.[7]

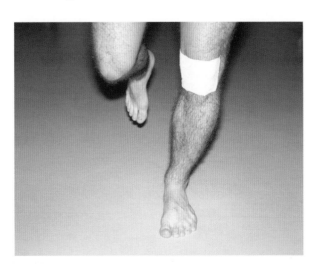

Figure CS4.3 Closed kinetic chain exercises with a patellar tape to decrease lateralization and pain and to improve sensorimotor control

When conservative treatment (over 6 months) fails, lengthening of the lateral retinaculum is done in combination with shortening of the medial patellofemoral ligament (*see* Case Study 6) (Biedert RM, in a presentation at the International Patellofemoral Study Group, Garmisch-Partenkirchen, Germany, 2000). Osteotomies (tibial tuberosity or lateral femoral condyle) are not indicated because there is no osseous pathology.

Summary

Increased patellofemoral pain under muscle strengthening or physical therapy is often caused by impaired biomechanical conditions. These include weakness of the vastus medialis obliquus, hypertrophy of the lateral structures and therefore lateralization of the patella with subluxation. Pain arises from hypercompression in the lateral patellofemoral joint, impingement of the lateral structures, and chronic synovitis caused chemically by cartilage destruction and wear particles.[8] Centralization of the patella is in most cases possible with adapted physical therapy. Surgical treatment is necessary only for dysplastic structures.

References

1. Biedert RM, Gruhl C (1997) Axial computed tomography of the patellofemoral joint with and without quadriceps contraction. *Arch Orthop Trauma Surg* **116**: 77–82
2. Guzzanti V, Gigante A, Di Lazzaro A, Fabbriciani C (1994) Patellofemoral malalignment in adolescents. Computerized tomographic assessment with or without quadriceps contraction. *Am J Sports Med* **22**: 55–60
3. Delgado-Martins H (1979) A study of the position of the patella using computerised tomography. *J Bone Joint Surg Br* **61-B**: 443–444
4. Pinar H, Akseki D, Karaoglan O, Genc I (1994) Kinematic and dynamic axial computed tomography of the patellofemoral joint in patients with anterior knee pain. *Knee Surg Sports Traumatol Arthrosc* **2**: 170–173

5. McConnell J (2002) The physical therapist's approach to patellofemoral disorders. *Clin Sports Med* **21**: 363–387

6. McConnell J (1986) The management of chondromalacia patellae: a long-term solution. *Aust J Physiother* **32**: 215–223

7. Hughston JC, Walsh WM, Puddu G (1984) *Patellar Subluxation and Dislocation. Saunders Monographs in Clinical Orthopaedics*, volume V. Philadelphia, PA, WB Saunders

8. Biedert RM, Kernen V (2001) Neurosensory characteristics of the patellofemoral joint: what is the genesis of patellofemoral pain? *Sports Med Arthrosc Rev* **9**: 295–300

Suggested reading

Biedert RM, Gruhl C (1997) Axial computed tomography of the patellofemoral joint with and without quadriceps contraction. *Arch Orthop Trauma Surg* **116**: 77–82

Guzzanti V, Gigante A, Di Lazzaro A, Fabbriciani C (1994) Patellofemoral malalignment in adolescents. Computerized tomographic assessment with or without quadriceps contraction. *Am J Sports Med* **22**: 55–60

McConnell J (1986) The management of chondromalacia patellae: a long-term solution. *Aust J Physiother* **32**: 215–223

CASE STUDY 5

Lateral patellar subluxation with dynamic reposition

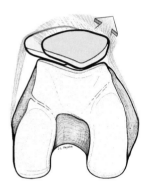

♦ What causes lateral subluxation with relaxed muscles?

♦ Why is a dynamic reposition possible?

♦ What are the consequences for the choice of treatment?

	Table CS5 Patellofemoral joint examination		
Diagnostic clues	Findings	Diagnostic clues	Findings
Pain	Peripatellar, lateral more than medial	Patellar apprehension	Normal
Tenderness	Peripatellar soft tissues	Q angle	Normal value
Effusion	None	Catching	Negative
Swelling	None	Locking	Negative
Patellar position, relaxed, 0°	Lateralization	Range of motion	Normal
Patellar position, contracted, 0°	Almost normal centralization, but patellar tilt	Radiographs	Normal
Patellar position, 30°	Normal centralization, patellar tilt		

Patellofemoral Disorders: Diagnosis and Treatment. Edited by Roland M. Biedert
© 2004 John Wiley & Sons, Ltd ISBN: 0-470-85011-6

History

A 19 year-old male suffered from patellofemoral pain in both knees, lateral more than medial. Sitting in a flexed position over a long time and going downstairs were especially painful. Pain relief was noted in extension. Effusion or swelling was never documented.

Comments

This case describes painful situations in knee flexion with a relief of pain near extension. Both knees had the same symptoms. We must therefore look for a pathology in mild knee flexion.

Course of action

Physical examination

The peripatellar soft tissues are painful on palpation, lateral more than medial. The tenderness is similar on both knees. The patella is lateralized in extension with relaxed quadriceps muscle. Medialization of the patella is noted, with active quadriceps contraction centring the patella almost normally into the trochlea but creating a patellar tilt. The medialization of the patella documents the dynamic reposition of the laterally subluxed patella. The gliding test of the patella shows decreased mobility to medial, with tight lateral structures. Performing the patellar tilt test in 30° of knee flexion, we find a well-centred patella in the trochlea with a mild lateral patellar tilt.

Radiographs

The standard radiographs showed mild lateralization of the patella in the anteroposterior and sagittal views. The trochlea was normal.

Axial CT evaluation

Lateralization of the patella was documented in both knees, on the left side more than on the

right, in extension and relaxation (Figure CS5.1). Contraction of the quadriceps muscle moved the patella to medial, with better centralization of the patella into the trochlea, but quadriceps contraction caused in addition a moderate patellar tilt, with hypercompression on the lateral patellofemoral joint (Figure CS5.2). The patella is well centred in 30° of knee flexion (Figure CS5.3).

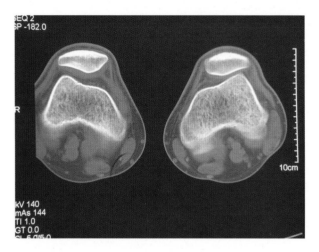

Figure CS5.1 Lateralization of the patella on both sides, left more than right. Normal trochlea and sulcus angle (axial view, extension, relaxed)

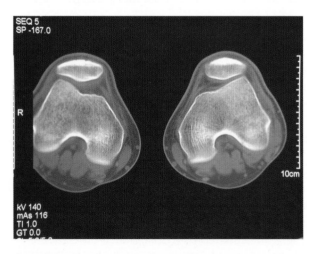

Figure CS5.2 The patella is positioned in the trochlea on both sides, but moderate lateral patellar tilt is documented (axial view, extension, contracted)

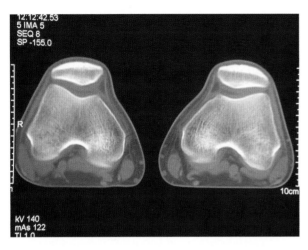

Figure CS5.3 Well-centred patella with only mild tilt and almost normal congruence of the patellofemoral joint. Note the normal congruence of the articular cartilage of patella and trochlea (axial view, 30°, relaxed)

Special considerations

This case outlines a better centralization of the patella performing quadriceps contraction than under relaxed conditions, where we find a laterally subluxed patella. This is called dynamic reposition.[1] These are good conditions for physical therapy and a strengthening programme. But quadriceps contraction also produces a patellar tilt. The lateral tilt documents tight lateral structures. These tight structures make a normal balancing of the patella impossible. In addition, patellar tightness causes impingement of the suprapatellar plica. The impingement is also responsible for the pain when the patient is sitting in a flexed position.

Plan

The goal of the treatment must be to eliminate the lateral patellar tilt and to improve the result of a strengthening programme. This needs lengthening of the lateral soft tissue structures, which can be achieved in most cases with physical therapy (Part IV). In the cases of unsuccessful conservative treatment, surgical intervention may be necessary after a certain time. Surgery consists of:

♦ Lengthening of the lateral retinaculum (*see* Case Study 3).

♦ Resection of a painful suprapatellar plica at the same time through short lateral arthrotomy or by arthroscopic treatment.

Postoperative care and rehabilitation

Goals

♦ Improved dynamic centring of the patella.

♦ Decrease of pain and postoperative swelling.

♦ Strengthening of the weak muscle groups.

Timeline

♦ Hospital	2–4 days	
♦ Mobilization	1st day	
♦ Weightbearing	Partial	10 kg for 1st and 2nd week
		20 kg for 3rd and 4th week
	Complete	After 4 weeks
♦ Sports	Depends on pain and swelling	
	Everything	After 2 months

Summary

This case outlines the positive situation where the patient is able to perform a dynamic reposition of a laterally subluxed patella, but the tight lateral structures make it impossible to achieve a completely normal balancing. The lateral structures must therefore be the target of the nonoperative or, in chronic cases, operative treatment. Lengthening of the tight lateral structures is the key to a successful outcome.

References

1. Biedert RM, Gruhl C (1997) Axial computed tomography of the patellofemoral joint with and without quadriceps contraction. *Arch Orthop Trauma Surg* **116**: 77–82

Suggested reading

Biedert RM, Gruhl C (1997) Axial computed tomography of the patellofemoral joint with and without quadriceps contraction. *Arch Orthop Trauma Surg* **116**: 77–82

Guzzanti V, Gigante A, Di Lazzaro A, Fabbriciani C (1994) Patellofemoral malalignment in adolescents. Computerized tomographic assessment with or without quadriceps contraction. *Am J Sports Med* **22**: 55–60

Additional reading

Biedert RM, Kernen V (2001) Neurosensory characteristics of the patellofemoral joint: what is the genesis of patellofemoral pain? *Sports Med Arthrosc Rev* **9**: 295–300

Delgado-Martins H (1979) A study of the position of the patella using computerised tomography. *J Bone Joint Surg Br* **61-B**: 443–444

Pinar H, Akseki D, Karaoglan O, Genc I (1994) Kinematic and dynamic axial computed tomography of the patellofemoral joint in patients with anterior knee pain. *Knee Surg Sports Traumatol Arthrosc* **2**: 170–173

CASE STUDY 6

Lateral patellar subluxation with dynamic impairment and normal trochlea

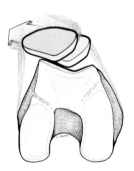

♦ What causes persistent lateral patellar subluxation?

♦ Why do we find a dynamic impairment?

♦ What is our treatment concept?

Table CS6 Patellofemoral joint examination

Diagnostic clues	Findings	Diagnostic clues	Findings
Pain	Lateral and medial, increased with muscle contraction or loading	Patellar gliding mechanism	Lateralization near extension
Tenderness	Lateral and medial soft tissues	Patellar apprehension	Mild positive to lateral
Effusion	None	Q angle	Decreased value
Swelling	Sometimes lateral	Catching	Sometimes
Patellar position, relaxed, 0°	Lateralization	Locking	Sometimes
Patellar position, contracted, 0°	Increased lateralization	Range of motion	Normal
Patellar position, 30°	Normal	Radiographs	Lateralization of the patella in the anteroposterior and sagittal views

Patellofemoral Disorders: Diagnosis and Treatment. Edited by Roland M. Biedert
© 2004 John Wiley & Sons, Ltd ISBN: 0-470-85011-6

History

A 19 year-old female complained about patello-femoral pain during the last 2 years when performing different sports activities. She also suffered from occasional locking and catching. Quadriceps muscle contraction (strengthening) and loading caused increased pain. Pharmacological (chondroitin) and nonpharmacological treatment (physical therapy, reduction of sports activities) were not helpful.

Comments

This case describes pain exacerbation under dynamic conditions, e.g. strengthening exercises. Locking and catching points disturbed the patellofemoral gliding mechanism.[1]

Course of action

Physical examination

The peripatellar lateral and medial soft tissue structures were painful on palpation. The patella was lateralized under relaxed conditions. Full quadriceps muscle activation increased the persisting lateralization and caused additional external rotation of the patella and the lateral soft tissue structures. Movements from extension into flexion centred the patella in the trochlea, with a mild medialization during the first 30° of knee flexion. The tubercle–sulcus angle was normal in 90° of flexion.

Radiographs

The standard radiographs in three planes showed mild lateralization of the patella in the anteroposterior and sagittal views. The trochlea was normal in sagittal view.

Axial CT Evaluation

In 0° of extension and relaxation, the patella was lateralized (Figure CS6.1). The trochlea was normal. Contraction of the quadriceps muscle in

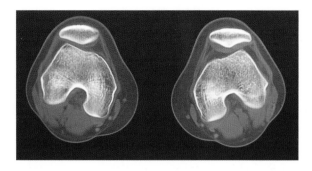

Figure CS6.1   Lateralization of the patella. Normal trochlea (axial view, extension, relaxed)

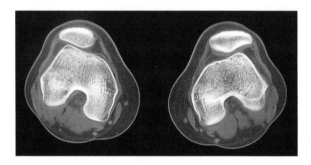

Figure CS6.2   Increased dynamic lateralization of the patella (axial view, extension, quadriceps contracted)

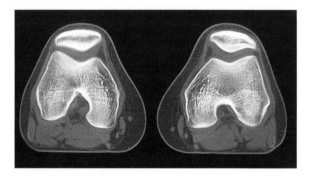

Figure CS6.3   Well-centred patella with normal sulcus angle and lateral trochlea (axial view, 30°, relaxed)

extension caused increased lateralization of the patella[2] (Figure CS6.2). The persisting distance between the osseous borders of the lateral patella and the lateral trochlea documented the height of the articular cartilage in the lateral patellofemoral joint. The patella was well-centred in 30° of knee flexion with a mild patellar tilt (Figure CS6.3).

Plan

In this case, we have to treat permanent lateralization of the patella. No osseous correction is necessary because the form of the trochlea is normal, the height of the patella is correct, and the torsion of the lower extremity is without pathology. The underlying pathoanatomies are the shortened lateral and lax medial structures. The permanent lateralization caused overstretching of the medial patellofemoral ligament and shortening of the lateral retinaculum. Soft tissue reconstruction is therefore necessary to centre the patella in the trochlea and to keep it well centred during the whole range of motion.

Surgery consists of two steps:

♦ Lengthening of the lateral retinaculum (*see* Case Study 3).

♦ Shortening of the medial patellofemoral ligament.

The reconstruction is performed using two short incisions (Figure CS6.4). The reconstruction begins on the lateral side with the incision and preparation of the retinaculum, with the option to perform a correct lengthening at the end of surgery. Inspection of the patellofemoral joint is possible through the short lateral arthrotomy.

The next step consists of identification of the medial patellofemoral ligament through the second incision medially (Figures CS6.5 and CS6.6). The ligament is cut and prepared close to the medial epicondyle. Three or four U-shaped sutures are set from posterior to anterior (Figure CS6.7). The sutures are provisionally put under tension (Figure CS6.8), pulling the patella into the centre of the trochlea. The knee joint is carefully flexed

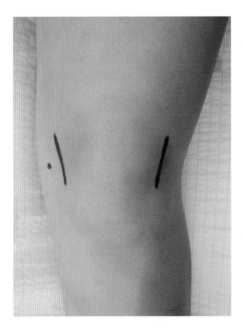

Figure CS6.4 Landmarks of the lateral and medial incisions as well as the medial epicondyle (point) (left knee)

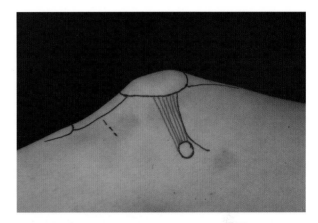

Figure CS6.5 Landmarks of the medial patellofemoral ligament

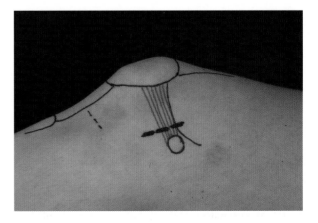

Figure CS6.6 Skin incision to prepare the medial patellofemoral ligament (0, medial epicondyle)

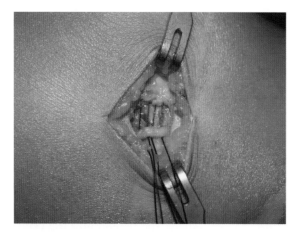

Figure CS6.7   Sutures in the dorsal part of the medial patellofemoral ligament (left knee)

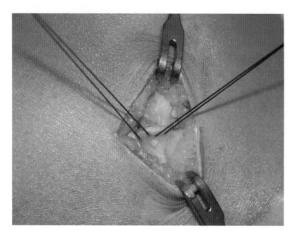

Figure CS6.8   Tightening of the sutures causes shortening and doubling of the medial patellofemoral ligament (left knee)

and the tension of the sutures adapted as necessary. Then the sutures are tightened (Figure CS6.9). The lengthening of the lateral retinaculum is performed in 60–80° of flexion to avoid shortening.

Postoperative care and rehabilitation

Goals

♦ Static and dynamic centring of the patella in the trochlea.

♦ Decreasing pain.

♦ Strengthening of the muscle groups.

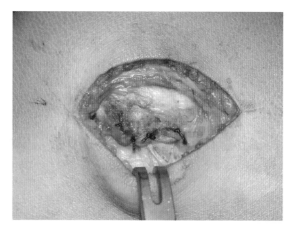

Figure CS6.9   Final result after medial reconstruction (left knee)

Timeline

Hospital	2–4 days	
♦ Mobilization	1st day	
♦ Weightbearing	Partial	Max. 20 kg for 4 weeks
	Complete	After 4 weeks
♦ Sports	Bicycle	After 2 weeks with more than 90° of flexion and no effusion
	Swimming	After 4 weeks, depends on muscle activity
	Everything	After 3 months

Summary

This case outlines permanent lateral patellar subluxation with impairment under dynamic conditions. Permanent subluxation causes shortening of the lateral and overstretching of the medial soft tissue structures. The trochlea is normal and cannot be the cause of subluxation. Only the soft tissue structures are pathological and must therefore be the target of the treatment. Surgical correction is necessary in chronic cases; long-term nonoperative treatment is not successful.

References

1. Biedert RM, Gruhl C (1997) Axial computed tomography of the patellofemoral joint with and without quadriceps contraction. *Arch Orthop Trauma Surg* **116**: 77–82

2. Guzzanti V, Gigante A, Di Lazzaro A, Fabbriciani C (1994) Patellofemoral malalignment in adolescents. Computerized tomographic assessment with or without quadriceps contraction. *Am J Sports Med* **22**: 55–60

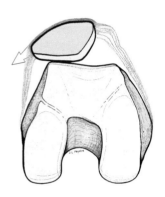

♦ What causes persistent lateral patellar subluxation?

♦ Which investigations are necessary?

♦ Do we need surgical correction?

Table CS7   Patellofemoral joint examination

Diagnostic clues	Findings	Diagnostic clues	Findings
Pain	Lateral and medial soft tissues	Patellar gliding mechanism	Lateralized with crepitations
Tenderness	Lateral and medial	Patellar apprehension	Positive and painful to lateral
Effusion	Sometimes	Q angle	Decreased value
Swelling	Sometimes	Catching	Sometimes
Patellar position, relaxed, 0°	Lateralized	Locking	Sometimes
Patellar position, contracted, 0°	Increased lateralization	Range of motion	Normal
Patellar position, 30°	Centred	Radiographs	Dysplastic trochlea
Patellar mobility	Increased to lateral, decreased to medial		

Patellofemoral Disorders: Diagnosis and Treatment.   Edited by Roland M. Biedert
© 2004 John Wiley & Sons, Ltd   ISBN: 0-470-85011-6

History

The history of a 22 year-old Judo player included two complete lateral patellar dislocations on the left side which required reduction in the emergency room. Two years after the second dislocation, he complained about chronic pain, weakness and a feeling of unsteadiness during his sports activities. Maximum quadriceps contraction was not possible because he was afraid of sustaining another dislocation.

Comments

Permanent lateral patellar subluxations are most commonly the result of initial dislocations.[1] The reason for the first patellar dislocation is often a dysplastic trochlea with a flat lateral condyle,[2-4] one of several causing factors. Dislocations of the patella disrupt the medial patellofemoral ligament and/or medial retinaculum and lead to insufficient stability of the medial soft tissue structures.[1] The vector of the quadriceps muscle is shifted from the straight into the superolateral direction.[5] Tightness of the lateral soft tissue structures with permanent increased lateral pull are the consequences.

The present history documents the chronic persisting lateral patellar instability. Valgus, flexion and external rotation mechanisms during Judo cause increased lateral patellar subluxation with pain and weakness.

Course of action

Physical examination

We examined the patient in the supine position. The patella was lateralized with the quadriceps relaxed. Therefore the Q-angle value was low and seemed to be 'normal'[6] (Figure CS7.1). Maximum quadriceps contraction pulled the patella even more laterally and increased the lateral subluxation (Figure CS7.2). In 30° of knee flexion, the patella was less lateralized but the persisting overhang caused a vacuum effect on the

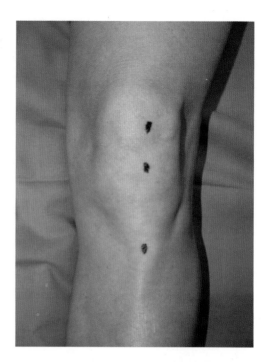

Figure CS7.1 'Normal' Q angle caused by lateral patellar subluxation (left knee, extension, quadriceps relaxed)

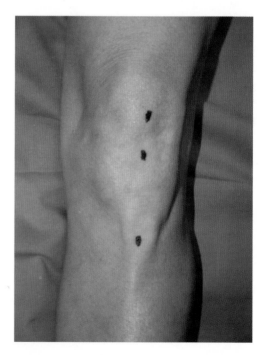

Figure CS7.2 Increased lateral patellar subluxation with tight lateral soft tissue structures (left knee, extension, quadriceps contracted)

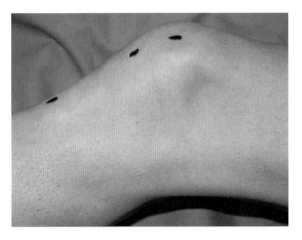

Figure CS7.3 Mild lateralization of the patella with vacuum effect between the lateral patellar facet and the femoral condyle (left knee, 30°, relaxed)

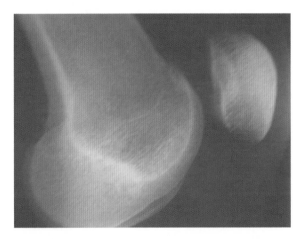

Figure CS7.4 Crossing sign with trochlear dysplasia (lateral view)

lateral structures (Figure CS7.3). The overhang was caused by tight lateral soft tissues. The apprehension test was positive and painful to the lateral, negative to the medial side. In testing the patellar mobility to lateral, no osseous resistance was noted. Patellar mobility was decreased medially.

Radiographs

The lateral radiograph showed trochlear dysplasia (Figure CS7.4). The anteroposterior radiograph revealed lateralization of the patella.

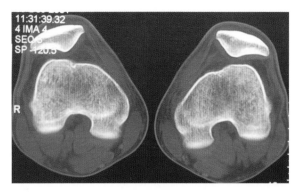

Figure CS7.5 Lateral subluxation of the patella on both sides with dysplastic trochlea and flat lateral condyle (only left side is injured). Pathological tilt (axial view, extension, relaxed)

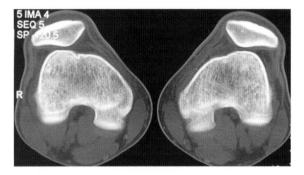

Figure CS7.6 Severe lateral subluxation with hypercompression in the lateral patellofemoral joint, tilt. Minimal central bump is noted (axial view, extension, contracted)

Axial CT evaluation

In axial CT scans in 0° extension, the patella was subluxed to lateral and tilted; the lateral trochlea was flat (Figure CS7.5). Axial CT confirmed the trochlear dysplasia. Quadriceps contraction increased lateral patellar subluxation (Figure CS7.6). In 30° of knee flexion, the patella was more centred but still lateralized (caused by the tight lateral structures) (Figure CS7.7).

Plan

The present case manifests three problems that need treatment – the flat lateral condyle with

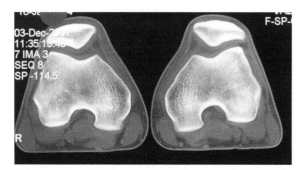

Figure CS7.7   Decreased lateral subluxation of the patella (axial view, 30°, relaxed)

dysplastic trochlea, the tight lateral soft tissues, and the insufficient medial stabilizing structures. Conservative treatment to solve these problems will not be successful, because it may not influence the structural failure with the trochlear dysplasia. Only surgical treatment may improve the pathoanatomy. The surgical procedure consists of three steps:

♦ Reconstructing (raising) the lateral condyle.

♦ Lengthening of the lateral structures.

♦ Shortening and imbrication of the medial structures.[7]

Surgery starts with a parapatellar lateral incision. The lateral retinacula are incised in the longitudinal direction and the superficial and oblique retinaculum separated (Figure CS7.8). The arthrotomy is performed posteriorly (*see* Case Study 3). The flat lateral condyle and the trochlea are inspected. The incomplete lateral osteotomy goes from the proximal edge of the trochlea to distal, always ending proximal to the sulcus terminalis (Figure CS7.9). The osteotomy is opened carefully with the use of a chisel. Fracture of the distal cartilage may occur and has no consequences; sharp edges must be smoothed. Then the lateral condyle is lifted up.[8] Cancellous bone (obtained from the lateral head of the tibia) is inserted and impacted (Figure CS7.10). The amount of raising depends on the form of the trochlea and the femoral condyle; in most cases 5–6 mm are sufficient. Overcorrection must be avoided. Additional fixation is possible

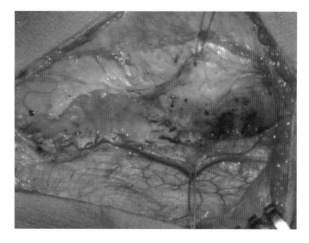

Figure CS7.8   The superficial retinaculum (held with the suture at the bottom) is separated from the oblique transverse retinaculum (suture at the top) (left knee)

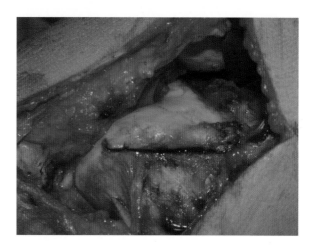

Figure CS7.9   Intraoperative lateral view showing the osteotomy and the flat lateral condyle. Note the distal end of the osteotomy, where the articular cartilage may fracture (left knee)

by using sutures. This reconstruction improves the osseous stability.

The last step consists of shortening and imbricating the medial patellofemoral ligament and, in some cases, also the medial retinaculum (*see* Case Study 6). The lateral retinacula are adapted in about 80° of knee flexion to guarantee lengthening and to eliminate the preoperatively increased lateral pull.

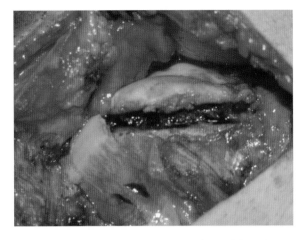

Figure CS7.10 Intraoperative view after raising the lateral femoral condyle and filling the osteotomy gap with cancellous bone taken from the lateral tibial head

Complications are possible. They include fracturing of the lateral condyle, too much thinning of the osteochondral flap of the lateral trochlea, lateral hypercompression and loosening of the cancellous bone.

Postoperative Care and Rehabilitation

Goals

♦ Persistent centring of the patella in the trochlea.

♦ Normal balancing of the soft tissue structures.

♦ Strengthening of the muscle groups.

Timeline

♦ Hospital	3–4 days	
♦ Mobilization	2nd day	
♦ Weightbearing	Partial	20 kg for 4 weeks
	Complete	After 4 weeks
♦ Sports	Bicycle	After 2 weeks, no resistance
	Swimming	After 3 weeks
	Everything	After 3 months

♦ Range of motion	Immediate	0–0–80° (continuous passive motion included), complete after 4 weeks

Summary

The dysplastic trochlea is one of the most important aetiological factors of permanent lateral patellar subluxation causing patellar instability.[9–12] Tightness of the lateral and weakness of the medial soft tissue structures are secondary effects. The treatment must therefore include all the structures involved and eliminate especially the underlying primary cause, the missing osseous stability of the patella in the trochlea. Only the combined reconstructions of all the pathological structures improves the postoperative outcome.

References

1. Sallay PI, Poggi J, Speer KP, Garrett WE (1996) Acute dislocation of the patella. A correlative pathoanatomic study. *Am J Sports Med* **24**: 52–60
2. Reider B, Marshall JL, Warren RF (1981) Clinical characteristics of patellar disorders in young athletes. *Am J Sports Med* **9**: 270–274
3. Atkin DM, Fithian DC, Marangi KS et al (2000) Characteristics of patients with primary acute lateral patellar dislocation and their recovery within the first 6 months of injury. *Am J Sports Med* **28**: 472–479
4. Arnbjornsson A, Egund N, Rydling O et al (1992) The natural history of recurrent dislocation of the patella. Long-term results of conservative and operative treatment. *J Bone Joint Surg Br* **74**: 140–142
5. Kolowich PA, Paulos LE, Rosenberg TD, Farnsworth S (1990) Lateral release of the patella: indications and contraindications. *Am J Sports Med* **18**: 359–365

6. Biedert RM, Warnke K (2001) Correlation between the Q angle and the patella position: a clinical and axial computed tomography evaluation. *Arch Orthop Trauma Surg* **121**: 346–349

7. Biedert RM (2000) Is there an indication for lateral release and how I do it. In: Proceedings of the International Patellofemoral Study Group, Garmisch-Partenkirchen, Germany

8. Albee FH (1915) The bone graft wedge in the treatment of habitual dislocation of the patella. *Med Rec* **88**: 257–259

9. Galland O, Walch G, Dejour H, Carret JP (1990) An anatomical and radiological study of the femoropatellar articulation. *Surg Radiol Anat* **12**: 119–125

10. Dejour H, Walch G, Nove-Josserand L, Guier C (1994) Factors of patellar instability: an anatomic radiographic study. *Knee Surg Sports Traumatol Arthrosc* **2**: 19–26

11. Dejour H, Walch G, Neyret P, Adeleine P (1990) [Dysplasia of the femoral trochlea]. *Rev Chir Orthop Reparatrice Appar Mot* **76**: 45–54

12. Carillon Y, Dejour D, Tavernier T, Dejour H (1997) Aspect scannographique de la trochlée fémorale en cas d'instabilité rotulienne objective. In: *XXIV Groupe d'Etude et de Travail d'Imagerie Osteo-articulatife*, University of Lyon, pp 215–225

Suggested reading

Arnbjornsson A, Egund N, Rydling O et al (1992) The natural history of recurrent dislocation of the patella. Long-term results of conservative and operative treatment. *J Bone Joint Surg Br* **74**: 140–142

Biedert RM, Warnke K (2001) Correlation between the Q angle and the patella position: a clinical and axial computed tomography evaluation. *Arch Orthop Trauma Surg* **121**: 346–349

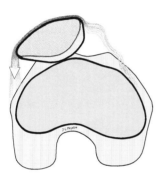

♦ What is the influence of patella alta on the patellar position?

♦ How can we document patella alta?

♦ What is our treatment plan?

Diagnostic clues	Findings	Diagnostic clues	Findings
Pain	Proximal–lateral	Patellar gliding mechanism	Lateralization
Tenderness	Lateral soft tissue structures	Patellar apprehension	Positive to lateral
Effusion	None	Q angle	Normal value
Swelling	None	Catching	Sometimes lateral
Patellar position, relaxed, 0°	Lateralization and proximalization	Locking	Sometimes lateral
Patellar position, contracted, 0°	Increased lateralization and proximalization	Range of motion	Free
Patellar position, 30°	Centred	Radiographs	Patella alta
Patellar mobility	Increased to lateral		

Table CS8 Patellofemoral joint examination

Patellofemoral Disorders: Diagnosis and Treatment.   Edited by Roland M. Biedert
© 2004 John Wiley & Sons, Ltd   ISBN: 0-470-85011-6

History

A 26 year-old male suffered from pain and occasional catching in his patellofemoral joint. He reported a weakness during movements close to full extension. Loading or sitting in higher degrees of flexion were pain-free.

Course of action

Physical examination

The physical examination in the present case showed that the patella was positioned lateral and very proximal (Figure CS8.1). Proximalization and lateralization were increased with full contraction of the quadriceps muscle. The mobility of the patella in extension was also increased to medial and lateral, indicating an instability. Manual mediolateral movements of the patella are loose, documenting the missing osseous stability and also a constitutional laxity. The stability improved in higher degrees of flexion. The improved stability also eliminated the lateralization and normalized the gliding mechanism of the patella in flexion.

Radiographs

Sagittal radiographs in 30° of flexion (Figure CS8.2) show patella alta measured according to the different indices.

Axial CT evaluation

In 0° extension with relaxed quadriceps muscle, the patella lies laterally with a mild tilt (Figure CS8.3). The flat trochlea and the missing Roman arch indicate that the CT scan was taken through the centre of the patella and through the proximal end of the trochlea. This documents the proximal position of the patella in the trochlea (patella alta). Contraction of the quadriceps muscle caused increased proximalization and

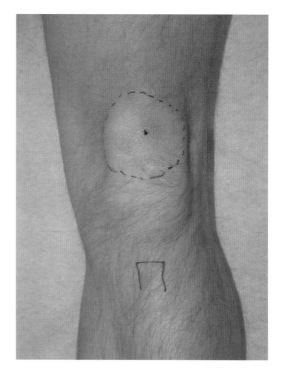

Figure CS8.1   The patella lies proximal and lateral

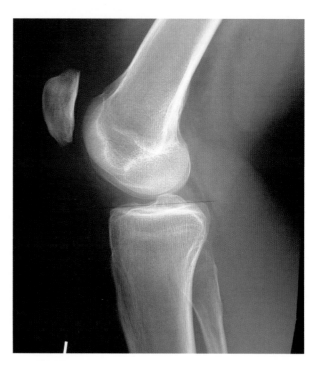

Figure CS8.2   Patella alta (lateral view, 30° flexion)

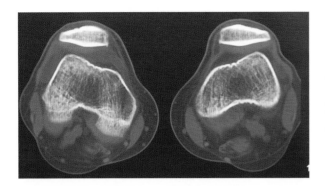

Figure CS8.3 Patella alta: patella positioned proximal in the trochlea (axial view, extension, quadriceps relaxed)

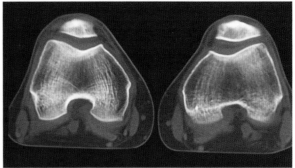

Figure CS8.5 Well-centred patella in flexion (axial view, relaxed, 30° flexion)

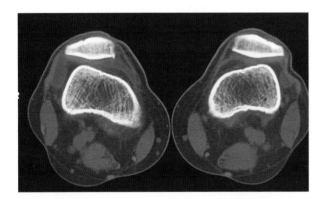

Figure CS8.4 Patella alta: increased lateral subluxation of the patella (axial view, extension, quadriceps contracted)

the patella with subluxation. Full active quadriceps contraction pulls the patella even more proximally and out of the trochlea, impairing the osseous stabilization even more. Improvement of stability is noted during flexion. The femur rolls and glides posteriorly on the tibia during knee flexion and the patella glides in accordance into the trochlea.[8,9] This enlarges the contact area between the patella and the trochlea and improves stabilization and centralization. This biomechanical behaviour is the cornerstone for the selection of the necessary treatment.

lateral subluxation of the patella (Figure CS8.4). CT scans taken in 30° of flexion showed correct centring of the patella (Figure CS8.5).

Plan

Special consideration

Patella alta is defined as pathological proximalization of the patella with reference to the tibia or the trochlea.[1–5] This means that the articular surface of the patella lies more tangentially to the distal femur, rather than in the trochlea. The contact surface is decreased in this position and therefore the passive osseous stabilization is low.[6,7] This allows increased lateralization of

The goal of the treatment is to improve patellofemoral contact and keep the patella in the trochlea. Excessive proximalization must be corrected. This can be achieved by distalization of the whole extensor apparatus. The amount of distalization is calculated on lateral radiographs according to the different indices to measure patellar height (Figure CS8.6). The osteotomy of the tibial tuberosity is performed in the horizontal plane (Figure CS8.7) with a distal oblique cut. The 8 mm-long piece of bone is removed after a second cut. The tibial tuberosity is finally fixed with two compression screws (Figures CS8.8 and CS8.9). Imbrication or lengthening of the medial or lateral soft tissue structures may be necessary. Osteotomy of the tibial tuberosity

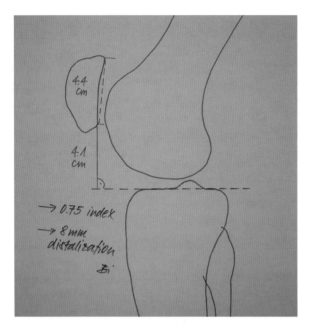

Figure CS8.6 Preoperative planning of the distalization in patella alta. The Blackburne–Peel index[2] is used for calculations to determine the amount of correction. The ratio in this case is almost 1.0. The correction to a ratio of 0.75 needs distalization of the tibial tuberosity of 8 mm

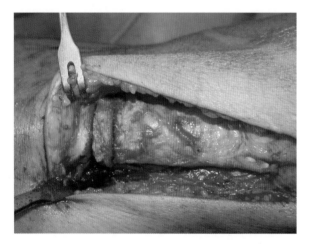

Figure CS8.7 Intraoperative view of the horizontal osteotomy of the tibial tuberosity and the two distal oblique cuts (left knee)

with distalization of the whole functional unit improves the osseous stabilization of the patella in the trochlea.

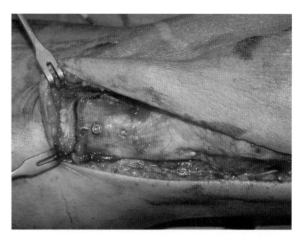

Figure CS8.8 Final situation after distalization and refixation of the tibial tuberosity with two screws

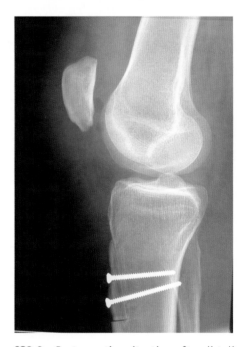

Figure CS8.9 Postoperative situation after distalization of the tibial tuberosity and with this of the patella (lateral view)

Postoperative care and rehabilitation

Goals

♦ Improving patellar stabilization.

♦ Balancing of the patella in the trochlea.

♦ Strengthening of the muscles.

Timeline

◆ Hospital	4–6 days	
◆ Mobilization	1st day	
◆ Weightbearing	Partial	Max. 10 kg for 6 weeks
	Complete	Depends on healing of the osteotomy documented on radiographs
◆ Sports	Defensive	After 8 weeks
	Aggressive	After 4 months

Summary

This case outlines possible negative effects of patella alta and additional laxity. Surgical correction is indicated only in patients with severe complaints and failure of conservative treatment. Nonsurgical treatment is the therapy of choice at the beginning (muscle strengthening, elastic sleeve, taping).

References

1. Grelsamer RP, Proctor CS, Bazos AN (1994) Evaluation of patellar shape in the sagittal plane. A clinical analysis. *Am J Sports Med* **22**: 61–66

2. Blackburne JS, Peel TE (1977) A new method of measuring patellar height. *J Bone Joint Surg Br* **59**: 241–242

3. Insall J, Salvati E (1971) Patella position in the normal knee joint. *Radiology* **101**: 101–104

4. Caton J, Deschamps G, Chambat P et al (1982) [Patella infera. A propos of 128 cases]. *Rev Chir Orthop Reparatrice Appar Mot* **68**: 317–325

5. Bernageau J, Goutallier D, Debeyre J, Ferrane J (1969) Nouvelle technique d'exploration de l'articulation fémoro-patellaire. Incindices axiales quadriceps contracté et décontracté. *Rev Chir Orthop Reparatrice Appar Mot* **61**(suppl 2): 286–290

6. Biedert RM, Gruhl C (1997) Axial computed tomography of the patellofemoral joint with and without quadriceps contraction. *Arch Orthop Trauma Surg* **116**: 77–82

7. Hille E, Schulitz KP, Henrichs C, Schneider T (1985) Pressure and contract-surface measurements within the femoropatellar joint and their variations following lateral release. *Arch Orthop Trauma Surg* **104**: 275–282

8. Goodfellow J, Hungerford DS, Woods C (1976) Patellofemoral joint mechanics and pathology. 2. Chondromalacia patellae. *J Bone Joint Surg Br* **58**: 291–299

9. Müller W, Wirz D (2000) Anatomie, Biomechanik und Dynamik des Patellofemoralgelenks. In: Wirth CJ, Rudert M (eds), *Das patellofemorale Schmerzsyndrom*. Darmstadt, Steinkopff-Verlag, pp 3–19

CASE STUDY 9

Habitual patellar dislocation with severe dysplastic trochlea in adolescents

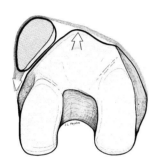

♦ What are the reasons for habitual dislocation of the patella?

♦ How can we document the pathoanatomy?

♦ What is our treatment concept?

Table CS9 Patellofemoral joint examination			
Diagnostic clues	Findings	Diagnostic clues	Findings
Pain	Diffuse patellofemoral joint	Patellar gliding mechanism	Lateralization, unstable
Tenderness	Lateral and medial	Patellar apprehension	Severely positive to lateral
Effusion	With overload	Q angle	'Normal' value
Swelling	With overload	Catching	Lateral. Under contraction between 0° and 30° of flexion
Patellar position, relaxed, 0°	Severe lateral subluxation	Locking	In flexion
Patellar position, contracted, 0°	Lateral dislocation	Range of motion	Decreased, painful
Patellar position, 30°	Severe lateral subluxation or dislocation	Radiographs	Dysplastic trochlea
Patellar mobility	Increased to lateral		

Patellofemoral Disorders: Diagnosis and Treatment.   Edited by Roland M. Biedert
© 2004 John Wiley & Sons, Ltd   ISBN: 0-470-85011-6

History

A 17 year-old female suffered from chronic bilateral patellofemoral pain and weakness. At the age of 13 years, she had an operation on the right knee, consisting of soft tissue reconstruction on the medial side (horizontalization and distalization of the vastus medialis obliquus muscle). This operation on the right side decreased the problems but did not eliminate them, because the epiphyseal cartilage was not yet closed and bony reconstruction was not possible. Surgical treatment on the left side was delayed until after epiphyseal fusion.

Comments

Chronic patellofemoral pain in combination with weakness is classic for patellar instability, such as subluxation or dislocation. Bilateral complaints beginning at the age of 10 years or younger are suggestive of severe dysplasia of the patellofemoral joint.

Course of action

Physical examination

The patient showed pain and anxiety on slight palpation of the patella during physical examination of the left knee. She moved her leg away from the examiner. The patella was subluxed laterally (Figure CS9.1). The patellar apprehension test was severely positive.

Radiographs

The lateral view showed a severely dysplastic trochlea with crossing sign (Figure CS9.2).

Axial CT evaluation

The severe lateral subluxation of the left patella could be documented with axial CT scans

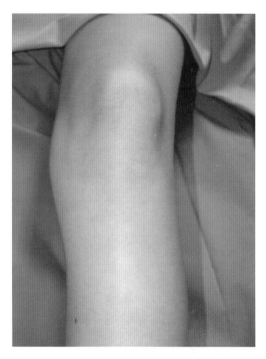

Figure CS9.1   Anterolateral view showing lateral subluxation of the patella

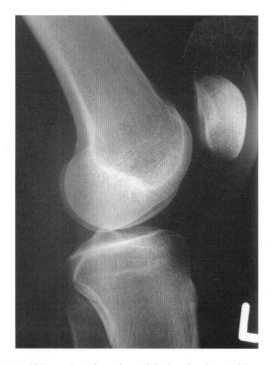

Figure CS9.2   Crossing sign with dysplastic trochlea (lateral view)

in extension and relaxed quadriceps muscle (Figure CS9.3). Quadriceps contraction caused complete dislocation of the patella (Figure CS9.4). Axial CT scans in extension documented the convex-shaped dysplastic trochlea with a central bump.

In 30° of flexion the patella was still dislocated.

Special considerations

Habitual dislocation of the patella in the younger age represents a severe problem. The aetiological factors also include patella alta and pathological torsion of femur or tibia, and especially dysplastic trochlea.[1-3] Trochlear dysplasia may

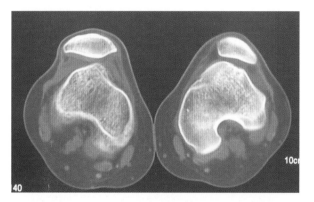

Figure CS9.3 Severe lateral subluxation of the left patella. Note the false joint between the patella and the lateral femoral condyle (axial view, extension, relaxed)

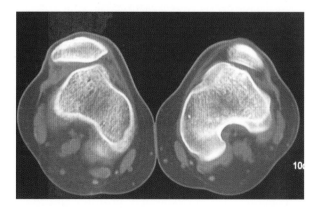

Figure CS9.4 Dislocation of the patella to lateral (axial view, extension, contracted)

consist of a flat lateral condyle, hypoplasia of the medial trochlea, or a central bump with convex shape of the trochlea. Patients with convex trochlear 'groove' have no osseous stability of the patella and dislocations may easily occur. The pathoanatomy of the form of the trochlea determines the necessary therapy. Habitual dislocation of the patella also causes tightness of the lateral structures and overstretching of the medial soft tissue structures. This has to be considered in the treatment concept.

Plan

The goal of the treatment must be to eliminate the habitual dislocation. This provides improved osseous stability of the patella in the femoral groove, lengthening of the lateral, and doubling of the medial structures. In detail, this surgical procedure consists of several steps:

◆ Lengthening of the lateral retinacula, the iliotibial tract and the vastus lateralis muscle–tendon unit.

◆ Doubling of the medial retinaculum and the medial patellofemoral ligament.

◆ Deepening of the trochlear groove (trochlearplasty).[4,5]

The surgical procedure begins with a parapatellar lateral incision and localization of the lateral retinacula (*see* Case Study 3). The superficial retinaculum is longitudinally incised and separated from the oblique part of the retinaculum in the posterior direction. This separation also includes the proximal attachment of the vastus lateralis tendon. The joint is opened after an osteotomy of the tibial tuberosity has been performed and the patella retracted to medial with hooks. Inspection of the joint shows the convex shape of the trochlea with the central bump (Figure CS9.5). The lateral articular part of the trochlea is too short and too flat (even falling off) in reference to the central part. A lateral

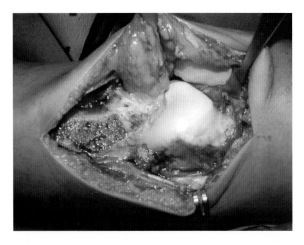

Figure CS9.5 Intraoperative lateral view showing the dysplastic trochlea with the central bump. The lateral part of the trochlea is falling off and is too short

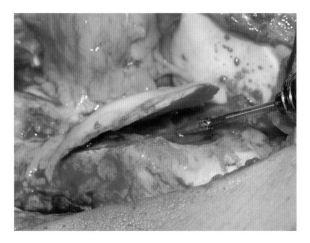

Figure CS9.7 Deepening of the anterior femoral cancellous bone using a burr

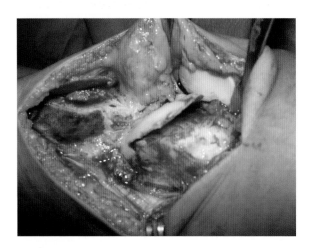

Figure CS9.6 Incomplete osteotomy of the trochlea from proximal to distal, creating an osteochondral flap

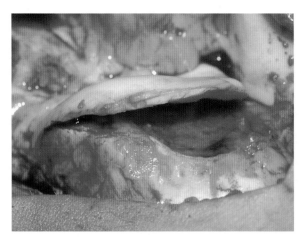

Figure CS9.8 The central rim is the deepest point, then rising slightly to lateral, proximal and medial

incision with the knife separates the articular cartilage from the synovial layer. Then the dysplastic trochlea is partially detached from the lateral condyle using a chisel, beginning proximally. The osteochondral flap remains attached distally (Figure CS9.6). It is extremely important not to break the distal attachment. Deepening of the cancellous femoral bone is now performed, using a high-speed burr (Figure CS9.7). It is important that the deepening is continued to proximal into the femoral shaft; this guarantees elimination

of the central bump.[5] The correct deepening is reached when the new surface is proximally on the same plane as the anterior femoral cortical bone (Figure CS9.8). The detached osteochondral flap of the trochlea is now thinned with a burr without removing all bone. Thinning is completed when the osteochondral flap is elastic and fits into the new form of the femur. This step is tested by carefully using a pestle. To keep the osteochondral flap in the new position and to guarantee deepening of the trochlea, the central part of the trochlea is fixed with a resorbable

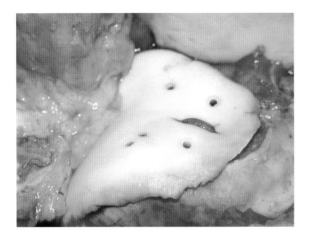

Figure CS9.9 Central fixation of the trochlea with a longitudinal suture. The drill holes are made from lateral using an aiming device. The sutures are tightened over the lateral femoral condyle

suture (Vicryl, 5 mm) (Figure CS9.9). Two lateral and two medial resorbable smart nails (length 16 mm) secure the reposition of the trochlea (Figure CS9.10). The osteotomy gap is filled with the removed cancellous bone. Single sutures adapt the synovial layer to the articular cartilage (Figure CS9.11). The final step consists of doubling the medial and lengthening the lateral structures. The tibial tuberosity is refixed with cancellous screws.

The risks of this technique include breaking of the osteochondral flap, distal detachment, and too much thinning of the flap, decreasing the blood supply.

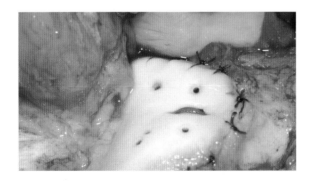

Figure CS9.10 Lateral view of the final result after trochlearplasty with deepening of the groove

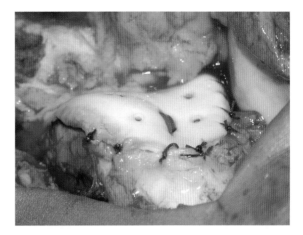

Figure CS9.11 Final result shows the new form of the trochlea. View from proximal

Postoperative care and rehabilitation

Goals

♦ Protection of the trochlea.

♦ Normalization of patellar balancing in the trochlea.

♦ Strengthening of the weak muscle groups.

Timeline

After the operation, the knee joint is placed on a continuous passive motion machine in 20° of flexion. This allows slight compression and stabilization of the new trochlea with the patella.[5]

♦ Hospital	4–6 days		
♦ Mobilization	2nd day		
♦ Weightbearing	Partial	Max. 20 kg for 6 weeks	
	Complete	After 6 weeks with correct healing of the osteotomy	
♦ Range of motion	0–20–90°	After 2 weeks unlimited	

♦ Sports	Bicycle, swimming	After 6 weeks
	Everything	After 6 months with optimal healing process and rehabilitation

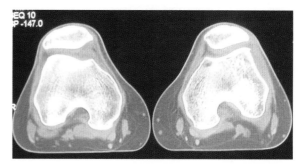

Figure CS9.13   Axial CT scan 3 months after troch-learplasty. Normal centralization of the patella (axial view, 30°, relaxed)

Discussion

The presented surgical procedure respects the underlying pathology. Deepening of the patello-femoral groove improves the osseous passive stability of the patella[2,4,5] (Figures CS9.12 and CS9.13). Soft tissue reconstruction alone is often not sufficient to stabilize the patella, especially in cases with severe trochlear dysplasia.[5] Transposition of the tibial tuberosity is not recommended in patients with dysplastic trochlea because it does not address the real pathoanatomy, but may create additional complaints.

Summary

Trochlearplasty offers a good modality to increase osseous stability of the patella. However, this procedure is strictly reserved for cases with severe dysplastic trochlea and habitual dislocation of the patella.

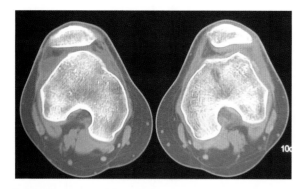

Figure CS9.12   Axial CT scan 3 months after troch-learplasty on the left side. Well-centred patella and 'normal' form of the trochlea. Note persisting subluxation on the right side after only soft tissue reconstruction (axial view, extension, relaxed)

References

1. Dejour H, Walch G, Nove-Josserand L, Guier C (1994) Factors of patellar instability: an anatomic radiographic study. *Knee Surg Sports Traumatol Arthrosc* **2**: 19–26
2. Dejour H, Walch G, Neyret P, Adeleine P (1990) [Dysplasia of the femoral trochlea]. *Rev Chir Orthop Reparatrice Appar Mot* **76**: 45–54
3. Dejour H, Walch G, Nové-Josserand L, Guier CA (1994) Diagnosis and treatment of ligament injuries about the knee. In: Feagin JA Jr (ed), *The Crucial Ligaments*. New York, Churchill Livingstone, pp 361–367
4. Bereiter H, Gautier E (1994) Die Trochleaplas-tik als chirurgische Therapie der rezidivierenden Patellaluxation bei Trochleadysplasie des Femurs. *Arthroskopie* **7**: 281–286
5. Bereiter H (2000) Die Trochleaplastik bei Trochlea-dysplasie zur Therapie der rezidivierenden Patel-laluxation. In: Wirth CJ, Rudert M (eds), *Das patellofemorale Schmerzsyndrom*. Darmstadt, Steinkopff-Verlag, pp 162–177

Suggested reading

Bereiter H, Gautier E (1994) Die Trochleaplastik als chirurgische Therapie der rezidivierenden Patellaluxation bei Trochleadysplasie des Femurs. *Arthroskopie* **7**: 281–286

Bereiter H (2000) Die Trochleaplastik bei Trochlea-dysplasie zur Therapie der rezidivierenden Patel-laluxation. In: Wirth CJ, Rudert M (eds), *Das patellofemorale Schmerzsyndrom*. Darmstadt, Steinkopff-Verlag, pp 162–177

CASE STUDY 10

Severe lateral patellar subluxation

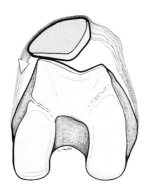

♦ What causes lateral patellar subluxation?

♦ Which structures are involved?

♦ How should we treat this problem?

Table CS10   Patellofemoral joint examination

Diagnostic clues	Findings	Diagnostic clues	Findings
Pain	Lateral more than medial	Patellar gliding mechanism	Lateralization, unstable
Tenderness	Lateral	Patellar apprehension	Positive to lateral
Effusion	None	Q angle	High value
Swelling	None	Catching	Negative
Patellar position, relaxed, 0°	Lateral subluxation with tilt	Locking	Sometimes lateral
Patellar position, contracted, 0°	Severe lateral subluxation with tilt	Range of motion	Normal
Patellar position, 30°	Well centred, minimal tilt	Radiographs	Lateral patellar subluxation
Patellar mobility	Increased to lateral	Tubercle–sulcus angle	10°, lateralization

Patellofemoral Disorders: Diagnosis and Treatment.   Edited by Roland M. Biedert
© 2004 John Wiley & Sons, Ltd   ISBN: 0-470-85011-6

History

This 18 year-old female suffered from chronic patellofemoral pain on both sides. She felt repetitive lateral subluxation of both patellae with weakness and giving-way symptoms. Complete dislocation of the patella was not reported. She was handicapped in daily life and sports activities. No trauma was documented.

Comments

Pain in combination with weakness and giving way are classic symptoms for patellar instability.[1-6] The complaints on both sides and the history support an atraumatic aetiology for the instability.

Course of action

Physical examination

The most obvious finding during physical examination was the lateral patellar subluxation with patellar tilt on both sides. Quadriceps contraction increased the lateral patellar subluxation and the tilt. The patella almost dislocated completely. A positive patellar apprehension test laterally was present. The Q angle value was nevertheless high because the tibial tubercle was lateral and the proximal tibia showed increased external rotation. This tibial external rotation causes a tubercle–sulcus angle of 10° to the lateral side. But the patella was well-centred in 30° of knee flexion and the patellar tilt was almost normal.

Radiographs

The anteroposterior and the lateral views showed mild lateral patellar subluxation.

Axial CT evaluation

The subluxation of the patella and the patellar tilt were documented in extension with relaxed

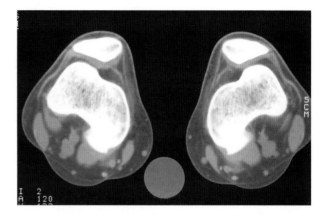

Figure CS10.1 Moderate lateral patellar subluxation with patellar tilt on both sides. The form of the trochlea and the sulcus angle are normal. The Roman arch is still visible but very low, documenting the proximal end of the femoral condyles (axial view, extension, relaxed)

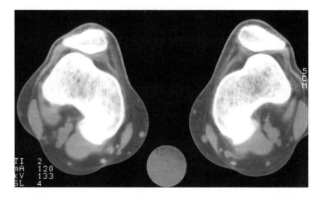

Figure CS10.2 Severe patellar subluxation to lateral with tilt. The trochlear groove is less deep, the Roman arch is still visible (axial view, extension, contracted)

quadriceps muscle (Figure CS10.1). Contraction of the quadriceps muscle caused severe patellar subluxation to lateral with tilt (Figure CS10.2). Reposition of the patella into the trochlear groove was documented in 30° of knee flexion (Figure CS10.3).

Special considerations

This severe lateral patellar subluxation is caused by different aetiological factors that can be revealed with physical examination and finally

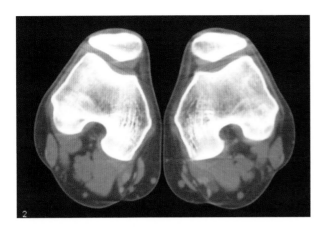

Figure CS10.3 Reposition of the left patella with normal centring in the trochlea. Mild persisting lateral subluxation with tilt of the patella on the right side. Roman arch and trochlea are normal (axial view, 30°, relaxed)

documented with axial CT scans. In particular, the following features are present (a) high Q-angle value with pathological tubercle–sulcus angle caused by high external tibial rotation;[7] (b) the patella lies in extension proximally in the trochlea, similar to a patella alta – this is documented with the shape of the Roman arch; therefore the patella has only minimal osseous stabilization in the trochlear groove;[8] and (c) normal (left side) or almost normal (right side) reposition of the patella is present in 30° of knee flexion.[8] In summary, the underlying pathoanatomy consists of two major parts: (a) increased pull of the patella to lateral, caused by the laterally positioned tibial tubercle in extension and 90° of flexion, with or without quadriceps muscle contraction; and (b) insufficient osseous stabilization of the patella in the trochlea, caused by the proximal position of the patella in a short trochlea. This must be respected in the treatment.

Plan

Treatment must eliminate lateral patellar subluxation and tilt. This can only be achieved by surgery. The surgical intervention consists of four steps:

♦ Mild medialization of the tibial tubercle in reference to the tubercle–sulcus angle (which should be 0°[7]).

♦ Lengthening of the lateral soft tissue structures; tightness is controlled in extension and flexion (in about 80°).

♦ Mild raising of the proximal lateral femoral condyle in combination with lengthening of the trochlea.

♦ Doubling of the medial soft tissue structures (retinaculum, patellofemoral ligament).

The surgical procedure begins with a parapatellar lateral incision and lateral arthrotomy, in consideration of the lengthening of the lateral soft tissue structures. The tibial tuberosity is partially detached, moved medially, and temporarily fixed with a Kirschner wire in the planned position (Figure CS10.4). The tubercle–sulcus angle must be controlled in 90° of knee flexion. When the tubercle–sulcus angle is 0°, then the tibial tubercle is fixed definitively with one or two screws (Figure CS10.5). The next step consists of the raising and lengthening of the lateral aspect of the trochlea (*see* Case Studies 7 and 18). The lateral soft tissue structures are temporarily adapted in 80° of knee flexion with some sutures.

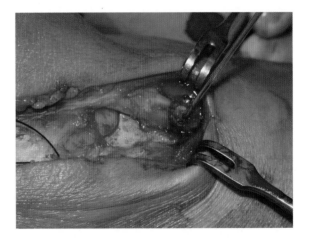

Figure CS10.4 Intraoperative view showing the temporary fixation of the tibial tuberosity and the control of the tubercle–sulcus angle

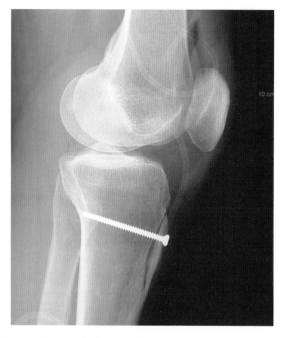

Figure CS10.5 Definitive fixation after mild and controlled medialization of the tibial tuberosity (radiograph, lateral view)

The position of the patella, the lateral displacement and the patellar glide are then controlled. The patella should remain in the trochlea, the displacement and glide of the patella to medial and lateral should be one to two quadrants.[7] If this is present, no doubling of the medial soft tissue structures is necessary. If the patellar glide or lateral patellar displacement are still pathological (i.e. more than two quadrants), then shortening of the medial patellofemoral ligament and the medial retinaculum may be necessary.

Postoperative care and rehabilitation

Goals

♦ Healing of the osteotomies of the tibial tuberosity and the lateral femoral condyle.

♦ Static and dynamic normalization of the patella balancing in the trochlea.

♦ Muscle strengthening.

Timeline

♦ Hospital	4–6 days	
♦ Mobilization	1st day	
♦ Weightbearing	Partial	Max. 15 kg for 4 weeks
	Partial	Max. 30 kg for weeks 5 and 6 postoperative
	Complete	After 6 weeks with healed osteotomies on radiographs
♦ Sports	Bicycle, swimming	After 4 weeks
	Everything	After 4 months

Summary

This case outlines the multi-aetiological problem of patellar instability. Correct evaluation needs axial CT scans. All the underlying pathologies must be taken into account in the treatment. Overcorrections (too much medialization or raising of the lateral condyle) must be strictly avoided.

References

1. Dandy DJ (1996) Chronic patellofemoral instability. *J Bone Joint Surg Br* **78**: 328–335
2. Papagelopoulos PJ, Sim FH (1997) Patellofemoral pain syndrome: diagnosis and management. *Orthopedics* **20**: 148–157; quiz 158–159
3. Dejour H, Walch G, Nove-Josserand L, Guier C (1994) Factors of patellar instability: an anatomic radiographic study. *Knee Surg Sports Traumatol Arthrosc* **2**: 19–26
4. Nove-Josserand L, Dejour D (1995) [Quadriceps dysplasia and patellar tilt in objective patellar instability]. *Rev Chir Orthop Reparatrice Appar Mot* **81**: 497–504
5. Boden BP, Pearsall AW, Garrett WE Jr, Feagin JA Jr (1997) Patellofemoral instability: evaluation and management. *J Am Acad Orthop Surg* **5**: 47–57

6. Madigan R, Wissinger HA, Donaldson WF (1975) Preliminary experience with a method of quadricepsplasty in recurrent subluxation of the patella. *J Bone Joint Surg Am* 57: 600–607
7. Kolowich PA, Paulos LE, Rosenberg TD, Farnsworth S (1990) Lateral release of the patella: indications and contraindications. *Am J Sports Med* 18: 359–365
8. Biedert RM, Gruhl C (1997) Axial computed tomography of the patellofemoral joint with and without quadriceps contraction. *Arch Orthop Trauma Surg* 116: 77–82

Suggested reading

Dejour H, Walch G, Nove-Josserand L, Guier C (1994) Factors of patellar instability: an anatomic radiographic study. *Knee Surg Sports Traumatol Arthrosc* 2: 19–26

CASE STUDY 11

Chronic patellar dislocation in adults

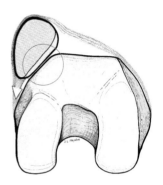

♦ What are the reasons for chronic dislocation?

♦ Which is the best imaging modality for documentation?

♦ How can we treat it?

Table CS11	Patellofemoral joint examination		
Diagnostic clues	Findings	Diagnostic clues	Findings
Pain	Diffuse patellofemoral joint	Patellar gliding mechanism	Unstable with lateral patellar dislocation near extension and partial reposition with knee flexion
Tenderness	Medial and lateral	Patellar apprehension	Severely positive to lateral
Effusion	With overload	Q angle	Normal value
Swelling	With overload	Catching	Lateral
Patellar position, relaxed, 0°	Severe lateral subluxation	Locking	Sometimes between extension and 30° flexion
Patellar position, contracted, 0°	Lateral dislocation	Range of motion	Decreased in flexion, painful
Patellar position, 30°	Lateralization, subluxation and patellar tilt	Radiographs	Dysplastic trochlea, severe patellar subluxation
Patellar mobility	Increased to lateral, decreased to medial	Other	Weakness

Patellofemoral Disorders: Diagnosis and Treatment. Edited by Roland M. Biedert
© 2004 John Wiley & Sons, Ltd ISBN: 0-470-85011-6

History

A 27 year-old female came to our clinic complaining about chronic patellofemoral pain, weakness and feelings of patellar instability. At the age of 14 years, she had had a surgical lateral release and purse-string sutures of the medial retinaculum on the left knee. She was disabled in daily life and sports activities.

Comments

The patient's history already revealed the problem of patellar instability with episodes of complete patellar dislocation. Complaints in both knees in young age are suggestive of severe dysplastic conditions of the patellofemoral joint.

Course of action

Physical examination

The physical examination of this patient revealed identical findings on both sides. The patella severely subluxed to the lateral side in extension with relaxed muscles (Figure CS11.1). Contraction of the quadriceps muscle caused complete patellar dislocation. The apprehension test was severely positive laterally. On moving the knee joint passively from extension to 30° of flexion, the patella reduced medially on the femur. The apprehension test was now negative and remained negative with increased flexion. Physical examination in the standing position showed normal static situation of the feet but excessive external rotation of the proximal tibia. Accordingly, the tibial tubercle was positioned extremely laterally. Examination of the hip joint was normal.

Radiographs

The anteroposterior view in extension showed severe lateral subluxation of the patella. The lateral views revealed a severe dysplastic trochlea.[1-4] The axial views, performed in 30° of knee flexion, showed well-centred patellae in the trochlea

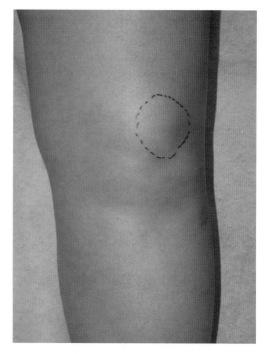

Figure CS11.1   Severe lateral patella subluxation (left knee, extension, relaxed)

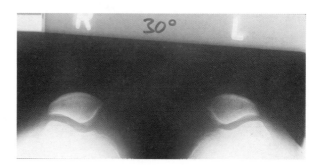

Figure CS11.2   Well-centred patellae on both sides (radiographs, axial views, 30°, relaxed)

on both sides (Figure CS11.2). This documented the significant difference of the patella position between extension and 30° of flexion.

Axial CT evaluation

Moderate lateral dislocation of the patella is documented with axial CT scans in extension (Figure CS11.3).[5,6] Quadriceps contraction even increases the amount of dislocation

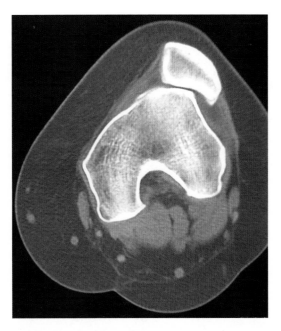

Figure CS11.3 Moderate lateral patellar dislocation on the left side (axial view, extension, relaxed)

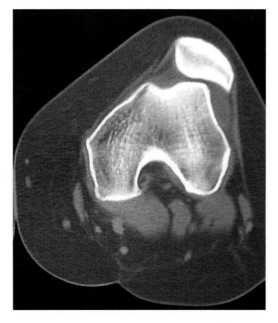

Figure CS11.5 Partial reduction of the patella with flexion (axial view, 30°, relaxed), left leg

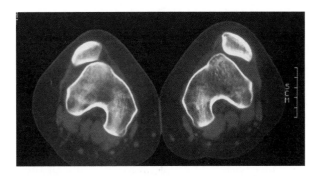

Figure CS11.4 Severe lateral patellar dislocation on both sides with quadriceps contraction. Note the dysplastic trochlea (missing trochlear groove). A neo-articulation is formed between patella and lateral condyle (axial views, extension, contracted)

but increased external rotation of the proximal tibia of 38° on the right and 34° on the left side.[2,4,8]

Special considerations

Chronic habitual patellar dislocation is a severe problem. A long history, beginning with complaints at a young age and persisting disability, documents this problem. A severe dysplastic trochlea is the underlying pathoanatomy in most of these cases and is the target of the treatment concept.

Plan

The goal of the treatment is to eliminate the dislocation of the patella. We must consider that a dysplastic trochlea is present, the medial soft tissue structures are overstretched, and the lateral structures are too tight. In addition, the patella is partially reduced in 30° of flexion during physical examination, when the femoral condyle moves

(Figure CS11.4). The trochlea is severely dysplastic and the sulcus angle cannot be measured.[7] Partial reposition of the patella on the trochlea is noted in 30° of flexion (Figure CS11.5). Additional CT scans to analyse the alignment of the lower extremity show normal femoral antetorsion

posteriorly on the tibia and the patella runs deeper into the trochlear groove.[9] The trochlea is dysplastic in the proximal part, but almost normal distally. These considerations determine the choice of the various surgical steps, which consist of:[8,10–13]

♦ Lengthening of the lateral retinacula, the iliotibial tract and the vastus lateralis tendon–muscle unit.

♦ Trochlearplasty with raising of the lateral condyle.

♦ Medialization and distalization of the tibial tuberosity.

♦ Doubling of the medial retinaculum and the medial patellofemoral ligament.

(*Note:* In 1999, Teitge, in a handout, endorsed these considerations and surgical steps.)

The intervention starts with a parapatellar lateral incision and osteotomy of the tibial tuberosity with a bone fragment of 8 × 1 × 1 cm. The pes anserinus remains attached at the tibial tuberosity. Then a lateral arthrotomy is performed, separating the lateral structures into two layers (*see* Case Study 3). Incomplete osteotomy of the lateral condyle is made with a curved chisel (*see* Case Study 6). The osteochondral flap is carefully raised 5–6 mm, using the chisel or an osteotome. Cancellous bone, which was taken at the beginning of surgery from the area of the tibial osteotomy, is put into the gap and carefully impacted (*see* Case Studies 6 and 18). This raises the lateral femoral condyle and forms the lateral trochlea. The bone fragment of the tibial tuberosity is moved medially and distally until the patella glides in the centre of the newly-shaped trochlea. It is important to control the position of the patella in extension and flexion. Temporary fixation of the tibial tuberosity using Kirschner wires allows precise corrections. The tibial tuberosity is finally fixed with two or three 4.0 cancellous screws (Figure CS11.6). The medial structures are

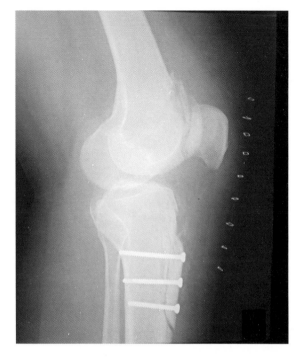

Figure CS11.6 Sagittal radiographs after reconstruction

shortened and doubled according to the new position of the patella and in reference to the patellar glide test. The lateral structures are reattached and lengthened in 80–90° of knee flexion. A diastasis remains in most cases. At the end of this individual reconstruction, the patella was 8 mm distalized and 12 mm medialized.

The risks of this technique include breaking of the osteochondral flap of the trochlea and too much distalization and medialization of the tibial tuberosity. The most difficult part is the correct balancing of the medial and lateral soft tissue structures.

Postoperative care and rehabilitation

Goals

♦ To keep the patella in the trochlea.

♦ To protect the healing of both osteotomies.

♦ To activate all stabilizing muscle groups and later to strengthen them.

Timeline

Hospital	7 days	
♦ Mobilization	2nd day	
♦ Weightbearing	Partial	10 kg for 6 weeks
	Complete	Depends on healing of osteotomies and quality of muscle control
♦ Sports	Bicycle, swimming	After 6 weeks
	Everything	Depends on final result

Discussion

The case study described represents one of the most difficult patellofemoral problems. The underlying pathoanatomy requires different surgical steps which must be adapted to each other. The correct balancing of the soft tissue structures and the amount of correction with the osteotomies need great experience. The long-term result of the present case was very positive at the

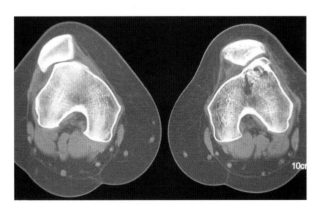

Figure CS11.7 Well-centred patella on the left side in extension. Note the healed osteotomy of the lateral femoral condyle. The lateral trochlea is raised in comparison to the nonoperated right side (axial views, extension, relaxed)

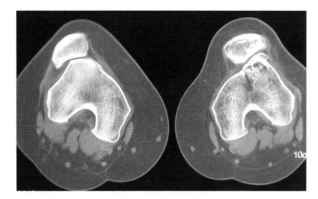

Figure CS11.8 Minimal lateralization of the patella under quadriceps muscle contraction (axial views, extension, contracted)

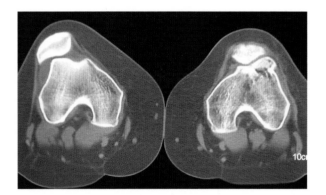

Figure CS11.9 Well-centred left patella in flexion. Note the severe lateral subluxation of the right patella, even in flexion (axial views, 30°, relaxed)

8 year follow-up, with correction of the left side only (Figures CS11.7, CS11.8 and CS11.9).

Summary

Multiple corrections and reconstructions at the same time in cases with most difficult pathologies can improve the problem but must remain in the hands of an experienced person to avoid impairment.

References

1. Walch G, Dejour H (1989) [Radiology in femoro-patellar pathology]. *Acta Orthop Belg* 55: 371–380

2. Dejour H, Walch G, Nove-Josserand L, Guier C (1994) Factors of patellar instability: an anatomic radiographic study. *Knee Surg Sports Traumatol Arthrosc* 2: 19–26

3. Dejour H, Walch G, Neyret P, Adeleine P (1990) [Dysplasia of the femoral trochlea]. *Rev Chir Orthop Reparatrice Appar Mot* 76: 45–54

4. Galland O, Walch G, Dejour H, Carret JP (1990) An anatomical and radiological study of the femoropatellar articulation. *Surg Radiol Anat* 12: 119–125

5. Biedert RM, Gruhl C (1997) Axial computed tomography of the patellofemoral joint with and without quadriceps contraction. *Arch Orthop Trauma Surg* 116: 77–82

6. Martinez S, Korobkin M, Fondren FB, Hedlund LW, Goldner JL (1983) Diagnosis of patellofemoral malalignment by computed tomography. *J Comput Assist Tomogr* 7: 1050–1053

7. Delgado-Martins H (1979) A study of the position of the patella using computerised tomography. *J Bone Joint Surg Br* 61-B: 443–444

8. Teitge RA, Faerber WW, Des Madryl P, Matelic TM (1996) Stress radiographs of the patellofemoral joint. *J Bone Joint Surg Am* 78: 193–203

9. Müller W, Wirz D (2000) Anatomie, Biomechanik und Dynamik des Patellofemoralgelenks. In: Wirth CJ, Rudert M (eds), *Das Patellofemorale Schmerzsyndrom*. Darmstadt, Steinkopff-Verlag, pp 3–19

10. Rillmann P, Dutly A, Kieser C, Berbig R (1998) Modified Elmslie–Trillat procedure for instability of the patella. *Knee Surg Sports Traumatol Arthrosc* 6: 31–35

11. Cash JD, Hughston JC (1988) Treatment of acute patellar dislocation. *Am J Sports Med* 16: 244–249

12. Hughston JC, Walsh WM, Puddu G (1984) *Patellar Subluxation and Dislocation. Saunders Monographs in Clinical Orthopaedics*, volume V. Philadelphia, PA, WB Saunders

13. Albee FH (1915) The bone graft wedge in the treatment of habitual dislocation of the patella. *Med Rec* 88: 257–259

Patellar pain and instability due to abnormal skeletal torsion

Robert Teitge

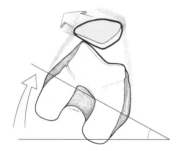

- ♦ What do we mean by 'abnormal skeletal torsion'?

- ♦ What causes patellar pain and instability?

- ♦ How can we document and treat this problem?

		Table CS12 Patellofemoral joint examination	
Diagnostic clues	Findings	Diagnostic clues	Findings
Pain	When attempting to squat	Patella gliding mechanism	Slight lateral patellar excursion
Tenderness	Medial and lateral retinaculum	Patella apprehension	Positive to medial
Effusion	Severe	Q angle	16°
Swelling	Moderate	Catching	Sometimes
Patella position, relaxed, 0°	Normal	Locking	None
Patella position, contracted, 0°	Normal	Range of motion	Normal
Patella position, 30°	Normal	Radiographs	Normal standard radiographs
Patella mobility	Increased to lateral	Other	Quadriceps atrophy, increased hip internal rotation and tibial external rotation, varus limb alignment

Patellofemoral Disorders: Diagnosis and Treatment.   Edited by Roland M. Biedert
© 2004 John Wiley & Sons, Ltd   ISBN: 0-470-85011-6

History

A 19 year-old girl presented in 1986 with complaints of painful giving-way of the left knee. She first developed the pain at age 16. An arthrogram was negative. Arthroscopic examination in 1983 revealed what appeared to be softness of the articular cartilage of the medial femoral condyle and chondroplasty was performed. There was no change in symptoms and 3 years later (3 months before consultation) she underwent a repeat arthroscopy which was nonrevealing.

The knee would give way with pain every 2 or 3 days. There was aching with sitting with the knee flexed (theatre sign) and stiffness when rising after sitting. She has not had a dislocation but she feels that the patella moves out of place. Occasionally she would manually move the patella from side-to-side to release it from a 'stuck' position. There was swelling, a sense of insecurity and a sense of weakness. She had no difficulty going up and down stairs and no limping. She was involved in no sports because of the knee.

Comments

This is one of the most common presentations of anterior knee pain. Activity-related pain is nonspecific and does not suggest either diagnosis or treatment. One must independently assess the skeletal geometry of the lower extremity, the patellofemoral ligament integrity, the condition of the articular cartilage and the musculotendinous unit. Complaints often present first in adolescence. These aspects are most likely due to growth, which increases both the length of lever arms and body mass, resulting in increased force transmission loads to a level exceeding biological tolerances. Coexisting trochlear dysplasia, patella alta, patellofemoral ligamentous laxity, excess internal femoral torsion, excess external tibial torsion, tight Achilles tendons and foot hyperpronation are common. The problem is deciding how much of each is present and which of the

variables present are the most likely offending factors. Physical examination and special studies give a clue to what may be responsible for the clinical syndrome, but in the final analysis there is no formula that gives a correct weight to each of the variables.

Course of action

Physical examination

She is 5 feet 7 inches (1.6 m) tall and weighs 128 lb (58.2 kg). The limb alignment appears to be varus, and nearly 3 inches (76 mm) separate the knees when the feet are together. The patellae point together and the feet appear to be straight. She was able to go up on her toes and back on her heels without difficulty. She could only squat to about 40° before complaining of pain. When standing on the flexed knee, the pain increased if the knee was pushed medially and decreased if the knee is pushed laterally. Motion was −5–150°; straight-leg raising was 90°; and a large effusion was present. There was no patellofemoral crepitation with active knee extension and no 'J' sign. There was a slight increase in lateral patellar excursion with side pressure applied but no apprehension; there was apprehension when the patella was pressed medially. Both patellae were equal in size. The Q angle was 16°.

There was tenderness in both the medial and lateral retinaculum. Significant atrophy of the quadriceps was present. Thigh girth at 5 inches (127 mm) above the superior pole of the left patella was 16 inches versus 18 inches (40.6 versus 45.7 cm) on the right side. The collateral and cruciate ligaments provided normal stability. McMurray and reverse McMurray tests were painful but the tests were not positive. The Ober test was zero. Prone knee flexion was 2 inches and bilaterally symmetrical. Hip internal rotation was 65° and external rotation was 20°. Foot–thigh axis was +5°.

Radiographs

Plain radiographs were considered 'normal'. The Insall ratio was 1; the trochlea on the lateral radiograph was normal. The patella was centred in the trochlea. The sulcus angle was 140° (Figure CS12.1).

Stress radiograph

Stress in the lateral direction measured 14 mm on the right side (Figure CS12.2) and 20 mm on the symptomatic left side (Figure CS12.3). Stress in the medial direction measured 14 mm on the right and 12 mm on the left.[1]

CT evaluation

CT arthrography revealed normal articular cartilage (Figure CS12.4).

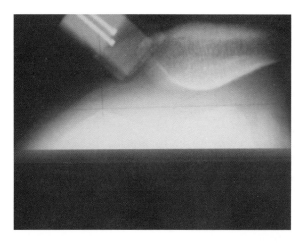

Figure CS12.3 Stress radiograph. Patella shows lateral displacement of 20 mm on the left side. The right–left difference is considered significant

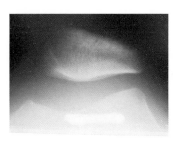

Figure CS12.1 Axial radiograph shows sulcus angle of 140° and congruence angle of 0°

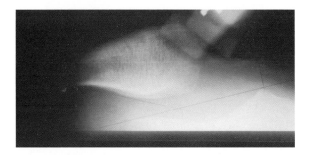

Figure CS12.2 Stress radiograph. Patella shows lateral displacement of 14 mm on the right side

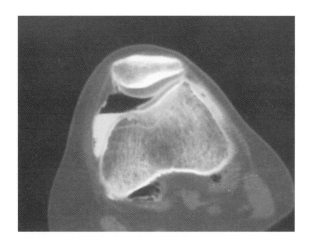

Figure CS12.4 CT arthrogram double contrast clearly images the articular cartilage. Here it is normal

Plan

Initial treatment was foot orthotics and a patellar stabilization brace. There was no improvement and 8 months later she underwent an imbrication of the medial patellofemoral ligament and medial retinaculum. At 3.5 years after surgery she stated she had been somewhat improved but then over the last 12 months, symptoms of swelling, catching and pain became worse. The reevaluation indicated that perhaps the torsional abnormality was contributing to the continuing symptoms. Further studies were ordered.

CT rotation evaluation

Measurements of the torsion of the femur revealed 26° on the right (Figure CS12.5) and 33° on the left. Tibial torsion measured 42° on the right and 51° on the left (Figure CS12.6).

Diagnosis

A diagnosis was made of lateral patellar instability associated with an excess of both femoral anteversion and an excess of external tibial torsion.

Treatment

At age 24 she underwent a 20° external rotation intertrochanteric femoral osteotomy (Figure CS12.7). At 1 year, postoperative symptoms were less than what had been present for the previous 9 years (Figure CS12.8). At 2.5 years after

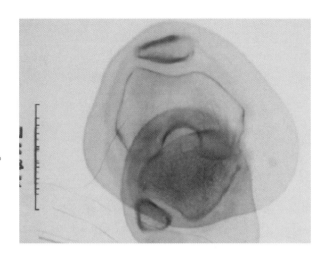

Figure CS12.6 Rotational study for tibial torsion overlaps the tibial plateau and the ankle joint. Here the external tibial torsion measures 42°. Yoshioka and Cooke[8] found that in females the normal external tibial torsion is 27°

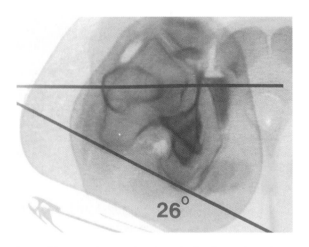

Figure CS12.5 CT rotational study for femoral torsion overlaps the femoral head, base of the neck of the femur and femoral condyles distally. Here the torsion (femoral anteversion) measures 26°. Yoshioka and Cooke[8] measured average anteversion in a set of femurs at 13°

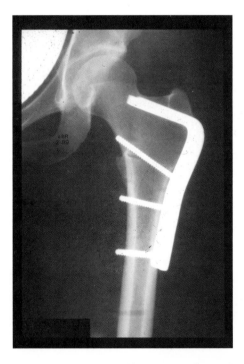

Figure CS12.7 Surgery to address excess femoral anteversion was an external femoral rotational osteotomy. This may be performed anywhere along the length of the femur. The intertrochanteric level avoids an acute angular change of the muscles which might occur if the osteotomy were performed distally

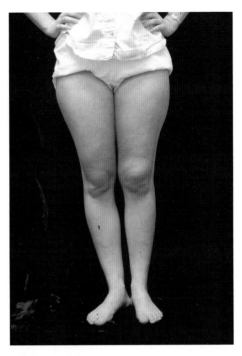

Figure CS12.8 Clinical photograph of the patient after surgery. The left femur has been externally rotated 13°. Note the apparent varus on the right, the inward pointing or squinting patella on the right and the apparent increase in outward rotation of the right foot. This is likely due to increased pronation, giving the appearance of external rotation. The left lower limb has a greater external femoral torsion

surgery she was definitely better than preoperatively and the plate was removed. Three weeks after plate removal she was able to do much more than at any time in the previous 11 years and had already returned to bowling. Five years after plate removal, she was still improved with no knee symptoms but with some soreness over the left greater trochanter.

Special considerations

This patient presented with a history and physical examination consistent with patellar subluxation (instability without dislocation). Two factors must exist for patellar instability: (a) a displacing force; and (b) a resistance to that displacing force.[1-5]

Either the normal displacing force is exerted on anatomically weak resistance structures, or an abnormally high displacing force is exerted on normal resisting structures, or a combination of both. The combination of both an increase in force and some weakness of anatomical resistance is the most common.

The displacement force is often an increase in twisting of the knee against a fixed or planted foot. The patellofemoral joint spins away from the line between the body centre of mass and the ground and the quadriceps muscle supporting knee pulls with more obliquity. If the knee is pointing inward the increased pull is lateral, and if the knee is pointing outward the increased pull is medial. Limb maltorsion produces a chronic oblique pull. The inward-pointing knee is the more common. Inward pointing of the knee occurs with an increase in femoral anteversion, external tibial torsion, pronation of the foot, tightness of the Achilles tendon and weak hip rotators (Figures CS12.9, CS12.10 and CS12.11).[6-10]

Correction of these abnormalities reduces the displacement force acting against the patella and reduces tension in the patellofemoral ligaments

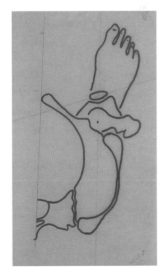

Figure CS12.9 Normal female limb torsion with a femur of 13° internal torsion and a tibia of 27° external torsion

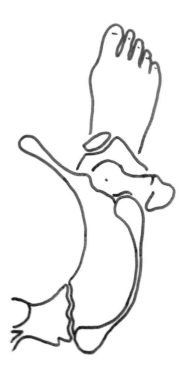

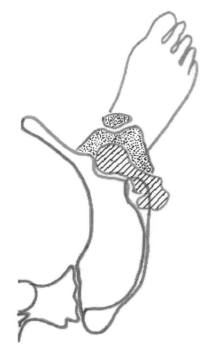

Figure CS12.10 With an increase in internal femoral torsion, the knee joint faces medially when the foot is in the position of normal foot progression angle. The foot would need to be turned outward during gait to have the knee joint moving forward. In this position the hip abductor muscles would be in a position of reduced mechanical advantage

Figure CS12.11 With an increase in external tibial torsion, the knee joint also faces medially when the foot is in the position of normal foot progression angle. The foot would need to be pointed outward to put the knee joint forward

and reduces load in the patellofemoral contact surface. Even in the presence of weak resistance to displacement, reduction of this force may eliminate instability and pain. It may be then possible to improve on instability symptoms with a femoral or tibial osteotomy without addressing the patellofemoral ligaments, trochlea or tibial tubercle. On the other hand, reconstruction of the patellofemoral ligaments may eliminate symptoms related to instability, which may or may not be sufficient to eliminate all symptoms of anterior knee pain. If maltorsion of the femur or tibia continues to exert abnormal shear forces, then these forces are not reduced through instability surgical procedures.

There are two primary anatomical structures which contribute to resist displacement:

(a) patellofemoral ligaments; and (b) bony trochlear congruence. Brattstrom[11] showed the association of trochlear dysplasia with recurrent dislocation of the patella. Dejour et al[3] expanded on this association and suggested a classification of increasing stages of dysplasia. On the other hand, Conlan et al[2] were the first to measure the contribution of ligaments to patellar stability and concluded that the medial patellofemoral ligament was the primary restraint. Secondary restraints are the medial meniscopatellar ligaments and the lateral retinaculum. Thus, releasing the lateral retinaculum would be expected to contribute to an increase in instability.

In the presence of strong resistance to displacement, the ligament may not fail, so instability does not result but continued excess force can result in the development of arthrosis, an association noted by Takai et al.[7]

There are two contributors to dislocation: (a) the dislocating force; and (b) the anatomical resistance structures. Addressing only one does not affect the other. Often in instability it is not useful to pull the patella onto the trochlea; it is necessary to rotate the trochlea back underneath the patella. Lack of awareness of this factor may account for an increased failure rate with surgery. When it is possible, addressing both factors may eventually yield better outcomes.

Summary

In the case presented here, anterior knee pain did not diminish when stability was restored, but pain was relieved after the femoral maltorsion was corrected.

References

1. Teitge RA, Faerber WW, Des Madryl P, Matelic TM (1996) Stress radiographs of the patellofemoral joint. *J Bone Joint Surg Am* 78: 193–203
2. Conlan T, Garth WP Jr, Lemons JE (1993) Evaluation of the medial soft-tissue restraints of the extensor mechanism of the knee. *J Bone Joint Surg Am* 75: 682–693
3. Dejour H, Walch G, Nove-Josserand L, Guier C (1994) Factors of patellar instability: an anatomic radiographic study. *Knee Surg Sports Traumatol Arthrosc* 2: 19–26
4. van Kampen A, Huiskes R (1990) The three-dimensional tracking pattern of the human patella. *J Orthop Res* 8: 372–382
5. Van Kampen A (1987) The Three-dimensional Tracking Pattern of the Patella. Thesis, University of Nijmegen, The Netherlands
6. Cooke TD, Price N, Fisher B, Hedden D (1990) The inward-pointing knee. *Clin Orthop* 260: 56–60
7. Takai S, Sakakida K, Yamashita F et al (1985) Rotational alignment of the lower limb in osteoarthritis of the knee. *Int Orthop* 9: 209–215
8. Yoshioka Y, Cooke TD (1987) Femoral anteversion: assessment based on function axes. *J Orthop Res* 5: 86–91
9. Yoshioka Y, Siu D, Cooke TD (1987) The anatomy and functional axes of the femur. *J Bone Joint Surg Am* 69: 873–880
10. Yoshioka Y, Siu DW, Scudamore RA, Cooke TD (1989) Tibial anatomy and functional axes. *J Orthop Res* 7: 132–137
11. Brattstrom H (1964) Shape of the intercondylar groove normally and in recurrent dislocation of the patella. *Acta Orthop Scand* Suppl 68: 1–148

Suggested reading

Teitge RA, Faerber WW, Des Madryl P, Matelic TM (1996) Stress radiographs of the patellofemoral joint. *J Bone Joint Surg Am* 78: 193–203

Yoshioka Y, Cooke TD (1987) Femoral anteversion: assessment based on function axes. *J Orthop Res* 5: 86–91

Dejour H, Walch G, Nove-Josserand L, Guier C (1994) Factors of patellar instability: an anatomic radiographic study. *Knee Surg Sports Traumatol Arthrosc* 2: 19–26

Acute patellar dislocation in children and adolescents

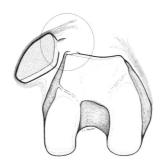

♦ What are the epidemiological factors of patellar dislocation?

♦ Which structures are injured after the initial dislocation event?

♦ What is our treatment plan?

Table CS13	Patellofemoral joint examination		
Diagnostic clues	Findings	Diagnostic clues	Findings
Pain	Medial retinaculum, medial patellofemoral ligament, adductor tubercle, vastus medialis obliquus muscle	Patellar gliding mechanism	Decreased, painful
Tenderness	Medial soft tissues, adductor tubercle	Patellar apprehension	Positive, painful to lateral
Effusion	Moderate to large	Q angle	Normal or 'abnormal'
Swelling	Moderate medial	Catching	None
Patellar position, relaxed, 0°	Moderate lateral subluxation	Locking	None
Patellar position, contracted, 0°	Increased lateral subluxation	Range of motion	Limited in flexion
Patellar position, 30°	Minimal lateralization	Radiographs	Normal or dysplastic. Sometimes avulsed osseous fragments
Patellar mobility	Increased to lateral	Other: MRI	Injuries to medial patellofemoral ligament, vastus medialis obliquus muscle, medial retinaculum, bone bruise

Patellofemoral Disorders: Diagnosis and Treatment. Edited by Roland M. Biedert
© 2004 John Wiley & Sons, Ltd   ISBN: 0-470-85011-6

History

A 12 year-old female suffered from acute patellar dislocation during alpine skiing with full giving-way. The dislocated patella required reduction in the emergency department. Effusion (haemarthrosis) and limited range of motion were present. The clinical examination revealed pain on the medial side of the patellofemoral joint and a lateral patellar instability with painful apprehension test.

Comments

Acute dislocation of the patella in children or adolescents is a severe injury that can lead to chronic pain, subluxations or recurrent dislocations.[1] Considerations about the essential pathoanatomy of the acute injury are necessary to avoid fair or poor results. Abnormalities of the lower extremity that are associated with familial or dysplastic risk factors must be assessed. The mechanism of the injury is important for treatment and prognosis. In addition, there exist numerous differences in patellar dislocation of children or adolescents in comparison to adults (due to continued development of the locomotor system).

An exact knowledge of the patient's history should be completed during the clinical examination, not only of the patellofemoral joint but also of the whole lower extremity (hips to feet).

Course of action

Physical examination

In young patients with primary acute lateral patellar dislocation we find (after reduction) effusion or haemarthrosis in over 80%,[1,2] swelling and tenderness over the adductor tubercle (Bassett's sign)[3] in 70%, tenderness along the medial retinaculum and vastus medialis obliquus,[1,2] and a positive painful apprehension test in 40%.[1]

Several anatomical alignment factors of the lower extremity must be examined at the same time: femoral and tibial torsion, foot pronation, quadriceps muscle, position (height), tilt, and mobility of the patella[1] (see Chapter 5).

Radiographs

The radiological evaluation includes three planes: anteroposterior, lateral and axial views in 30° of knee flexion. Loose bodies or avulsed fragments are noted medial to the patella in 20% of patients, and fractures of the patella itself in about 21%[1] (Figure CS13.1). Signs of trochlear dysplasia are depicted in lateral radiographs (Figure CS13.2).

Axial CT evaluation

In 0° extension with relaxed quadriceps muscle, the patella lies laterally with a mild tilt.

When the patella is subluxed, contraction of the quadriceps causes increased lateral subluxation.

As we know at this time, CT scans are not really helpful in determining the exact diagnosis, the existence of a trochlear dysplasia or the necessary treatment. MRI is a better investigative tool. It has several advantages.

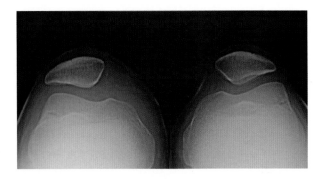

Figure CS13.1 Axial radiographs in 30° of knee flexion, showing increased lateralization of the patella on the right side after dislocation and an avulsed osseous fragment medially

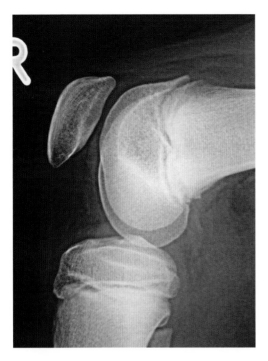

Figure CS13.2 Lateral view showing trochlea dysplasia with a present crossing sign

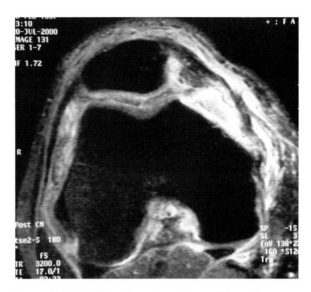

Figure CS13.3 Situation after primary dislocation, as visualized on MRI

MRI evaluation

MRI is an excellent means of investigation, with characteristic findings of injured structures after patellar dislocation.[1] A tear of the medial patellofemoral ligament from the femoral origin, at the level of the medial epicondyle, is frequent (94%).[1] The torn edge of the ligament is found deep to the distal edge of the vastus medialis obliquus muscle. Injury to the vastus medialis obliquus muscle occurs in the majority of the cases, showing cephalad displacement of the distal muscle belly. Increased signal can be present in the lateral femoral condyle or in the medial patella (bone bruises).

MRI is sensitive in visualizing the patho-anatomy of the primary dislocation (Figure CS13.3). Acute patellar dislocation is associated in most cases with a tear of the medial patellofemoral ligament–vastus medialis obliquus muscle complex from the femoral origin at the adductor tubercle. During patellar dislocation, the vastus medialis obliquus muscle is stripped away from the adductor magnus tendon, the medial patellofemoral ligament is torn, and the capsule with the patellotibial ligament is also damaged.[1] Avulsion of the medial retinaculum from the patella is rare; normally that site is not the location of the injury. This has important clinical implications for treatment.

Special considerations

First, the injury mechanism must be clear. We must differentiate between a direct blow to the knee (direct traumatic dislocation) and an indirect, self-luxating (atraumatic dislocation) valgus, flexion and external rotation mechanism of injury.[1,4] This is important for the necessary initial therapy and the long-term outcome. Traumatic dislocations have a low risk of redislocation, whereas atraumatic indirect dislocations continue to have episodes of subluxation or dislocation. The reason is the association of indirect dislocations with predisposing factors.[2,4] These factors are found in children and adolescents, such as increased femoral (antetorsion) and tibial torsion, foot pronation and genu valgum,

Table CS13.1   Differences on the lower extremity between children/adolescents and adults with regard to predisposing factors for patellar dislocation[4]

Localization	Differences	Factors		Age
		In general	Specific patellofemoral joint	
Proximal femur	Increased antetorsion angle ♦ Children: 30–40° ♦ adults: ca. 12–15°	Internal rotation lower extremity	Internal rotation of distal femur with lateral patellar subluxation	Newborn, normalization during growth in most cases
Distal femur	Open epiphysis	Femoral condyle not modified	Flat trochlea, no osseous stabilization	Trochlea deepened and lateral femoral condyle is formed during adolescence
Foot/ankle	Increased internal rotation, minus torsion of the bi-malleolar axis	Increased foot pronation	Increased internal rotation proximal tibia	Normalization in most cases during growth
Complete axis of the leg	Newborn with varus axis, increased valgus axis, especially in females	Increased valgus axis	Tendency for lateral patellar subluxation	Normalization depending on different factors

tight lateral retinaculum, patella alta, dysplastic trochlea, generalized ligament laxity and vastus medialis muscle deficiency.[1,2,4–8] It is important to know the differences of the predisposing factors between children, adolescents and adults (Table CS13.1).

Damage to the medial capsuloligamentous structures, including the vastus medialis obliquus muscle, occurs if the patella has dislocated.[1,3] Conlan et al,[9] Burks et al,[10] and Desio et al[11] found that the medial patellofemoral ligament is the major medial soft tissue restraint preventing lateral displacement of the patella. It contributes an average of 53% of the total restraining force. This underlines the importance of the medial patellofemoral ligament and that repair of this ligament restores stability in the majority of cases.[1] In addition, repair of this ligament seems to restore the normal orientation of the vastus medialis obliquus muscle, reestablishing its normal posterior insertion to the medial epicondyle. Sallay et al[1] believe that the medial patellofemoral ligament is dynamized by the vastus medialis obliquus muscle and that the two function as a complex that acts to prevent patellar dislocation. The repair of the injured structures, i.e. the real pathological anatomy, is the key for successful treatment. Isolated lateral release, distal advancement of the medial insertion of the vastus medialis obliquus muscle (a different biomechanical vector than the medial patellofemoral ligament), midretinacular placation, and distal bony realignment may all fail because they do not address the primary pathological entity associated with patellar dislocation, especially the posterior rupture of the medial patellofemoral ligament close to the medial epicondyle.[1] Lengthening of the lateral retinaculum (not release) may be indicated, in conjunction with medial patellofemoral ligament repair in cases with a very tight lateral structure.

Plan

Treatment after patellar dislocation is conservative or operative. Conservative treatment includes partial weightbearing, stabilization of the patella with an elastic bandage, brace or posterior splint,[12] and physical therapy. Nevertheless, the results are not good enough, with 63% having continued episodes of subluxation or dislocation and 50% with fair or poor subjective results.[1,12]

In contrast, short-term results with acute repair of the injury are promising.[13–15] In the study performed by Sallay et al,[1] none of the surgically treated patients have experienced recurrent dislocations. It must be considered that in children and adolescents only soft-tissue reconstruction is possible. This is a major difference in comparison with adults.

In cases with multiple lesions (present case), surgery is performed using a lateral incision. In isolated injuries, surgery may be performed through a medial incision. In the present case, the exposed joint showed an avulsed bony fragment, fissuring of the lateral condyle and a dysplastic trochlea (Figure CS13.4). Inspection of the medial side revealed complete rupture of the medial patellofemoral ligament near the medial epicondyle and of the vastus medialis obliquus complex (Figure CS13.5).

After removal of the detached fragment, the reconstruction consisted of three steps. First, moderate raising of the lateral condyle distal to the epiphysis was performed by an osteotomy

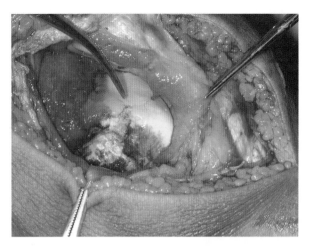

Figure CS13.4 Lateral intraoperative view showing the avulsed fragment, cartilage fissuring, flat trochlea and thickened suprapatellar plica (right knee)

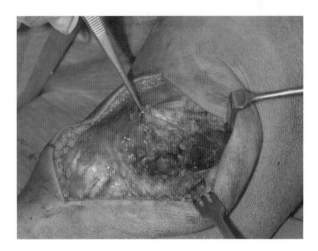

Figure CS13.5 Intraoperative findings on the medial side. The medial patellofemoral ligament–vastus medialis obliquus complex is ruptured close to the medial epicondyle. The torn medial patellofemoral ligament is lifted with forceps (right knee, view from anteromedial)

and insertion of cancellous bone to correct the dysplastic flat trochlea and to create a nearly normal sulcus angle (Figure CS13.6). Second, the lateral retinaculum was adapted with lengthening at the same time. Third, anatomical reconstruction on the medial patellofemoral ligament–vastus medialis oblique complex was performed (Figure CS13.7). When raising the lateral

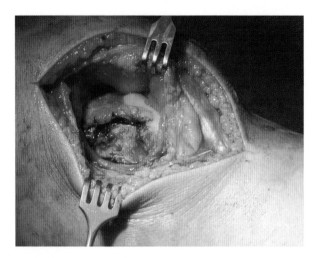

Figure CS13.6   Lateral view showing the lateral condyle after raising the trochlea

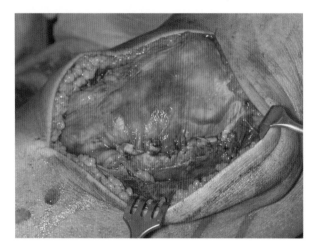

Figure CS13.7   Medial side after the reconstruction with sutures. Note the relatively posterior rupture line of the medial patellofemoral ligament and vastus medialis obliquus

condyle, caution is absolutely mandatory not to damage an open epiphysis. If there is any doubt, only soft tissue reconstruction is recommended.

An open exploration of the isolated injured medial patellofemoral ligament is performed after an oblique incision (about 4 cm) is made directly over the medial epicondyle[1] (*see* Case Study 6). The covering fascia is incised carefully so as not to injure the branches of the saphenous nerve. The distal belly of the vastus medialis obliquus muscle and the torn edge of the medial patellofemoral ligament are identified deep to the covering fascia and retracted superiorly and anteriorly. When a residual stump of the ligament in the area of the medial epicondyle is present, direct suture repair of the ligament is possible. With an area of bare bone where the ligament was avulsed, suture anchors (metallic or biodegradable) or drill holes placed vertically along the anterosuperior border of the tubercle facilitate repair of the ligament directly to bone.

Postoperative care and rehabilitation

Goals

♦ Stabilization of the patella in the trochlea.

♦ Avoidance of recurrent dislocations.

♦ Strengthening of the stabilizing muscles.

Timeline

♦ Hospital	3–5 days	
♦ Mobilization	2nd day	
♦ Weightbearing	Partial	4–6 weeks
	Complete	After 6 weeks
♦ Sports	Bicycle, crawl	After 4 weeks
	Everything	After 4 months; depends on final result

Early functional rehabilitation with immediate range of motion between 0–0–80° and muscle activation is recommended. All braces or sleeves are optional.

Summary

Acute primary lateral patellar dislocation leads to an injury of the medial patellofemoral ligament at the medial epicondyle in more than 90% of cases.[1,13] This is therefore the real place of the pathoanatomy. Surgical treatment of patellar dislocation has not been very successful up to now because it did not address to the true location of injury.

Nonoperative treatment also has had a high failure rate.[1,4] Acute and precise repair of the medial patellofemoral ligament and elimination of predisposing factors improve the postoperative outcome.[1,13–15] A different approach and plan of treatment seems to be necessary, especially in children and adolescents.

References

1. Sallay PI, Poggi J, Speer KP, Garrett WE (1996) Acute dislocation of the patella. A correlative pathoanatomic study. *Am J Sports Med* **24**: 52–60
2. Atkin DM, Fithian DC, Marangi KS et al (2000) Characteristics of patients with primary acute lateral patellar dislocation and their recovery within the first 6 months of injury. *Am J Sports Med* **28**: 472–479
3. Bassett FH (1976) Acute dislocation of the patella, osteochondral fractures, and injuries to the extensor mechanism of the knee. *Instr Course Lect* **25**: 40–49
4. Biedert RM (2002) Patellaluxation beim Kind und Jugendlichen. *Sportorthopädie-Sporttraumatologie* **18**: 164–168
5. Hughston JC, Walsh WM, Puddu G (1984) *Patellar Subluxation and Dislocation. Saunders Monographs in Clinical Orthopaedics*, volume V. Philadelphia, PA, WB Saunders
6. Reider B, Marshall JL, Warren RF (1981) Clinical characteristics of patellar disorders in young athletes. *Am J Sports Med* **9**: 270–274
7. Cash JD, Hughston JC (1988) Treatment of acute patellar dislocation. *Am J Sports Med* **16**: 244–249
8. Arnbjornsson A, Egund N, Rydling O, Stockerup R, Ryd L (1992) The natural history of recurrent dislocation of the patella. Long-term results of conservative and operative treatment. *J Bone Joint Surg Br* **74**: 140–142
9. Conlan T, Garth WP Jr, Lemons JE (1993) Evaluation of the medial soft-tissue restraints of the extensor mechanism of the knee. *J Bone Joint Surg Am* **75**: 682–693
10. Burks RT, Desio SM, Bachus KN et al (1998) Biomechanical evaluation of lateral patellar dislocations. *Am J Knee Surg* **11**: 24–31
11. Desio SM, Burks RT, Bachus KN (1998) Soft tissue restraints to lateral patellar translation in the human knee. *Am J Sports Med* **26**: 59–65
12. Mäenpää H, Matti U, Lehto UK (1997) Patellar dislocation. The long-term results of nonoperative management in 100 patients. *Am J Sports Med* **25**: 213–217
13. Tuxoe JI, Teir M, Winge S, Nielsen PL (2002) The medial patellofemoral ligament: a dissection study. *Knee Surg Sports Traumatol Arthrosc* **10**: 138–140
14. Boden BP, Pearsall AW, Garrett WE Jr, Feagin JA Jr (1997) Patellofemoral instability: evaluation and management. *J Am Acad Orthop Surg* **5**: 47–57
15. Vainionpaa S, Laasonen E, Silvennoinen T et al (1990) Acute dislocation of the patella. A prospective review of operative treatment. *J Bone Joint Surg Br* **72**: 366–369

Suggested reading

Sallay PI, Poggi J, Speer KP, Garrett WE (1996) Acute dislocation of the patella. A correlative pathoanatomic study. *Am J Sports Med* **24**: 52–60

CASE STUDY 14

Acute patellar dislocation in adults

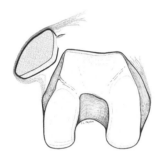

♦ What are the reasons for the first acute dislocation?

♦ How can we document the pathoanatomy?

♦ What is our treatment concept?

	Table CS14 Patellofemoral joint examination		
Diagnostic clues	Findings	Diagnostic clues	Findings
Pain	Diffuse patellofemoral joint	Patellar apprehension	Severely positive to lateral
Tenderness	Diffuse, medial more than lateral	Q angle	Normal value
Effusion	Haemarthrosis	Catching	Sometimes
Swelling	Diffuse	Locking	Sometimes with osteo-chondral fragment
Patellar position, relaxed, 0°	Lateralization after reposition	Range of motion	Flexion decreased
Patellar position, contracted, 0°	Lateralization	Radiographs	Normal or dysplastic trochlea, bone fragment
Patellar position, 30°	Often not enough flexion	Other	Weakness of the quadriceps muscle
Patellar mobility	Increased to lateral		
Patellar gliding mechanism	Unstable, painful		

Patellofemoral Disorders: Diagnosis and Treatment. Edited by Roland M. Biedert
© 2004 John Wiley & Sons, Ltd ISBN: 0-470-85011-6

History

This 26 year-old male sustained a direct trauma to his left patella from the medial side, thus producing a first complete patellar dislocation to lateral. Reposition of the patella was necessary under anaesthesia in the emergency room.

Comments

Even moderate violence may be sufficient to cause an inherently weak patellofemoral joint to dislocate. Often it is difficult to state whether pathological conditions, such as patella alta, dysplastic trochlea, torsional abnormalities of the lower extremity or ligament laxity, are responsible for the resultant instability of the joint.[1-3] Physical examination and additional investigations help to determine the underlying pathoanatomy.

Course of action

Physical examination

Before repositioning, the dislocated patella lay laterally beside the femoral condyle and the trochlear groove was empty. After repositioning, the patella was slightly lateralized. Excessive haemarthrosis is frequent (Figure CS14.1). This, together with the pain, weakens the quadriceps activity and severely decreases knee flexion. Palpation is especially painful over the injured medial soft tissue structures.

Radiographs

Before repositioning, anteroposterior and axial views showed a completely dislocated patella. After repositioning, the anteroposterior view may show slight lateralization of the patella (ruptured medial structures). The lateral view may reveal a dysplastic trochlea (Figure CS14.2).The axial view may show an osteochondral fragment (Figure CS14.3).

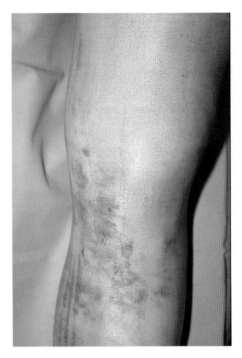

Figure CS14.1   Excessive haematoma after complete lateral patellar dislocation (anteroposterior view, left knee)

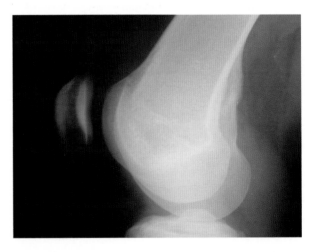

Figure CS14.2   Dysplastic trochlea with crossing sign (lateral view)

Axial CT evaluation

Axial CT scans are helpful to analyse the congruence of the patellofemoral joint and the form of

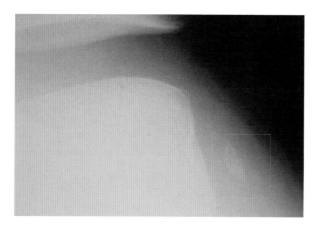

Figure CS14.3 Osteochondral fragment lateral to the femoral condyle after complete patellar dislocation (radiograph, axial view, left knee)

the trochlea.[3-5] In cases with severe soft tissue injuries on the medial side documented by MRI, CT scans are not mandatory for surgery, because the indication for open revision and reconstruction is already given.

Special considerations

Acute and first complete patellar dislocations may be treated conservatively or operatively. Indications for a surgical intervention are excessive soft tissue injury on the medial side, such as rupture of the medial patellofemoral ligament, retinaculum and aponeurosis of the vastus medialis obliquus muscle, osteochondral fractures, massive haemarthrosis and dysplastic trochlea. Nonsurgical treatment often leads to unsuccessful healing and habitual patellar dislocations.[3,6,7] However, the results of the nonoperative treatment depend on the quality of conservative management and the underlying pathoanatomy.[8,9]

Plan

The aim of the treatment is to stabilize the patella and to eliminate the risk of further dislocations. The radiographs of this patient showed a dysplastic trochlea and an osteochondral fragment on the lateral side. These were the indications for the surgical intervention.

After a lateral parapatellar incision, the patellofemoral joint was already open on the medial side, caused by the complete ruptures of the retinaculum and the medial patellofemoral ligament (Figure CS14.4). This facilitated access to the joint through the medial posttraumatic gap. Inspection of the joint revealed a dysplastic trochlea with a completely flat lateral femoral condyle (Figure CS14.5). These findings determined the following surgical steps:

♦ Raising the lateral femoral condyle (Figure CS14.6).

♦ Removing the osteochondral fragment.

♦ Suturing and reconstructing the medial stabilizing structures (*see* Case Studies 6 and 13).

♦ Lengthening the lateral retinaculum (*see* Case Studies 6, 8, 13 and 18).

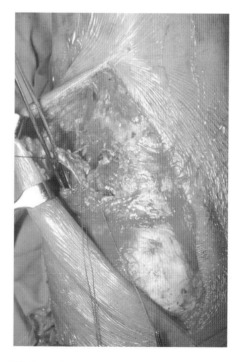

Figure CS14.4 Intraoperative anteroposterior view showing the ruptured soft tissue structures on the medial side (left knee)

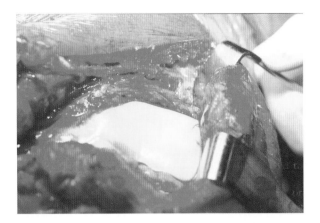

Figure CS14.5 Intraoperative anterolateral view showing the flat dysplastic trochlea (patella retracted with hooks to lateral; left knee)

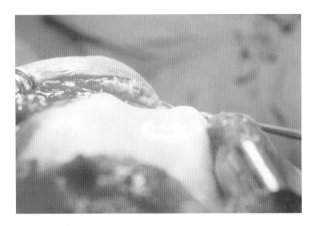

Figure CS14.6 Intraoperative anterolateral view of the reconstructed trochlea after raising the lateral femoral condyle. Note the 'normal' trochlear groove, improving the osseous stability of the patella

Postoperative care and rehabilitation

Goals

♦ Stabilization of the patella.

♦ Protection of the healing of the medial and lateral soft tissue structures and the osteotomy.

♦ Dynamic muscular balancing of the patella in the trochlea.

Timeline

♦ Hospital	5–7 days	
♦ Mobilization	2nd day	
♦ Weightbearing	Partial	10 kg for 4 weeks
	Complete	After 6 weeks, depending on healing of osteotomy and muscular control
♦ Brace	Sometimes	With excessive soft tissue injuries
♦ Sports	Bicycle	After 4 weeks
	Everything	Depends on final result but not before 4 months

Summary

The presented case describes a clear diagnostic situation. The keypoints are the predisposing factors. Precise evaluation of the real pathoanatomy is mandatory for the selection of treatment and the prevention of redislocations. Surgical treatment is recommended when an obvious pathology is documented and the risk for the development of habitual patellar dislocations is high.[3,8,9]

References

1. Macnicol MF (1986) *The Problem Knee.* London, William Heinemann Medical Books
2. Hutchinson MR, Ireland ML (1995) Patella dislocation. *Physician Sportsmed* **23**: 53–60
3. Biedert RM (2002) Patellaluxation beim Kind und Jugendlichen. *Sportorthopädie-Sporttraumatologie* **18**: 164–168
4. Biedert RM, Gruhl C (1997) Axial computed tomography of the patellofemoral joint with and without quadriceps contraction. *Arch Orthop Trauma Surg* **116**: 77–82

5. Martinez S, Korobkin M, Fondren FB et al (1983) Diagnosis of patellofemoral malalignment by computed tomography. *J Comput Assist Tomogr* **7**: 1050–1053

6. Vainionpää S, Laasonen E, Silvennoinen T et al (1990) Acute dislocation of the patella. A prospective review of operative treatment. *J Bone Joint Surg Br* **72**: 366–369

7. Mäenpää H, Matti U, Lehto UK (1997) Patellar dislocation. The long-term results of nonoperative management in 100 patients. *Am J Sports Med* **25**: 213–217

8. Arnbjornsson A, Egund N, Rydling O et al (1992) The natural history of recurrent dislocation of the patella. Long-term results of conservative and operative treatment. *J Bone Joint Surg Br* **74**: 140–142

9. Atkin DM, Fithian DC, Marangi KS et al (2000) Characteristics of patients with primary acute lateral patellar dislocation and their recovery within the first 6 months of injury. *Am J Sports Med* **28**: 472–479

Suggested reading

Mäenpää H, Matti U, Lehto UK (1997) Patellar dislocation. The long-term results of nonoperative management in 100 patients. *Am J Sports Med* **25**: 213–217

Vainionpää S, Laasonen E, Silvennoinen T et al (1990) Acute dislocation of the patella. A prospective review of operative treatment. *J Bone Joint Surg Br* **72**: 366–369

CASE STUDY 15

Local chondral damage of the trochlea

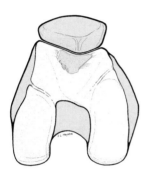

♦ What is the cause of the local damage?

♦ What is the reason for the effusion?

♦ What is our treatment plan?

Table CS15	Patellofemoral joint examination		
Diagnostic clues	Findings	Diagnostic clues	Findings
Pain	None or only mild	Patellar apprehension	Normal
Tenderness	Suprapatellar pouch	Q angle	Normal
Effusion	Moderate to severe	Catching	Possible
Swelling	Moderate to severe	Locking	Possible
Patellar position, relaxed, 0°	'Dancing' patella	Range of motion	Limited in flexion
Patellar position, contracted, 0°	Normal	Radiographs	Normal
Patellar position, 30°	Normal	CT	Normal
Patellar mobility	Normal or increased (effusion)	MRI	Local cartilage damage
Patellar gliding mechanism	Normal with crepitations	Other	Decreased activity quadriceps, decreased strength and tone

Patellofemoral Disorders: Diagnosis and Treatment.   Edited by Roland M. Biedert
© 2004 John Wiley & Sons, Ltd   ISBN: 0-470-85011-6

History

A 32 year-old male soccer player suffered from acute knee joint effusion. Pain was only present in the suprapatellar pouch when the knee was maximally flexed. All meniscal or stability tests were normal. No serious trauma was noted.

Comments

Acute knee joint effusion represents a significant sign of intraarticular derangement. The clinical signs for meniscal injuries or instability are missing, but the effusion focuses on a present cartilage problem. Chondral debris leads to irritation of the synovial membrane and causes the joint effusion. Supraphysiological loading or chondral damage may cause intraarticular debris.

It is helpful to know under which conditions the effusion was noted. Was it after trauma or atraumatic, painful or free of pain, was it the first time or repetitive?

Course of action

Physical examination

Patients with isolated cartilage damage have moderate to severe effusion without real pain. They complain about pressure or tension in the suprapatellar pouch during forced flexion and weakness in the joint. The quadriceps contraction is decreased. Patients even have problems stimulating the muscle. Palpation reveals liquid in the joint, without a localized painful area. All rotational movements and stability are normal.

Radiographs

The radiological evaluation in three planes shows no osseous abnormality. Signs of joint effusion are depicted (capsule distension).

Axial CT evaluation

This evaluation is not necessary except in specific situations, such as patellar subluxation.

MRI evaluation

MRI is the best means of documenting localized chondral damage. The present knee joint effusion gives sufficient contrast to depict cartilage fissuring or destruction (Figure CS15.1). Cuts at different levels may show partially detached chondral flaps at the border of the central damage (Figure CS15.2).

In the absence of joint effusion, contrast medium (diluted gadolinium) may be injected intraarticularly (MR arthrotomography) or intravenously [gadolinium-diethylenetriamine

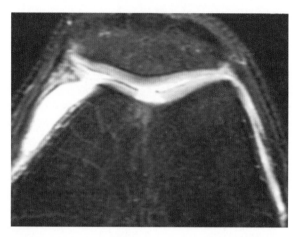

Figure CS15.1 Axial MRI scan showing localized cartilage destruction in the centre of the trochlea (T2-weighted, left knee, extension)

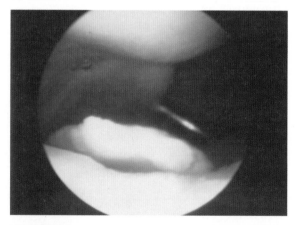

Figure CS15.2 Arthroscopic view showing chondral damage in the centre of the trochlea. Note the partially detached chondral flaps using a probe

penta-acetic acid (Gd-DTPA)] to depict minimal chondral lesions.

Plan

Isolated damage to the central area of the trochlea occurs relatively often during the second part of a sports career. The aetiological factors are unclear in many cases. Also, we have observed local chondral destruction in patients with normal patellofemoral alignment and balance. Direct anterior trauma to the patella or repetitive increased maximal loading in flexion may lead to cartilage fissuring, a sign of the beginning of chondral destruction. Once chondral flaps are partially detached, mechanical loading causes cartilage debris and irritation of the synovial membrane. At this moment, the risk of enlarging the area of destruction is high. This risk determines the necessary therapy. Treatment should stop the effusion and slow down cartilage destruction. This may be achieved by arthroscopic debridement.

Arthroscopy consists of general inspection of the joint and washing out of the effusion. A precise evaluation of the amount of cartilage damage is needed, using a probe. Unstable chondral flaps are removed carefully with a full-radius resector.[1] It is important to debride all loose cartilage to form a stable border of healthy cartilage around the defect (Figure CS15.3).

To enhance chondral resurfacing, the microfracture technique is a common and successful procedure.[1,2] This treatment provides a suitable environment for new tissue formation by the body's own healing potential. Microfracture is done using specially designed cartilage awls (chondropics) to produce multiple perforations, or microfractures, into the subchondral bone plate[1] (Figure CS15.4). Perforations are made approximately 3–4 mm apart to avoid one perforation breaking into another. The subchondral plate is left intact, thus preserving the load-bearing cortical bone.[2] The correct depth of perforation is reached (2–4 mm) when fat droplets and blood can be seen coming from the

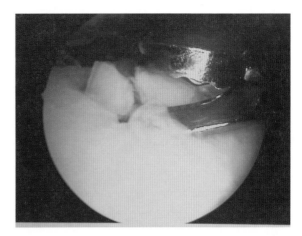

Figure CS15.3 Arthroscopic view showing removal of chondral flaps from the trochlea

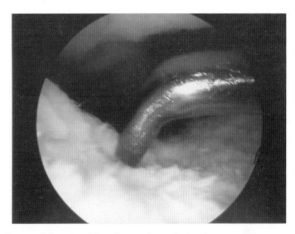

Figure CS15.4 Microfracturing of the destruction zone using chondropics. Perforation of the subchondral zone is needed

marrow cavity.[1] Microfracture starts in the periphery of the defect, then the holes are made towards the centre. The released marrow elements include mesenchymal stem cells, growth factors and other healing proteins, and form a surgically induced superclot that provides an enriched environment for new tissue formation.[1] No intraarticular drains are placed because the marrow elements should cover the lesion.

Postoperative care and rehabilitation

The rehabilitation programme after microfracture is crucial for successful treatment of chondral defects. Protection of the immature clot is the cornerstone of postoperative care. Avoidance of axial, torsional and shear stress to the defect is mandatory. Nonweightbearing is required for 6 weeks postoperatively.[2] The use of a brace is recommended to avoid the compression of the regenerating surfaces. The allowed range of motion depends on the location of the defect. Continuous passive motion (CPM) is prescribed for 8 weeks postoperatively, 6–8 hours a day.[1,2] Complete rehabilitation time after surgery is 4–9 months.

Goals

♦ Protection of the regenerating surface.

♦ Continuous passive motion.

♦ Elimination of the joint effusion.

Timeline

♦ Hospital	2–3 days	
♦ Mobilization	1st day	
♦ Weightbearing	None	For 6 weeks
	Partial	For weeks 7–10
♦ Sports	Bicycle, swimming	After 3 weeks
	Everything	Not before 4 months, depends on final result

Summary

Acute pain-free joint effusion is suggestive of chondral damage. The central trochlea represents a frequent area of localized and isolated cartilage destruction. The aetiological cause is unclear in most cases; repetitive overloading or direct trauma on the patella are possible. Continued detachment of chondral pieces must be avoided. Arthroscopic debridement in combination with microfracture is the recommended treatment to attain sufficient results, but structural damage is always present.

References

1. Steadman JR, Rodkey WG, Rodrigo JJ (2001) Microfracture: surgical technique and rehabilitation to treat chondral defects. *Clin Orthop* **391** (suppl): 362–369
2. Sledge SL (2001) Microfracture techniques in the treatment of osteochondral injuries. *Clin Sports Med* **20**: 365–377

Suggested reading

Steadman JR, Rodkey WG, Rodrigo JJ (2001) Microfracture: surgical technique and rehabilitation to treat chondral defects. *Clin Orthop* **391** (suppl): 362–369

CASE STUDY 16

Secondary medial patellar instability following lateral retinacular release

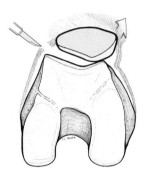

- ◆ Does the lateral retinacular release cause medial instability?

- ◆ How can we document medial patellar instability?

- ◆ Is there a surgical solution?

Table CS16	Patellofemoral joint examination

Diagnostic clues	Findings	Diagnostic clues	Findings
Pain	Diffuse around the patella	Patellar gliding mechanism	Unstable
Tenderness	More medial than lateral	Patellar apprehension	To medial more positive than to lateral, painful
Effusion	None	Catching	Walking downstairs
Swelling	Moderate	Locking	None
Patellar position, relaxed, 0°	Normal	Range of motion	Normal
Patellar position, contracted, 0°	Mild medialization	Radiographs	Normal
Patellar position, 30°	Normal	Other: manual pressure applied to patella	Severe medial patellar subluxation
Patellar mobility	Markedly increased to medial		

Patellofemoral Disorders: Diagnosis and Treatment.   Edited by Roland M. Biedert
© 2004 John Wiley & Sons, Ltd   ISBN: 0-470-85011-6

History

A 24 year-old female rowing athlete suffered from bilateral patellofemoral pain. Surgery was performed on both sides. Lateral retinacular release was performed 2 years ago, which caused additional pain and weakness. She was unable to compete or even to strengthen her muscles by performing squats. Moderate impairment in daily life resulted and loss of strength of the quadriceps muscles occurred.

Comments

The performed surgical treatments could not eliminate the initial pain and complaints. Surgery created additional weakness and discomfort.

Course of action

Physical examination

Clinical examination revealed diffuse tenderness and pain on palpation around the patellofemoral joint. No effusion but moderate swelling was noted. The mobility of the patella to medial was markedly increased and extremely painful. Medial patellar dislocation was almost possible when applying manual pressure from the lateral side (Figure CS16.1).

The apprehension, patellar relocation and gravity subluxation tests[1] were severely positive. Muscle atrophy and functional weakness were present during manual muscle testing. Both knees showed the same findings.

Axial CT evaluation

Axial CT scans in 0 degrees extension with and without quadriceps contraction showed no obvious pathology. Severe medial subluxation/dislocation of the patella was noted when applying a medially directed manual pressure on the lateral patellar facet (Figures CS16.1 and CS16.2). Secondary medial patellar instability is

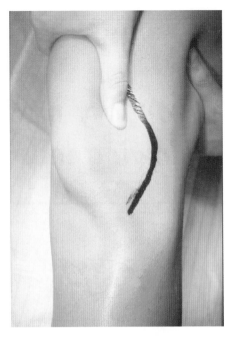

Figure CS16.1   Lateral manual pressure subluxates the patella to medial (left knee). Continued line shows the incision of the lateral retinacular release

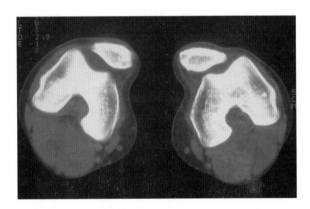

Figure CS16.2   Severe medial subluxation/dislocation on both sides following lateral retinacular release (extension, relaxed, manual pressure from lateral)

documented using stress CT scans[2] (Chapter 8). This gives the unequivocal proof of secondary medial patellar instability.[2–6]

Special considerations

Lateral retinacular release is a procedure widely performed to eliminate patellar tilt, to release tight lateral soft tissue structures, and to reduce the tendency of lateral patellar subluxation or dislocations. It is described as an effective surgical procedure to alleviate pain particularly in patients with lateral patellar compression syndrome.[7–10] However, some patients experience a secondary and different patellofemoral pain after surgery. Increased mobility of the patella with a tendency for medial subluxation is present in such patients and has led to the assumption that medial instability is a possible sequel of the lateral release operation. Kolowich et al[9] found an incorrect technique with over-release or preoperative subluxation and increased tilt to be associated with a poor postoperative result. Biedert and Friederich[3] described the poor clinical outcome of failed lateral release. Wrong indications (unspecific patellofemoral pain) and incorrect surgical procedures were the main reasons for failure. Hughston and Deese[11] reported the development of medial patellar subluxation in 50% of their patients who failed to improve after arthroscopic lateral retinacular release. All cases with medial subluxation demonstrated an atrophy of the vastus lateral muscle. Nonweiler and DeLee[1] found increased medial subluxation associated with a disturbed integrity of the vastus lateralis muscle-tendon unit. They ascribed the instability to the failure of the quadriceps to pull the patella into the patellofemoral groove due to the detached tendon.

The lateral retinaculum is an important static structure which, in complex interplay with the intraarticular components and the dynamic structures, ensures patellofemoral stability and correct balancing of the patella in the trochlea.[3] The position of the patella, the central pivotal point of the knee extensor mechanism, is thus controlled also by the passive lateral patellar structures.[3,11–16]

The release of the lateral retinaculum results in biomechanical changes of the position of the patella and of its gliding behavior in the trochlea.[2,3,7–9,11,17–20] Medial subluxation of

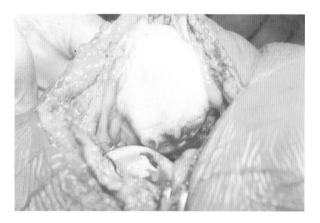

Figure CS16.3 Cartilage damage only on the medial patellar facet, caused by secondary medial patellar instability with medial subluxations (left knee)

the patella may cause cartilage destruction (Figure CS16.3).

The therapeutic effects of lateral retinacular release are not clear and still a matter of controversy. Some suggest that reduction of the pressure in the patellofemoral joint may lead to a temporary recovery of the cartilage resulting from a shift of the contact surface area.[21] Some believe that the incision of the lateral retinaculum interrupts, in chronic cases, the pain transmission from possible neuroma documented in patients with patellofemoral malalignment.[22–26]

Plan

Elimination of the medial subluxation of the patella is the goal to strive for. Normal stability and mobility with gliding mechanism of the patella must be regained. This requires open revision with secondary reconstruction of the lateral structures using the present scar tissue or, if insufficient, a quadriceps tendon graft[2,12] (see Case Study 19). (Figures CS16.4, CS16.5 and CS16.6).

The lateral retinaculum is reconstructed with respect to a normal patella mobility of 1 to 2 quadrants.[9,12]

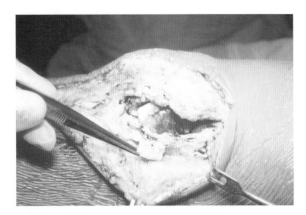

Figure CS16.4 Preparation of the scar tissue for the secondary reconstruction of the lateral retinaculum

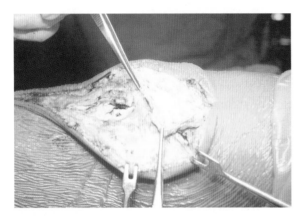

Figure CS16.5 Check of the possible closure

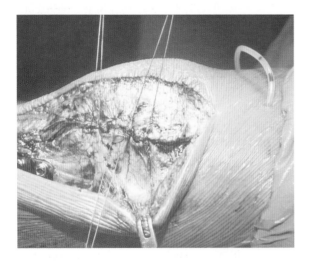

Figure CS16.6 Final result of the secondary reconstruction of the lateral retinaculum. The knots are definitively tied in about 80° of knee flexion

Postoperative care and rehabilitation

Goals

♦ Decrease of swelling and pain.

♦ Strengthening of the weak muscles.

♦ Regain normal patellar mobility.

Timeline

♦ Hospital　　　　3–4 days
♦ Mobilization　　1st day
♦ Weightbearing　4 weeks from 10 kg to
　　　　　　　　　　20 kg
♦ Sports　　　　　Everything after 3 months

Summary

This case outlines the secondary medial patellar instability with medial subluxations of the patella following lateral retinacular release. Subsequent muscular weakness with passive medial instability (Case Study 17) are additional problems in patients' history.

These observations must be a warning for the generalized noncritical use of lateral retinacular release in patients with unspecific patellofemoral pain. Clear indications for lateral retinacular release are rare. Unique patellar tilt without any other pathology may be one indication. Instead of lateral retinacular release, we recommend lengthening of the lateral retinaculum to avoid medial patellar subluxation (Case Studies 3 and 6).

References

1. Nonweiler DE, DeLee JC (1994) The diagnosis and treatment of medial subluxation of the patella after lateral retinacular release. *Am J Sports Med* **22**: 680–686
2. Teitge RA, Faerber WW, Des Madryl P, Matelic TM (1996) Stress radiographs of the patellofemoral joint. *J Bone Joint Surg Am* **78**: 193–203
3. Biedert RM, Friederich NF (1994) Failed lateral retinacular release: clinical outcome. *J Sports Traumatol* **16**: 162–173

4. Biedert RM (2000) Is there an indication for lateral release and how I do it. In: Proceedings of the International Patellofemoral Study Group, Garmisch-Partenkirchen, Germany

5. Biedert RM (2003) Complicated case studies. In: Sanchis-Alfonso V (ed), *Anterior Knee Pain and Patellofemoral Instability in the Active Young. The Black Hole of Orthopaedics*. Medica Panamericana, Madrid, Spain, 287–301 (in press)

6. Biedert RM (2000) 124 operations to treat 10 patients suffering from patellofemoral pain. What was wrong? In: Proceedings of the International Patellofemoral Study Group, Garmisch-Partenkirchen, Germany

7. Larson RL, Cabaud HE, Slocum DB et al. (1978) The patellar compression syndrome: surgical treatment by lateral retinacular release. *Clin Orthop* **134**: 158–167

8. Metcalf RW (1982) An arthroscopic method for lateral release of subluxating or dislocating patella. *Clin Orthop* **167**: 9–18

9. Kolowich PA, Paulos LE, Rosenberg TD, Farnsworth S (1990) Lateral release of the patella: indications and contraindications. *Am J Sports Med* **18**: 359–365

10. Henry JH, Goletz TH, Williamson B (1986) Lateral retinacular release in patellofemoral subluxation. Indications, results, and comparison to open patellofemoral reconstruction. *Am J Sports Med* **14**: 121–129

11. Hughston JC, Deese M (1988) Medial subluxation of the patella as a complication of lateral retinacular release. *Am J Sports Med* **16**: 383–388

12. Biedert RM, Gruhl C (1997) Axial computed tomography of the patellofemoral joint with and without quadriceps contraction. *Arch Orthop Trauma Surg* **116**: 77–82

13. Terry GC (1989) The anatomy of the extensor mechanism. *Clin Sports Med* **8**: 163–177

14. Ficat P (1970) *Pathologie Fémorale-Patellaire*. Paris, Masson

15. Müller W (1982) *Das Knie*. Heidelberg, Springer-Verlag

16. Busch MT, DeHaven KE (1989) Pitfalls of the lateral retinacular release. *Clin Sports Med* **8**: 279–290

17. Dzioba RB (1990) Diagnostic arthroscopy and longitudinal open lateral release. A four-year follow-up study to determine predictors of surgical outcome. *Am J Sports Med* **18**: 343–348

18. McGinty JB, McCarthy JC (1981) Endoscopic lateral retinacular release: a preliminary report. *Clin Orthop* **158**: 120–125

19. Betz RR, Magill JT III, Lonergan RP (1987) The percutaneous lateral retinacular release. *Am J Sports Med* **15**: 477–482

20. Ceder LC, Larson RL (1979) Z-plasty lateral retinacular release for the treatment of patellar compression syndrome. *Clin Orthop* **144**: 110–113

21. Hille E, Schulitz KP, Henrichs C, Schneider T (1985) Pressure and contract-surface measurements within the femoropatellar joint and their variations following lateral release. *Arch Orthop Trauma Surg* **104**: 275–282

22. Biedert RM, Kernen V (2001) Neurosensory characteristics of the patellofemoral joint: what is the genesis of patellofemoral pain? *Sports Med Arthrosc Rev* **9**: 295–300

23. Biedert RM, Sanchis-Alfonso V (2002) Sources of anterior knee pain. *Clin Sports Med* **21**: 335–347

24. Sanchis-Alfonso V, Rosello-Sastre E, Monteagudo-Castro C, Esquerdo J (1998) Quantitative analysis of nerve changes in the lateral retinaculum in patients with isolated symptomatic patellofemoral malalignment. A preliminary study. *Am J Sports Med* **26**: 703–709

25. Fulkerson JP (1982) Awareness of the retinaculum in evaluating patellofemoral pain. *Am J Sports Med* **10**: 147–149

26. Fulkerson JP, Tennant R, Jaivin JS, Grunnet M (1985) Histologic evidence of retinacular nerve injury associated with patellofemoral malalignment. *Clin Orthop* **197**: 196–205

Suggested reading

Biedert RM, Friederich NF (1994) Failed lateral retinacular release: clinical outcome. *J Sports Traumatol* **16**: 162–173

Hughston JC, Deese M (1988) Medial subluxation of the patella as a complication of lateral retinacular release. *Am J Sports Med* **16**: 383–388

CASE STUDY 17

Secondary medial patellar instability following lateral retinacular release documented by gait analysis

Roland M. Biedert and **I. A. Kramers-de Quervain**

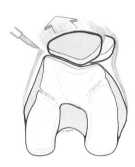

♦ What causes medial patellar instability?

♦ Which investigations are necessary for documentation?

♦ What is our treatment plan?

Table CS17	Patellofemoral joint examination		

Diagnostic clues	Findings	Diagnostic clues	Findings
Pain	Diffuse around the patella	Patellar gliding mechanism	Unstable
Tenderness	Moderate medial and lateral	Patellar apprehension	Positive to lateral and especially painful to medial
Effusion	None	Catching	Walking downstairs
Swelling	Mild	Locking	None
Patellar position, relaxed, 0°	Normal	Range of motion	Normal
Patellar position, contracted, 0°	Normal	Radiographs	Normal or mild osteoarthritis
Patellar position, 30°	Normal	Other: gait analysis	Abnormal medial translation of the patella. Functional weakness
Patellar mobility	Markedly increased to medial and lateral		

Patellofemoral Disorders: Diagnosis and Treatment.   Edited by Roland M. Biedert
© 2004 John Wiley & Sons, Ltd   ISBN: 0-470-85011-6

History

Lateral retinacular release combined with medio-patellar plica resection was performed on the left side in this 22 year-old woman due to anterior knee pain. The previous symptoms disappeared with surgery, but a different type of knee pain developed around the patella. A knee rehabilitation programme did not help to reduce the pain. With regard to the results of the physical examination and patient's history, a gait analysis was used as a diagnostic tool to look for patellar instability 3 years after surgery.[1]

Comments

This history reveals a special problem – the surgical treatment eliminated the initial pain but, with time, created a different secondary pain and disorder.

Course of action

Physical examination

Range of motion was normal for all lower extremity joints. The left knee joint was tender around the patella. A mild swelling was present, but no effusion. The mobility of the patella, both medial and lateral, was markedly increased compared with the opposite asymptomatic side. The apprehension sign and gravity subluxation test were positive. The thigh circumference on the affected side was smaller (by 2 and 1 cm as measured 10 and 15 cm, respectively, above the superior border of the patella) than on the noninvolved side. Functional weakness was present during manual muscle testing. The opposite knee was without symptoms.

Radiographs

The standard radiographs did not reveal obvious pathology.

Axial CT evaluation

In 0° extension and relaxed, the left patella showed mild lateralization with a normal right side (Figure CS17.1). The trochlea was normal on both sides. Lateralization increased with quadriceps contraction (Figure CS17.2). The lateral subluxation of the patella was combined on the right side with patellar tilt, on the left side with lateral joint space narrowing. In 30° of flexion, normal centralization was noted on both sides (Figure CS17.3).

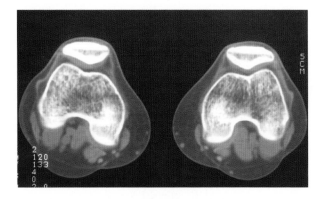

Figure CS17.1 Normal trochlea on both sides. The right patella is well-centred, the left patella is minimally lateralized (axial view, extension, relaxed)

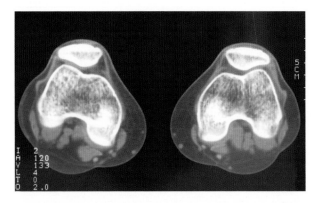

Figure CS17.2 Quadriceps contraction increases the lateralization of the patella on both sides, combined with a mild patellar tilt on the right side. Note the narrowing of the osseous contours of patella and trochlea on the left side (axial view, extension, contracted)

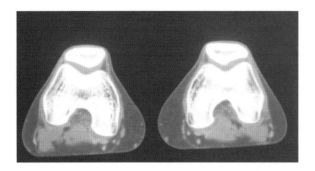

Figure CS17.3 Normal centralization of both patellae with increased flexion. Minimal tilt on the right side (axial view, 30°, relaxed)

We found a discrepancy between the findings in the physical examination (patellar instability to medial) and the results of the axial CT evaluation. With normal CT scans, we could not document medial patellar instability, only mild dynamic lateralization of the patella. Documentation of patellar instability requires stress CT scans[2] (*see* Case Study 16 and Chapter 8).

This patient felt functional weakness, instability of the patella, and catching going down the stairs. Therefore, we decided to perform a gait analysis to gain more insight into the functional balancing of the patella during walking.

Gait analysis

Gait performance was assessed at the Laboratory for Biomechanics of the Swiss Federal Institute of Technology (ETH), Zürich, Switzerland. Three-dimensional motion analysis was performed using a five-camera VICON System (Oxford Metrics Ltd) for data capture. A dynamic eight-channel electromyographic system with surface electrodes (Laboratory for Biomechanics) was used for dynamic electromyography. The ground reaction forces were recorded by four three-dimensional Kistler force plates (Kistler Instrumente AG, Winterthur). Kinematic, kinetic- and electromyographic data were collected simultaneously while the patient walked over a 25 m walkway. The patient was asked to walk at her most comfortable speed (self-selected free gait velocity). Regular video recordings were performed in addition to the computer-assisted and instrumented gait analysis.

Video recordings were performed with a Sony EVO-9100P Hi 8 camera using a shutter speed of 1/1000 s. A strict frontal view of several trials of free walking was recorded, focusing on the lower extremities. The position of the patella was marked (circled) on the skin while the knee was extended (in the standing position) (Figure CS17.4). For data analysis, the patella position and translation beneath the skin were monitored by watching the video in slow motion and comparing the affected side with the opposite side. By observing the movements 'frame by frame', it was possible to recognize the phase of the gait cycle during which abnormal patellar translation occurred.

For kinematic analysis data capture, 21 spherical retroreflective markers (diameter 25 mm) were

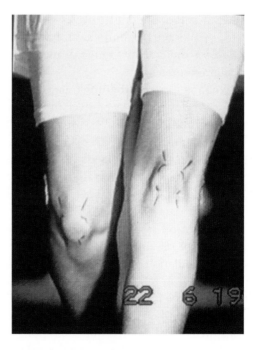

Figure CS17.4 Images taken from the video recordings, focusing on the knee with medial patellar instability. Loading of the affected left leg. The patella remains within the skin marks on both sides

placed over anatomical landmarks of the trunk and the upper and lower extremities. The five phase-locked and strategically placed VICON cameras recorded the marker position coordinates bilaterally at a sampling rate of 60 Hz. This recording technique allowed a simultaneous assessment of motion of both lower extremities as well as the trunk and arm positions. With a calibrated measuring volume of $4 \times 2 \times 2$ m it was possible to record two sequential gait cycles (four steps) during each trial.

Further data processing was performed by the biomechanical analysis package ANALYZE, written by Meglan[3] and adapted by our laboratory. The kinematic analysis was based upon the principles of three-dimensional rigid body mechanics. Segment position and orientation were calculated relative to a global coordinate system, using the recorded marker-based information and anthropometric data. Individual joint angles were then calculated relative to a joint-centred coordinate system, referenced to the proximal segment. Mean values of six gait cycles were computed for peak knee flexion in stance and swing phase and for the dynamic range of motion during weight acceptance.

For dynamic electromyographic data capture, surface electrodes were placed over the following muscle groups bilaterally – vastus medialis and vastus lateralis, rectus femoris, medial and lateral hamstrings, and the medial head of the gastrocnemius. The sampling rate for the electromyographic signal was 480 Hz. The raw electromyographic data were filtered by a high-pass filter with a cut-off frequency of 30 Hz. Onset and duration of the individual activity phases as well as modulation of the activity amplitude were interpreted in relation to the simultaneously recorded motion data.

For kinetic analysis data capture, the ground reaction forces were recorded at a sampling rate of 240 Hz by four three-dimensional Kistler force plates, which were embedded in the floor in the middle of the 25 m walkway. The vertical, mediolateral and fore–aft forces were all mapped, normalized to body weight. The force plate recordings were further analysed by a parameter analysis programme, developed at the Laboratory. Specific parameters, such as the peak values of the vertical ground reaction forces and the loading and unloading rates, were used for side-to-side comparison. Eight trials were analysed.

The following time/distance parameters were calculated from kinematic and force plate readings: velocity, cadence, stride length, step length, and the relative and absolute duration of the individual gait phases. The gait phases are total stance time, single-limb stance time, and double-limb stance time of each side.

Results

Video recording

During weight acceptance (loading response), the patella position remained within the circle marked on the skin on both sides (Figure CS17.4). In late stance phase, however, during rapid knee flexion prior to toe-off, a fast translation of the patella towards medial occurred on the affected left side. The contour of the patella moved 'beneath' the skin mark towards medial and back again (Figure CS17.5). Such a patellar translation could not be observed on the opposite side.

Time/distance parameters

The patient walked at a free-gait velocity of 1.42 m/s with a cadence of 115 steps/min and a stride length of 1.49 m (ratio of stride length/leg length = 1.65). She had a slightly longer right-step length (right-step length, 0.76 m; left-step length, 0.73 m). The timing of the individual gait phases was normal and symmetrical, without indication of a limp.

Kinematic analysis

Motion pattern was normal at the hip, knee and ankle on the affected side. In particular,

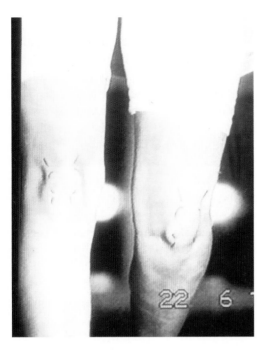

Figure CS17.5 Taken during unloading of the affected left leg, demonstrating the marked patellar translation toward medial beneath the skin marks on the affected side

normal loading-response knee flexion was seen, indicating a sufficient function of the active extensor mechanism during level gait. On the opposite side she had slightly more knee flexion during stance, with a side difference of peak knee flexion during weight acceptance of 5°.

Dynamic electromyography

Affected left side

All parts of the quadriceps muscle studied (rectus femoris, vastus medialis and vastus lateralis) on the affected side showed a normal timing during gait; the activity period started during the second half of the swing phase and lasted into weight acceptance. During single-limb stance and weight release, no quadriceps activity was observed. Activity of the hamstrings was normal.

Contralateral right side

On the right side the activity period of the quadriceps was prolonged into single-limb stance (rectus femoris and vastii). The activity period of the hamstrings was normal, lasting throughout weight acceptance. The gastrocnemius and tibialis anterior had normal activity patterns on both sides.

Kinetic analysis

Analysis of the ground reaction forces revealed a normal and symmetrical dynamic behaviour during level gait, without indication of a limp or favouring of one side.

Special considerations

Medial patellar instability is a known complication after lateral release surgery. Typical symptoms and clinical findings have been described by several authors.[4–9] A possible objective investigation method was used by Teitge (Teitge RA, handout, 1988), performing patellofemoral stress radiographs. Miller et al[7] and Biedert and Friederich[4] described documentation by computed tomography. Shellock[9] assessed the patellar alignment by kinematic magnetic resonance imaging. However, all these examination techniques investigate the patellar laxity in a passive situation, without considering the functional activity period of the muscles acting around the knee. Kramers-de Quervain et al[1] first described the relationship of patellar instability to the activity period of the quadriceps muscle group during a given function. The muscles may be imbalanced or the quadriceps may fail to pull the patella into the patellofemoral groove due to the detached tendon. Knowledge about this activity period is crucial for further treatment planning, particularly if muscle strengthening is considered as a treatment method.

Instrumented gait analysis revealed a normal gait pattern, reflected by motion, electromyographic and force-plate recordings. It demonstrated a sufficient function of the active extensor mechanism (quadriceps) on the affected side during level gait, with a normal loading response knee flexion. There was no evidence of a quadriceps avoiding pattern. The patient examined was able to walk at a high self-selected gait velocity, compared with accepted normal values, consisting of a normal-to-high cadence and stride length.

Except for a slight asymmetry of step length, no evidence of a limping gait pattern was present. The force plate recordings in particular demonstrated a normal dynamic behaviour without favouring one side. The medial patellar instability, documented by the video recording, occurred during unloading of the leg in late stance and preswing, prior to toe-off. This was seen without change in the overall motion pattern and without a limping behaviour. While the knee was rapidly bending in preparation for the swing phase, an increased medial translation of the patella occurred. This is a period during the gait cycle when the muscles around the knee are usually silent.[10,11] This was also the case in our subject, as documented by the dynamic electromyographic recordings in combination with motion analysis. During the regular activity period of the quadriceps (end of swing phase and weight acceptance) we observed a normal motion pattern, with a normal loading response knee flexion in the kinematic analysis and a centred position of the patella seen in the video recording.

Plan

In reference to the documented medial patellar instability, secondary reconstruction of the lateral retinacula was performed, using mobilized local scar tissue (*see* Case Study 16). The patient returned to full sports activity level 3 months after surgery.

Summary

The global gait performance of our subject was quantified by instrumented gait analysis techniques with graphical and numerical documentation of the motion pattern in relation to the activity periods of the muscles around the knee. The

patellar instability itself was documented qualitatively by video recordings and by comparison of the two sides. Due to the relative skin motion, it was not possible to quantify further this fast translational movement of the patella using surface markers. The selected method, involving circling the patella position on the skin, allowed a visual documentation of the patella translation beneath the skin. Documentation of this abnormal patella translation was possible because the instability was severe enough to be visible on the video recording.

This case demonstrates that even in the presence of a medial patellar instability, the active quadriceps mechanism can be sufficient to allow a high gait velocity with a normal loading response knee flexion and with a centred patella during loading. It also demonstrates that visible patellar instability can occur while the patella is guided by the passive structures only. Our finding of the timing of the medial subluxation stresses the importance of the integrity of the passive restraining structures and weakens the argument of muscular imbalance as a major cause for failed lateral release surgery. This also explains why an exercise rehabilitation programme was unsuccessful in improving the symptoms in our patient. We conclude, therefore, that treatment of failed lateral release surgery not only has to address the muscle imbalance but also imbalance of the passive structures.[1]

References

1. Kramers-de Quervain IA, Biedert R, Stüssi E (1997) Quantitative gait analysis in patients with medial patellar instability following lateral retinacular release. *Knee Surg Sports Traumatol Arthrosc* 5: 95–101
2. Teitge RA, Faerber WW, Des Madryl P, Matelic TM (1996) Stress radiographs of the patellofemoral joint. *J Bone Joint Surg Am* 78: 193–203
3. Meglan DA (1991) Enhanced Analysis of Human Locomotion. Thesis, The Ohio State University, Columbus, OH

4. Biedert RM, Friederich NF (1994) Failed lateral retinacular release: clinical outcome. *J Sports Traumatol* **16**: 162–173

5. Hughston JC, Deese M (1988) Medial subluxation of the patella as a complication of lateral retinacular release. *Am J Sports Med* **16**: 383–388

6. Nonweiler DE, DeLee JC (1994) The diagnosis and treatment of medial subluxation of the patella after lateral retinacular release. *Am J Sports Med* **22**: 680–686

7. Miller PR, Klein RM, Teitge RA (1991) Medial dislocation of the patella. *Skeletal Radiol* **20**: 429–431

8. Holmes PF, Henry JH (1989) The results of extensor mechanism realignment following failed lateral retinacular releases. *Clin Sports Med* **8**: 291–296

9. Shellock FG, Mink JH, Deutsch A et al (1990) Evaluation of patients with persistent symptoms after lateral retinacular release by kinematic magnetic resonance imaging of the patellofemoral joint. *Arthroscopy* **6**: 226–234

10. Kadaba MP, Ramakrishnan HK, Wootten ME et al (1989) Repeatability of kinematic, kinetic, and electromyographic data in normal adult gait. *J Orthop Res* **7**: 849–860

11. Murray MP, Mollinger LA, Gardner GM, Sepic SB (1984) Kinematic and EMG patterns during slow, free, and fast walking. *J Orthop Res* **2**: 272–280

Suggested reading

Kramers-de Quervain IA, Biedert R, Stüssi E (1997) Quantitative gait analysis in patients with medial patellar instability following lateral retinacular release. *Knee Surg Sports Traumatol Arthrosc* **5**: 95–101

CASE STUDY 18

Secondary distal medial subluxation with osteoarthritis and persisting proximal lateral subluxation

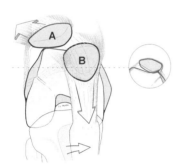

♦ What are the reasons for lateral and medial subluxation?

♦ Which structures are involved in the problem?

♦ Which treatment may be successful?

Diagnostic clues	Findings	Diagnostic clues	Findings
Pain	Lateral proximal and distal medial patellofemoral joint, medial femorotibial joint	Patellar gliding mechanism	Unstable, crepitations, pain
Tenderness	Diffuse	Patellar apprehension	Positive to medial and to lateral
Effusion	Following overload	Catching	Proximal lateral and distal medial
Swelling	Chronic	Locking	Sometimes near 30° flexion
Patellar position, relaxed, 0°	Normal	Range of motion	Normal
Patellar position, contracted, 0°	Lateral subluxation	Radiographs	Osteoarthritis, patellofemoral joint and medial femorotibial joint
Patellar position, 30°	Medial subluxation	Other	Varus axis lower extremity
Patellar mobility	Increased to medial and lateral		

Table CS18   Patellofemoral joint examination

Patellofemoral Disorders: Diagnosis and Treatment.   Edited by Roland M. Biedert
© 2004 John Wiley & Sons, Ltd   ISBN: 0-470-85011-6

History

This 42 year-old female patient suffered from habitual lateral patellar dislocations. The first dislocation occurred when she was a 15 year-old adolescent. She underwent numerous surgical procedures with repetitive releases of the lateral retinaculum and three times increased medialization of the tibial tuberosity. Medialization of 28 mm from the normal tibial shaft axis finally resulted, but the proximal lateral patellar subluxations and even lateral dislocations continued to occur. The major complaints included pain on the medial patellofemoral and femorotibial side, muscular weakness, swelling, and impairment in daily activities.

Comments

Even excessive medialization of the tibial tuberosity could not eliminate the persisting lateral patellar dislocations. But in addition, severe pain on the whole medial side of the knee was created over the years.

Course of action

Physical examination

The physical examination revealed pain and tenderness on palpation on the medial aspect of the patellofemoral and femorotibial joints as well as proximal lateral on the patellofemoral joint.

Effusion with chronic swelling was noted. The patella was spontaneously subluxed to medial with relaxed muscles, but pulled superolaterally with subluxation under quadriceps contraction. The apprehension test was severely positive medially and laterally. The patellar mobility increased to medial and lateral. Positive signs for meniscal pathology were noted on the medial side. Varus axis was present in the one-leg standing position.

Radiographs

The long monopodal anteroposterior view documented different pathologies (Figures CS18.1 and CS18.2).

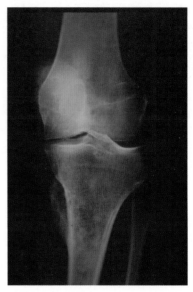

Figure CS18.1 Anteroposterior view shows varus axis with lateral thrust of the head of the tibia, severe osteoarthritis on the medial femorotibial joint, medial subluxation of the patella, and excessive medialization of the tibial tuberosity (monopodal)

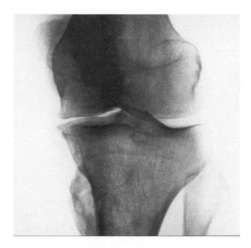

Figure CS18.2 Same patient, documenting the excessive medialization of the tibial tuberosity and the degenerative changes on the medial femorotibial joint compartment. Note the spontaneous medial subluxation of the patella (anteroposterior view, monopodal)

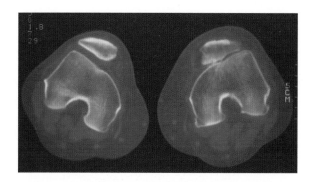

Figure CS18.3 Severe medial osteoarthritis of the patellofemoral joint with medial subluxation of the patella (left side). Trochlear dysplasia is present on both sides (axial views, extension, relaxed)

Axial CT evaluation

Severe medial subluxation of the patella with osteoarthritis was documented in normal axial CT scans (Figure CS18.3). Osseous narrowing documented destruction of the cartilage in the medial patellofemoral joint. Osteophytes, especially on the medial femoral condyle, documented femorotibial osteoarthritis.

Special considerations

Excessive medialization of the tibial tuberosity caused overloading of the medial patellofemoral and femorotibial joints, resulting in severe degenerative changes with osteoarthritis.[1,2] The medial subluxation of the patella increased the destruction of the medial part of the patellofemoral joint. Medial overload also caused destruction of the medial meniscus and changed the force vector of the whole extensor mechanism. In time, this overload caused varus alignment with opening instability of the lateral femorotibial joint by overstretching the lateral active and passive structures.

In spite of the distal excessive medializations of the tibial tuberosity, the proximal patellar subluxations and dislocations persisted. This documents that the dysplastic trochlea with the flat lateral condyle is still the persisting pathoanatomy causing the instability.[3-5]

This case reveals several major problems at the same time as a consequence of the initial underlying pathoanatomy and the secondarily caused pathology.

♦ Varus alignment with bicompartmental medial osteoarthritis.

♦ Overcorrection of the tibial tuberosity (medialization).

♦ Dysplastic trochlea.

♦ Distal medial patellar subluxation.

♦ Proximal lateral patellar subluxation or dislocation.

♦ Medial meniscal injury.

Plan

The treatment must eliminate the different problems described. The specific steps are summarized in Table CS18.1.

Postoperative care and rehabilitation

Goals

♦ Centring and stabilizing the patella in the trochlea.

♦ Decreasing the pain.

♦ Improving neuromuscular control.

Timeline

♦ Hospital	7 days	
♦ Mobilization	2nd day	
♦ Weightbearing	Partial	10 kg for 6 weeks
	Complete	After 8 weeks
♦ Full recovery time	4 months	
♦ Sports	Bicycle, swimming	After 4–6 weeks
	Everything	After 6 months

Table CS18.1 Surgical steps to treat the documented pathologies

Pathology	Surgical procedure
♦ Excessive medialization of the tibial tuberosity (Figures CS18.4 and CS18.5), distal medial patellar subluxation	→ Re-Elmslie with complete osteotomy of the tibial tuberosity and reposition according to the normal anatomy (Figure CS18.6)
♦ Trochlear dysplasia (Figure CS18.7), proximal lateral patellar subluxation	→ Reconstruction of the lateral trochlea by raising the lateral condyle (Figure CS18.8)
♦ Varus alignment with medial osteoarthritis (Figures CS18.1 and CS18.2)	→ High tibial valgization osteotomy (Figure CS18.6)
♦ Medial meniscal injury	→ Arthroscopic meniscus resection
♦ Insufficient lateral retinaculum, medial patellar instability	→ Secondary reconstruction of the lateral structures using scar tissue

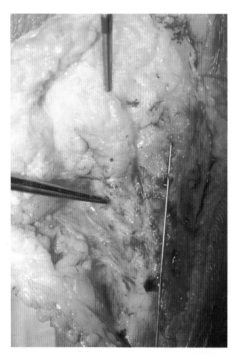

Figure CS18.4 Intraoperative anterior view showing the excessive medialization of the tibial tuberosity (left forceps indicates the centre), the normal axis of the tibial shaft (K wire), and the lateral border of the patella (forceps at the top) (left knee)

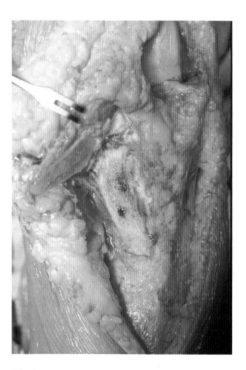

Figure CS18.5 Intraoperative anterior view shows the excessive medialization after osteotomy of the tibial tuberosity (detached and retracted with a hook) (left knee)

The patient had a physical examination and axial CT scans 6 years after the surgical procedures described. Medial and lateral patellar subluxations and dislocations had disappeared and medial pain was markedly reduced. She had almost free range of motion. CT evaluation

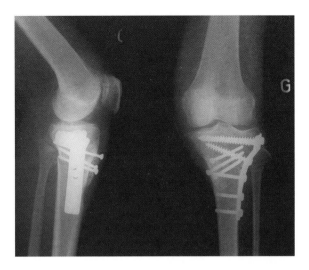

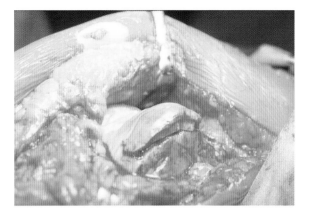

Figure CS18.8 Situation after reconstruction of the lateral condyle. The osteotomy is filled with bone from the tibial head. Note the subsequent 'normal' sulcus angle after raising the lateral condyle in comparison to the initial situation (*see* Figure CS18.7) (left knee)

Figure CS18.6 Sagittal and anteroposterior radiographs after reposition of the tibial tuberosity and high tibial valgization osteotomy (monopodal, left knee). Note the valgus axis with decreased load in the medial femoro-tibial compartment

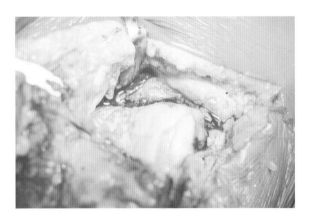

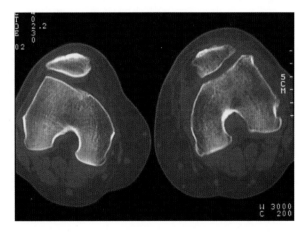

Figure CS18.9 Same patient as Figure CS18.3, 6 years after surgery. Axial CT scan shows well-centred patella, normal distance between patella and trochlea, healed osteotomy of the lateral condyle and normal sulcus angle (left side operated, extension, relaxed)

Figure CS18.7 Intraoperative anterolateral view of the trochlea. Degenerative changes on the medial side (overload) and osteophytes on the lateral side (patellar subluxation) are obvious. Note the flat dysplastic trochlea (left knee)

documented improved balancing of the patella (Figure CS18.9).

Summary

This case outlines the consequences of excessive medialization of the tibial tuberosity in a patient with dysplastic trochlea. The overcorrection could not even eliminate the lateral patellar subluxations and dislocations, because this treatment did not respect the initial underlying pathology (trochlear dysplasia). In addition, it created severe secondary complications.

The case documents that the treatment should, whenever possible, focus on the present pathology and not create additional pathological situations (medialization) to try to compensate for the real pathoanatomy.

References

1. Biedert RM, Friederich NF (1994) Failed lateral retinacular release: clinical outcome. *J Sports Traumatol* **16**: 162–173
2. Teitge RA, Faerber WW, Des Madryl P, Matelic TM (1996) Stress radiographs of the patellofemoral joint. *J Bone Joint Surg Am* **78**: 193–203
3. Hughston JC (1968) Subluxation of the patella. *J Bone Joint Surg Am* **50**: 1003–1026
4. Hughston JC, Deese M (1988) Medial subluxation of the patella as a complication of lateral retinacular release. *Am J Sports Med* **16**: 383–388
5. Hughston JC, Walsh WM, Puddu G (1984) *Patellar Subluxation and Dislocation. Saunders Monographs in Clinical Orthopaedics*, volume V. Philadelphia, WB Saunders

Suggested reading

Biedert RM (2000) 124 operations to treat 10 patients suffering from patellofemoral pain. What was wrong? In: *Proceedings of the International Patellofemoral Study Group*, Garmisch-Partenkirchen, Germany

CASE STUDY 19

Secondary medial osteoarthritis with medial subluxation of the patella

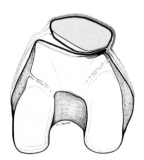

♦ What is the reason for medial subluxation?

♦ How important is medial osteoarthritis?

♦ What is our treatment concept and how can we make the decisions?

Table CS19 Patellofemoral joint examination

Diagnostic clues	Findings	Diagnostic clues	Findings
Pain	Severe medial patellofemoral joint	Patellar gliding mechanism	Unstable, crepitations
Tenderness	Medial patellofemoral joint, anterior knee pain	Patellar apprehension	Positive medial and lateral
Effusion	Only with overload	Catching	Medial and lateral
Swelling	Only with overload	Locking	Partially, between 20° and 40° flexion
Patellar position, relaxed, 0°	Medial subluxation	Range of motion	Free
Patellar position, contracted, 0°	Mild lateralization	Radiographs	Medial osteoarthritis
Patellar position, 30°	Mild medialization	Other	Patellar tendon stuck to the head of the tibia, excessive anterolateral vacuum, loss of power of the whole extensor mechanism
Patellar mobility	Increased to medial and lateral		

Patellofemoral Disorders: Diagnosis and Treatment. Edited by Roland M. Biedert
© 2004 John Wiley & Sons, Ltd ISBN: 0-470-85011-6

History

A 19 year-old female patient suffered from unspecific bilateral anterior knee pain. Surgery was performed only on the right side. The first operation was performed at the age of 19 years and consisted of an enlarged Roux procedure. By the age of 43 years she had undergone a total of 24 operations on the right side. In addition to numerous arthroscopic debridements, a lateral retinaculum release was redone six times. Also, different osteotomies (valgization, flexion, varization) were performed and numerous procedures at the tibial tuberosity (Roux, Bandi, Elmslie) were added. None of the steps ever improved the situation. The major problems included pain in all loaded flexion positions, pain during the night, effusion and swelling following increased load, loss of strength, and inability to perform most sports. The unspecific bilateral anterior knee pain impaired her daily life.

Comments

Surgical treatment of unspecific anterior knee pain in the young female patient is a controversial problem. The described excessive high number of contradictory operative procedures documents the inaccuracy of existing therapeutic concepts in resolving this pain problem surgically.

Course of action

Physical examination

The physical examination of this patient showed tenderness and pain on palpation on the proximal lateral aspect of the patella, the medial facet of the patella and the medial femoral condyle, the tibial tuberosity and the patellar tendon. A mild chronic effusion could be documented. The range of motion was unlimited. The patella apprehension test was positive, especially to the medial side but also laterally, with pain and crepitation. The patella was locking during flexion and extension movements between 20° and 40° of flexion. The patellar tendon was stuck to the head of the tibia. The patellar tendon adhesions and excessive resection of the Hoffa fat pad caused a vacuum effect on the lateral side during knee flexion (Figure CS19.1). In addition this caused significant restriction of patellar mobility, especially impaired patellar rotation.

The Q angle (measured in extension) was 8° (Figure CS19.2) on the right side and 15° on the left side (Figure CS19.3). One-legged standing in flexion, such as going down stairs, was painful and created continued limping.

Axial CT evaluation

The medial subluxation with osteoarthritis could be documented with normal axial CT scans (Figure CS19.4). Axial CT scans through the head of the tibia (Figure CS19.5) documented the present position of the tibial tuberosity (in comparison to the normal left side) and with this the axis of the vector of the quadriceps muscle and the whole extensor apparatus.[1,2] The usually performed CT evaluation was completed with three-dimensional CT scans (Figures CS19.6 and CS19.7).

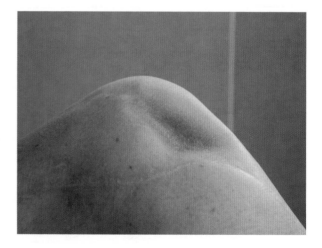

Figure CS19.1 Anterolateral view showing the important vacuum effect

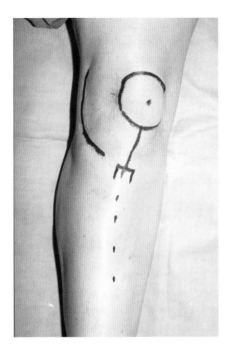

Figure CS19.2 Medial subluxation of the patella (circle with point), following medialization of the tibial tuberosity and excessive release of the lateral structures (marked line lateral incision). Decreased Q angle value

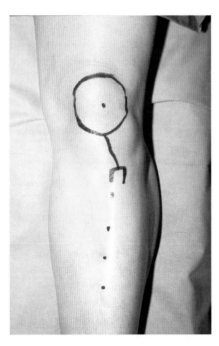

Figure CS19.3 Normal, nonoperated left knee with well-centred patella and higher Q angle value

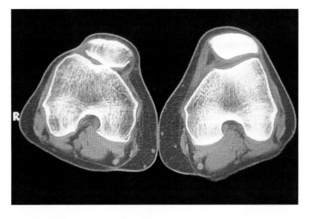

Figure CS19.4 Medial osteoarthritis of the patellofemoral joint with medial subluxation of the patella (extension, relaxed)

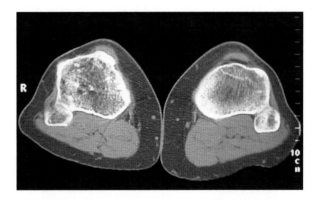

Figure CS19.5 Increased medialization of the tibial tuberosity on the right side (view from distal to proximal)

Special considerations

Increased medialization of the tibial tuberosity shifts the mechanical and loading axis of the extensor apparatus to medial. The potential problem associated with this is hyperpressure on the medial sides of the knee, both tibiofemoral and patellofemoral. Medialization of the tibial tuberosity is combined in most cases with a release of the lateral structures, especially the retinacula. This creates a secondary medial subluxation of the patella with increased pressure on the medial trochlea, causing overuse with degenerative changes.[3,4] This destructive process in the

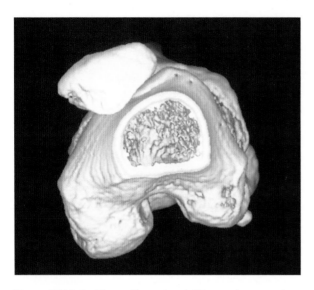

Figure CS19.6   Three-dimensional CT scan documenting medial subluxation of the patella in the view from proximal to distal (right knee, extension, relaxed)

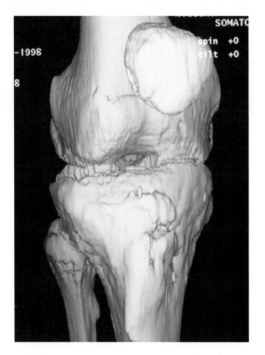

Figure CS19.7   Three-dimensional CT scan, showing medial subluxation of the patella with overcorrection of the tibial tuberosity to medial (right knee, extension, relaxed)

cartilage may release pieces of matrix components and wear particles, which may initiate a painful inflammatory reaction in the synovium.[5,6] Pain decreases muscle activity and limits training capabilities and effects. Strengthening of the vastus medialis obliquus muscle, as a dynamic stabilizer of the patella, cannot be successful, as this increases the medial subluxation of the patella with painful hyperpressure. In such cases, muscular weakness becomes more and more important.

Plan

The goal of the treatment must be to eliminate the medial subluxation of the patella and to decrease the hyperpressure in the medial patellofemoral joint. The passive stability of the patella in the femoral groove must be improved. The missing lateral structures must be replaced and the vacuum eliminated (Figure CS19.8).

The first step of the surgical procedure must include the recentring of the patella in the trochlea in combination with improved ligament stabilization. This can only be achieved by a re-Elmslie procedure and a secondary reconstruction of the lateral retinaculum, using either local scar tissue or a tendon graft, e.g. the quadriceps tendon.[4,7]

To decide how much we have to relateralize the tibial tuberosity, we can use measurements and alignment of the nonoperated knee (if possible) or we can respect the tubercle–sulcus angle.[7–9] After the bony realignment has been performed (*see* Case Study 18), the lateral retinaculum is reconstructed with respect to a normal patella mobility of one to two quadrants.[7,9]

When the remaining scar tissues of the lateral structures are not sufficient for a strong secondary reconstruction, then the quadriceps tendon provides an excellent graft.

First, the whole insertion of the quadriceps tendon on the patella is prepared. The graft is removed, along with a bone fragment from the

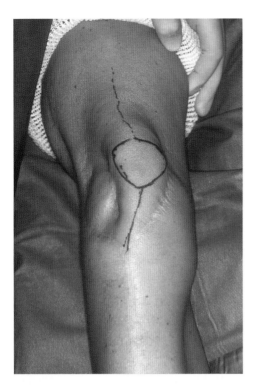

Figure CS19.8 Multiple pathological areas preoperatively

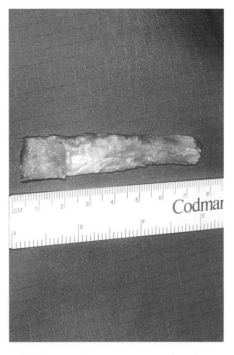

Figure CS19.9 Quadriceps tendon graft with bone fragment

patella (Figure CS19.9). Then holes are drilled from the defect side to the lateral side of the patella. A suture is passed through the hole and fixed on a K-wire. With the K-wire, it is possible to define the anatomical ('isometric') point on the lateral condyle where the graft will be attached (Figure CS19.10). The length of the suture gives the correct length of the graft. The form of the bony fragment is marked on the lateral condyle with a chisel to guarantee optimal press-fit. The cortical bone is removed from the condyle. The osseous part of the graft is inserted and fixed with a cancellous screw (Figure CS19.11). The graft is then pulled through the hole in the lateral aspect of the patella. It runs over the defect on the medial side of the patella. To determine the correct tension of the graft, the knee is moved carefully through the range of motion and the balancing of the patella is

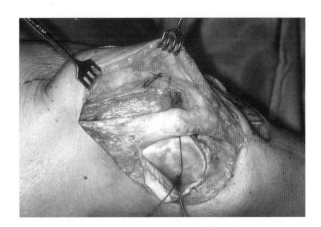

Figure CS19.10 Lateral view showing the suture fixed on a K-wire running from the proximal–medial part of the patella over the graft excision site, through the lateral holes in the patella to the lateral condyle to find the 'isometric point'

observed (Figure CS19.12). Finally, the graft is fixed proximally and medially with sutures

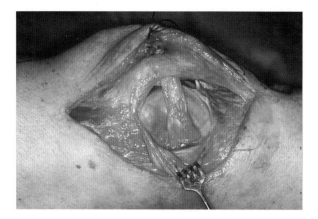

Figure CS19.11   Graft fixation with a screw on the lateral femoral condyle

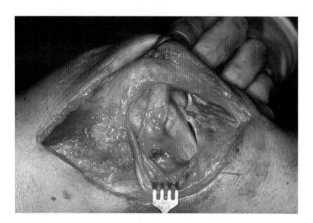

Figure CS19.12   Testing the tension of the graft through the whole range of motion

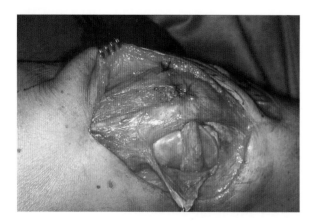

Figure CS19.13   Final fixation proximal and medial with closure of the graft donor area

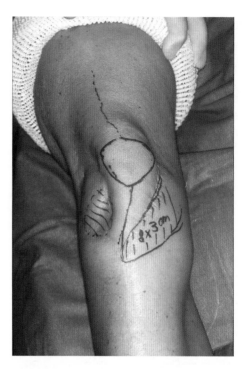

Figure CS19.14   Landmarks of the sliding flap medially (8 × 3 cm) and the lateral vacuum defect

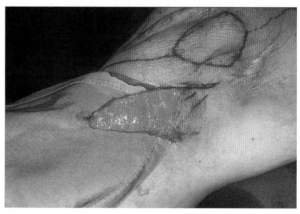

Figure CS19.15   Sliding flap after removal of the skin

(Figure CS19.13). Normal patellar mobility in extension of one and two quadrants medially and laterally is mandatory.

The anterolateral hole of the vacuum effect is filled with a sliding flap from the medial side, using subcutaneous tissue (Figures CS19.14, CS19.15, CS19.16 and CS19.17). The goal of

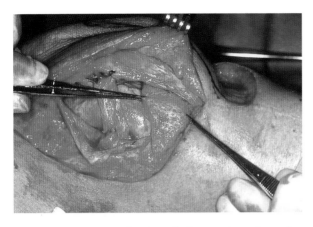

Figure CS19.16 The flap is pulled anterolaterally under the patellar tendon to replace the missing fat pad

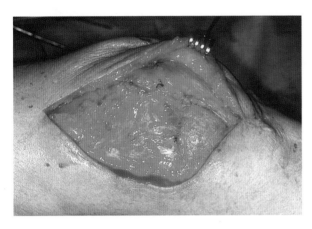

Figure CS19.17 Situation at the end of the reconstruction with a 'new Hoffa fat pad' filling the former anterolateral cavity

this surgical step is to prevent new patellar tendon adhesions and to preserve the corrected patellar mobility.

Postoperative care and rehabilitation

Goals

♦ Decrease of pain, inflammation, and locking

♦ Improvement of dynamic centring of the patella in the trochlea

♦ Strengthening weak muscle groups

Timeline

♦ Hospital	4–6 days	
♦ Mobilization	1st day	
♦ Weightbearing	Partial	Max. 20 kg for 6 weeks
	Complete	Depends on quality of muscular stabilization
♦ Sports	Bicycle, swimming	After 4–6 weeks
	Everything	Never possible; only low-demanding activities

Summary

This case outlines the severe complications following medial transposition of the tibial tuberosity with repetitive lateral retinaculum releases and additional overrelease in a patient with initial unspecific anterior knee pain. Secondary severe instability of the patellar gliding mechanism and degenerative changes occur with overuse of the medial patellofemoral joint. These are major problems, creating chronic pain and disability – problems that can no longer be corrected sufficiently.

References

1. Biedert RM (2000) 124 operations to treat 10 patients suffering from patellofemoral pain. What was wrong? In Proceedings of the International Patellofemoral Study Group, Garmisch-Partenkirchen, Germany

2. Biedert RM (2002) Complicated case studies. In: Sanchis-Alfonso V (ed), *Anterior Knee Pain and Patellofemoral Instability in the Active Young. The Black Hole of Orthopaedics*. Medica Panamericana, Madrid, Spain, 287–301

3. Biedert RM, Friederich NF (1994) Failed lateral retinacular release: clinical outcome. *J Sports Traumatol* **16**: 162–173

4. Teitge RA, Faerber WW, Des Madryl P, Matelic TM (1996) Stress radiographs of the patellofemoral joint. *J Bone Joint Surg Am* **78**: 193–203

5. van den Berg WB (1999) The role of cytokines and growth factors in cartilage destruction in osteoarthritis and rheumatoid arthritis. *Z Rheumatol* **58**: 136–141

6. Biedert RM, Kernen V (2001) Neurosensory characteristics of the patellofemoral joint: what is the genesis of patellofemoral pain? *Sports Med Arthrosc Rev* **9**: 295–300

7. Biedert RM, Gruhl C (1997) Axial computed tomography of the patellofemoral joint with and without quadriceps contraction. *Arch Orthop Trauma Surg* **116**: 77–82

8. Biedert RM (2000) Korrelation zwischen Q-Winkel und Patellaposition. In: Wirth CJ, Rudert M (eds), *Das patellofemorale Schmerzsyndrom*. Darmstadt, Steinkopff-Verlag

9. Kolowich PA, Paulos LE, Rosenberg TD, Farnsworth S (1990) Lateral release of the patella: indications and contraindications. *Am J Sports Med* **18**: 359–365

Suggested reading

Biedert RM, Friederich NF (1994) Failed lateral retinacular release: clinical outcome. *J Sports Traumatol* **16**: 162–173

Teitge RA, Faerber WW, Des Madryl P, Matelic TM (1996) Stress radiographs of the patellofemoral joint. *J Bone Joint Surg Am* **78**: 193–203

CASE STUDY 20

Lateral retinacular over-release

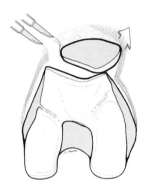

♦ What does 'over-release' mean?

♦ What are the causes for over-release?

♦ How can we treat it?

		Table CS20	Patellofemoral joint examination	

Diagnostic clues	Findings	Diagnostic clues	Findings
Pain	Chronic, diffuse, suprapatellar	Patellar gliding mechanism	Unstable, medialization
Tenderness	Lateral	Patellar apprehension	Severely positive to medial
Effusion	With overload	Q angle	Normal
Swelling	With overload	Catching	Sometimes, medial
Patellar position, relaxed, 0°	Centred	Locking	Sometimes, medial
Patellar position, contracted, 0°	Medialization	Range of motion	Normal
Patellar position, 30°	Medialization	Radiographs	Normal
Patellar mobility	Increased to medial and lateral	Other	Excessive defect of the lateral soft tissue structures, quadriceps weakness

Patellofemoral Disorders: Diagnosis and Treatment.   Edited by Roland M. Biedert
© 2004 John Wiley & Sons, Ltd   ISBN: 0-470-85011-6

History

This 31 year-old patient suffered from chronic patellofemoral pain, severe weakness and instability on his left knee. At the age of 21 years he had his first surgical intervention, with open revision and abrasion of the retropatellar cartilage. The second operation was performed 4 years later, repeating the abrasion and adding a lateral retinacular release. Because of persisting and increasing pain, the third surgical intervention was performed, extending the lateral retinacular release. After this operation, the condition (pain, weakness and instability) of his left knee continued to worsen.

Comments

Increasing and chronic patellofemoral pain, in combination with weakness and feeling of instability, document a combination of severe symptoms and a disquieting condition of the knee. Every time, the different surgical procedures caused additional complaints (weakness, instability). They did not eliminate the initial problem (pain).

Course of action

Physical examination

Visual inspection of the left knee confirmed the excessive persisting problem (Figure CS20.1). A parapatellar lateral incision reached from the tibial tuberosity to the vastus lateralis muscle and ended 10 cm proximal to the proximal edge of the patella. An extensive defect with a hole was present proximal and lateral to the patella (Figure CS20.2). At the site of the defect, the tendon and muscle belly of the vastus lateralis muscle no longer existed. In 30° of knee flexion, the defect remained and the quadriceps tendon (anterior) and the posterior part of the iliotibial band (posterolateral) became more visible

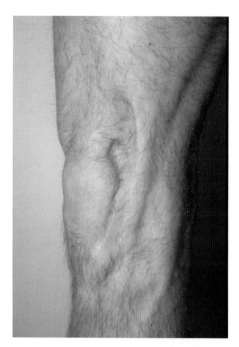

Figure CS20.1 Anterolateral view showing an impressive defect of the lateral soft tissue structures after three operations

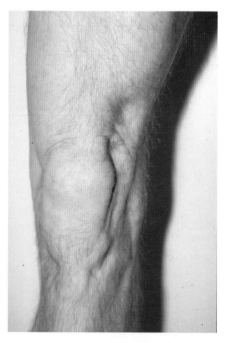

Figure CS20.2 Anterior view with the defect in the distal part of the musculotendinous unit of the vastus lateralis

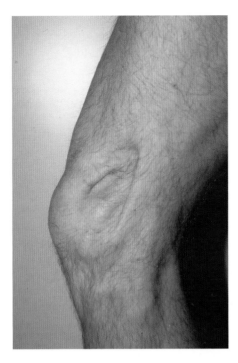

Figure CS20.3 Defect of the lateral soft tissue structures in flexion

(Figure CS20.3).The physical examination documented a severe instability of the patella to medial and lateral, with pathological patellar glide and stability tests. Activation of the quadriceps was inhibited and caused medialization of the patella. In addition, a very painful suprapatellar plica was palpated.

Radiographs

The standard radiographs showed no pathology of the patellofemoral joint. Only dystrophy of the patellar osseous structure with demineralization caused by inactivity was found.

Axial CT evaluation was not performed because the radiographs were normal and the pathology clear.

Special considerations

The continued impairment of the condition of the left knee with the extensive defect of the lateral

Table CS20.1 Complications following lateral retinacular release and over-release[1-10]
♦ Medial patellar instability (subluxations, dislocations)   ♦ Quadriceps muscle weakness   ♦ Loss of power of the extensor mechanism   ♦ Atrophy and retraction of the vastus lateralis muscle*   ♦ Loss of dynamic lateral stabilization of the patella*

*Complication following over-release.

soft tissue structures was caused by the various steps of surgery. It is well described that lateral retinacular release may cause secondary problems and complications (see Table CS20.1).[1-11] Excessive superior extension of the lateral release, which also severs the tendon of the vastus lateralis muscle, results in retraction and atrophy of the muscle.[6] This is combined with loss of power to the extensor mechanism and eliminates its function as a dynamic lateral stabilizer of the patella. The present patient suffered from all of these disabling complications. The initial cause of his pains was an inflamed suprapatellar plica that was never excised.

Plan

The goal of the treatment must be to eliminate the medial patellar instability and pain. In cases without over-release, lateral retinacular reconstruction using local scar tissue is often possible and recommended [3,7] (*see* Case Studies 16 and 18). In cases with severe over-release, secondary reconstruction of the lateral retinaculum and the vastus lateralis musculotendinous unit with a quadriceps graft is recommended (RA Teitge, Handout, 1988). The bone block of the graft is screwed to the lateral femoral condyle at the most isometric point; the tendinous part of the graft is passed through a transverse tunnel in the patella, then turned onto the superficial surface of the patella and anchored there with sutures (*see* Case Study 19). The inflamed suprapatellar plica is removed during the lateral reconstruction.

Postoperative care and rehabilitation

See Case Studies 16, 18 and 19.

Discussion

The lateral retinaculum is a normal anatomical structure with possible variations.[3,8] It is 'abnormal' when it is too short, tight or too thick. This may cause passive patellar tilt. Lateral retinacular release [12] may not be the only option. Some complications cannot always be eliminated, even when using correct surgical techniques. Therefore, instead of release, we recommend a lengthening of the lateral retinaculum (*see* Case Studies 3, 5 and 6).

Over-release with transection of the musculotendinous unit of the vastus lateralis is the most serious complication. The vastus lateralis muscle is composed of a vastus lateralis and a vastus lateralis obliquus component.[7,13] Over-release of both parts change the stability and alignment of the patellar balancing and should therefore absolutely be avoided.[3,6,7] The physiological function of the vastus lateralis muscle must be respected.

Summary

Over-release is the worst form of lateral retinacular release with the most serious complications. It absolutely must be avoided. Although the reconstruction may be structurally possible, the physiological function of the lateral structures can never be achieved again.

References

1. Kramers-de Quervain IA, Biedert R, Stüssi E (1997) Quantitative gait analysis in patients with medial patellar instability following lateral retinacular release. *Knee Surg Sports Traumatol Arthrosc* **5**: 95–101

2. Kolowich PA, Paulos LE, Rosenberg TD, Farnsworth S (1990) Lateral release of the patella: indications and contraindications. *Am J Sports Med* **18**: 359–365

3. Biedert RM, Friederich NF (1994) Failed lateral retinacular release: clinical outcome. *J Sports Traumatol* **16**: 162–173

4. Teitge RA, Faerber WW, Des Madryl P, Matelic TM (1996) Stress radiographs of the patellofemoral joint. *J Bone Joint Surg Am* **78**: 193–203

5. Hughston JC, Walsh WM, Puddu G (1984) *Patellar Subluxation and Dislocation. Saunders Monographs in Clinical Orthopaedics*, volume V. Philadelphia, PA, WB Saunders

6. Hughston JC, Deese M (1988) Medial subluxation of the patella as a complication of lateral retinacular release. *Am J Sports Med* **16**: 383–388

7. Nonweiler DE, DeLee JC (1994) The diagnosis and treatment of medial subluxation of the patella after lateral retinacular release. *Am J Sports Med* **22**: 680–686

8. Busch MT, DeHaven KE (1989) Pitfalls of the lateral retinacular release. *Clin Sports Med* **8**: 279–290

9. Henry JH, Goletz TH, Williamson B (1986) Lateral retinacular release in patellofemoral subluxation. Indications, results, and comparison to open patellofemoral reconstruction. *Am J Sports Med* **14**: 121–129

10. Marumoto JM, Jordan C, Akins R (1995) A biomechanical comparison of lateral retinacular releases. *Am J Sports Med* **23**: 151–155

11. Johnson DP, Wakeley C (2002) Reconstruction of the lateral patellar retinaculum following lateral release: a case report. *Knee Surg Sports Traumatol Arthrosc* **10**: 361–363

12. Arendt EA, Fithian DC, Cohen E (2002) Current concepts of lateral patella dislocation. *Clin Sports Med* **21**: 499–519

13. Javadpour DP, Finegan PJ, O'Brien M (1991) The anatomy of the extensor mechanism and its clinical relevance. *Clin J Sport Med* **1**: 229–235

Suggested reading

Nonweiler DE, DeLee JC (1994) The diagnosis and treatment of medial subluxation of the patella after lateral retinacular release. *Am J Sports Med* **22**: 680–686

PART IV

Physical Therapy

Mario Bizzini, Stephan Meyer, René de Vries and Roland M. Biedert

Disorders of the patellofemoral joint remain one of the most challenging pathologies encountered by physical therapists working in orthopaedic and sports medicine clinics. Patients suffering from patellofemoral pain present a large variety of signs and symptoms. Pain is the symptom common to all patients, but they also experience other symptoms.[1]

The individual presentation of patellofemoral pain needs an individual approach. A complete history, examination and evaluation and familiarity with the medical records permit the therapist to adapt an individual impairment-based treatment approach. Theoretical-, research- and evidence-based knowledge, combined with clinical experience, are the keys to implementing the most appropriate interventions for a specific problem in a specific situation. This corresponds to the practice of evidence-based medicine.[2] Specific knowledge of the anatomy, biomechanics, pathophysiology and any previous therapeutic interventions related to patellofemoral pain are necessary for the individual management of these patients.

Evidence-based therapy implicates selective thinking by the physical therapist, far away from the rigid nonoperative and postoperative rehabilitation protocols. The patient must be evaluated at each visit. Only the objective findings and the patient's unique treatment response lead us to adapt and modify the interventions to help the patient progress through rehabilitation.

To develop a feeling for the patient's Envelope of Function[3] is also crucial. This approach allows a safe functional progression towards the patient's own goals (activities of daily living and sports).

The following sections of this chapter aim to describe in detail the principles of physical therapy for patellofemoral pain. After a summary of our review of the published randomized clinical trials, we present rehabilitation protocols. Then we share with the reader a section on the therapeutic interventions that physical therapists use to treat the patients. The last part of this chapter emphasizes some of the biomechanical and motor-learning principles physical therapists incorporate in the nonoperative treatment of patients with patellofemoral pain.

Patellofemoral Disorders: Diagnosis and Treatment. Edited by Roland M. Biedert
© 2004 John Wiley & Sons, Ltd ISBN: 0-470-85011-6

Review of randomized controlled trials*

Several classification systems have been developed to assist in the diagnosis and treatment of patellofemoral pain.[4,5] Most often, these groupings are based on the medical model of disease, where identification of some pathology directs treatment.[6] However, patients frequently have no identifiable pathology. Their patellofemoral pain is classified as 'unspecific' (see Case Study 1).

Many physical therapy approaches have been used to treat the impairments associated with patellofemoral pain.[1,7] The Philadelphia Panel Evidence-based Clinical Practice Guidelines stated:[8]

> ... there is a lack of evidence at present regarding whether to include or exclude the use of thermotherapy, therapeutic massage, EMG biofeedback, therapeutic ultrasound, electrical stimulation, and combined rehabilitation interventions in the daily practice of physical rehabilitation for knee pain.

What should a physical therapist do to offer effective therapy to patients with patellofemoral pain?

Our systematic review* shows that although general exercises are helpful to reduce pain and improve short-term function, there is inconclusive evidence to support the superiority of one particular physical therapy intervention compared to another.[9] We searched the indexed literature for controlled clinical trials. We found only 20 articles to review.[10-29] We classified the trials by intervention, based on the primary goal of the intervention. We found that the studies fell into seven groups – orthotics (including foot orthoses, patellar braces, elastic sleeves, patellar taping), manual therapy, modalities, medications, acupuncture, strength-training methods, and combined interventions (e.g. education and taping, or exercise, taping and education).

---

*Adapted from an article by Bizzini et al (2003) J Orthop Sports Phys Ther 33:4–20[9]

We developed a scoring system to evaluate the quality of the controlled clinical trials. When we scored each of the trials, the scores ranged from 19 to 83 points. The percentage of studies meeting the minimum quality for each criterion scored is given in Table PT.1.

Conclusion of systematic review of controlled trials

Based on the results of trials that met or exceeded the level we defined for minimum quality,

Table PT.1 Scoring scale used to grade trial and percentage of trials meeting minimum quality* for each criterion

Criterion	Points	Trials meeting minimum quality* (%)
Population	25	
Inclusion	5	90
Exclusion	5	80
Adequate number	10	60
Homogeneity	5	65
Intervention	25	
Standardized and described	10	95
Control and placebo adequate	10	80
Co-interventions avoided	5	45
Effect size	25	
Relevant outcome	10	60
Blinded outcome	10	35
Follow-up period adequate	5	30
Data presentation and analysis	25	
Randomization described	5	25
Drop-outs accounted for	5	70
Intention to treat	5	50
Proper statistical procedures	10	75

*Minimum quality was operationally defined as a trial scoring at least half of the maximum possible score for criterion under review. Table adapted from Bizzini et al.[9]

treatments that decreased pain and improved function in patients with patellofemoral pain were acupuncture, quadriceps strengthening, the use of a resistive brace, and the combination of exercises with patellar taping and biofeedback. The use of soft foot orthotics in patients with excessive foot pronation appears to decrease pain. At a short-term follow-up, patients who received exercise programmes were more likely to be discharged from physical therapy.

Most randomized clinical trials we reviewed contained qualitative flaws that may bring the validity of the results into question, thus diminishing our ability to generalize the results into clinical practice. These flaws were primarily in the areas of randomization procedures, duration of follow-up, control of co-interventions, assurance of blinding, accountability and proper analysis of drop-outs, number of subjects, and relevance of the outcomes.

Trials of high quality will support the clinical decision-making process in the care of our patients and help to provide strong evidence that can contribute to the recognition of the value of physical therapy. Currently, there is a lack of evidence regarding the nonoperative treatment of patellofemoral pain. One of the main problems is the difficulty of performing high-quality studies in this field. Therefore, the clinician must consider all other information from the peer-reviewed literature (non-randomized studies, case reports), from non-peer reviewed literature (textbooks, continuing education) and from clinical experience.

Rehabilitation protocols

Pathology and surgery of the musculoskeletal system can lead to several impairments for the patient. The classical scheme of Nagy[30] shows how an active pathology can affect the overall body functions. As an example, if a patient has a painful swollen anterior part of the knee, impairments (e.g. inability to activate the quadriceps), functional limitations (e.g. inability to

descend stairs in a normal manner) and possibly social limitations (e.g. inability to work or to perform sport activities) will follow. Rehabilitation should focus on the physical and functional limitations. A complete physical examination of the patellofemoral joint is described in Chapter 5, while specific additional musculoskeletal examination will be described in this chapter. The combination of these examinations helps the physical therapist to choose the most appropriate therapeutic intervention and to predict the individual patient's functional outcome. This is often not a simple task, because the result of rehabilitation depends on several factors. Rehabilitation and surgery represent external factors; motivation and lifestyle are among the individual's characteristics; age, gender and healing potential are part of the risk factors. The individual's motivation is a determining factor for success – one that is frequently neglected in rehabilitation protocols.

Time-based protocols versus criterion-based protocols

In the last decade there was a trend towards accelerated knee rehabilitation programmes,[31] mostly with *time-based protocols*. Subsequently, individualized protocols – *criterion-based* – have been described in the literature.[32,33]

Time-based rehabilitation is a restrictive programme, based on pathology or surgical procedure and on expected healing times, where all patients receive the same amount of therapeutic interventions, independent of their treatment response. A time-based rehabilitation protocol does not take into account the individual characteristics of the patient, and therefore cannot target functional limitations.

Criterion-based rehabilitation is dictated by the patient's achievement of specific functional goals. The level of therapy is based on the patient's response to treatment. The goals of rehabilitation are determined by teamwork between patient and physical therapist. Criterion-based protocols are based on six basic principles of rehabilitation:[32]

♦ Healing tissue should never be overstressed.

♦ The deleterious effect of immobilization must be prevented.

♦ The patient must fulfil specific criteria to progress from one stage to the next.

♦ The rehabilitation programme must be based on current clinical and scientific research.

♦ The rehabilitation programme must not be a cookbook formula; it should be tailored to the patient's goals and response to treatment.

♦ Successful outcome is directly related to a team effort, with the orthopaedist, physical therapist, the family and the patient all working together. Effective communication plays a key role.

The patient is the main protagonist in rehabilitation. The patient is responsible for rehabilitating the knee. The team, including the orthopaedist, physical therapist and the family will direct, follow and monitor the patient's rehabilitation. Information and education are crucial; attitude and motivation can be positively influenced. The physical therapist should guide the patient in a functional and individual progression towards active daily living and chosen sports.

The rehabilitation programme and the treatment procedure should be based on scientific knowledge. Despite the research on some biomechanical aspects of knee exercises,[34] the overall knowledge and basic science on the effects of rehabilitation are still missing in the literature.

Phases of rehabilitation

In the rehabilitation of the lower extremity, not only is an adequate range of motion of the knee necessary, but also the regaining of neuromuscular control. Rehabilitation should focus on improving range of motion, muscle function, loading tolerance in the weight-bearing situations, sensorimotor control, and the functional activity level. Rehabilitation is divided into three phases – acute, subacute and chronic.

Phase I: Acute

During this first phase, pain management and the control of swelling must be taken into account in the rehabilitation protocol. Therapeutic interventions (discussed later in this chapter), activity modification and muscle training are among the best choices for treatment.

Phase II: Subacute

During this second phase, the neuromuscular stabilization of the knee and lower extremity during activities of daily living is crucial. The muscle groups are trained to support partial to full weightbearing, according to the knee's loading response (pain, swelling, muscle activity). The physical therapist must monitor the patient accurately to help the patient progress safely. Beside objective parameters (e.g. the physical therapist's observation of the patient's knee, leg and body stabilization while descending stairs), the subjective feelings of the patient must also be considered (e.g. the patient feels sure while descending stairs and accomplishing other activities of daily living).

Phase III: Chronic

The goals of rehabilitation during this third phase are focused on the patient's own goals (job, hobby and sport). The experience and knowledge of the rehabilitation team are important to help the patient achieve these goals. Often these goals are obtained only after specific and controlled training (sensorimotor, coordination, strength and endurance training).

Documentation

During rehabilitation, different measurement instruments can help the physical therapist document the patient's progress. Measures of impairment of the musculoskeletal system include findings from the examination (range of motion, muscle function, joint stability). Measures of functional limitations and disability include performance-based assessments (e.g. hop test),[33] isokinetic strength tests[35] and patient-reported measures of function (e.g. knee-specific questionnaire).[36]

Summary of pertinent points

The following points should be considered in the development of rehabilitation protocols for patients with patellofemoral pain:

♦ A criterion-based rehabilitation programme should be designed for each patient.

♦ The physical therapist's responsibilities include the appropriate interventions, patient's education, documentation of rehabilitation, and monitoring for progress or evidence of potential complications.

♦ Volume and length of rehabilitation are based on the patient's response to treatment.

♦ Communication between patient, physician, physical therapist and others (e.g. family, fitness trainer) is crucial.

Therapeutic interventions

In this section, we outline the therapeutic interventions for pain management by the physical therapist for the nonoperative treatment of patients with patellofemoral pain.

Pain in or around the knee produces reflex inhibition of the surrounding muscles, in particular the vastus medialis. Pain and swelling have an earlier and possibly greater effect on the vastus medialis obliquus muscle than on the vastus lateralis muscle.[37,38] This has the potential of leading to an imbalance of the soft tissue forces, causing lateral tracking of the patella,[39]

and may therefore predispose to the development of patellofemoral pain. With pain and swelling, exercises may be contraindicated.

Pain management

The initial priority of treatment is to reduce acute inflammation or pain. This is achieved with a combination of rest from aggravating activities, ice application, taping and electrotherapeutic modalities.[40,41]

Rest

The natural history of patellofemoral pain treated with rest only has attracted little research. It can be assumed that if all activity ceases, many symptoms will also cease. The course of patellofemoral pain is frequently chronic. Rest may need to be long-term to be effective.[19]

Ice

Local ice application is supported by empirical and clinical experience. Ice decreases pain and inflammation associated with patellofemoral pain.[42] Cryokinetics, a combination of cold and exercise, is an effective form of ice application to decrease pain and promote healing.[43] Exercise-induced vasodilatation during cryokinetics is greater than that induced by heat application. Exercise during cryokinetics activates the lymphatic system to help reduce swelling, retards development of adhesions, stimulates fibroblast activity and promotes fibre alignment.

Heat

Heat applications are not as effective as cold applications as an adjunct to exercise rehabilitation. There is some evidence that pain syndromes may increase with the use of heat.[43,44]

Taping

Patellar taping can provide short-term pain relief for patients with patellofemoral pain.[45] Some recent studies[11,20] have failed to find any benefits of using patellar tape in addition to physical therapy interventions (for practical use of taping, *see* Principles of training and rehabilitation, below).

Neuromuscular electrical stimulation

This may be helpful for patients who find it difficult to self-activate the vastus medialis obliquus muscle due to pain, oedema or weakness. The electrical stimulation indirectly elicits muscle contraction by activating the motor nerves that innervate muscles.[46] Its effectiveness is primarily determined by the intrinsic tissue properties of the individual. Studies[47,48] show that strengthening of hypotrophic muscles is more easily achieved with neuromuscular electrical stimulation than with voluntary exercises. This leads to the assumption that the stimulation can preferentially initiate faster-contracting motor units, normally only trained at high exercise intensities under voluntary conditions.[49] Thus, neuromuscular electrical stimulation may allow painless muscle strengthening while tissue homeostasis and healing occur.

Transcutaneous electrical nerve stimulation (TENS)

TENS has been used effectively in different pain conditions.[50,51] There have been no controlled trials on its effect on patellofemoral pain.[9] TENS sends messages through myelinated afferent nerve fibres to activate local inhibitory circuits within the dorsal horn of the spinal cord; endogenous opioids are released.[52] Thus, increased inhibition of pain is transmitted to the brain. Often it takes some time to determine optimal stimulation levels, pulse frequencies, electrode placements and lengths of stimulation time. This necessitates the skills of an experienced physical therapist or physician. The optimal frequency for activation of large-diameter fibres appears to be 50–100 Hz. These high pulse-rate settings should be felt as a tingling or prickling but not as an unpleasant sensation. The treatments may last at least 1 hour and sometimes several hours continuously. Patients who do not respond to conventional high-frequency TENS may benefit from low-frequency types of stimulation, i.e. acupuncture-like TENS. This has a similar analgesic effect but a shorter duration. Thus, it is effective in reducing chronic and acute knee pain and for treating osteoarthritic knee conditions.[53,54] It uses low pulse-rate settings and should be felt quite firmly (high intensity), almost like a pulsing sensation, at 2 pulses/second during a 30–60 minute treatment time. Often the electrode is placed on a trigger or suitable acupuncture point likely to maximize intrinsic opiate response.[55] Acupuncture points specified for patellofemoral pain are Spleen 9, Spleen 10 (which is also a motoric point) on the medial site, Gallbladder 33 and Stomach 35 on the lateral site. TENS is simply applied, safe, low-cost, has minimal or no side-effects and is suitable for self-management.

Ultrasound

This is frequently used to treat pain and influence soft tissue healing in musculoskeletal injuries. However, there is a lack of evidence of its clinical effectiveness as an therapeutic intervention in patellofemoral pain.[56]

Manual therapy for joints

Manual therapy is a cornerstone of the therapeutic interventions. It focuses not only on the patellofemoral joint itself, but also on the spine, hip, pelvis and associated joints.

Spine, pelvis, hip

Manipulative physical therapists test the spine (and any associated joints) for factors that could

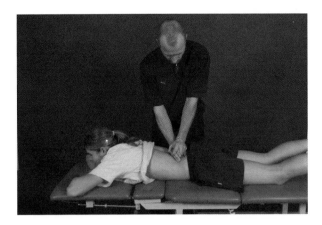

Figure PT.1 Segmental lumbar mobilization

influence the treatment of peripheral structures. Patellofemoral pain may be influenced by lumbar spine pathology (Figure PT.1).

In a randomized controlled trial,[26] sacroiliac joint manipulation decreased immediate quadriceps muscle inhibition. Longer-term effects of this technique are unknown. For patients suffering from knee, anterior thigh, hip and upper lumbar problems, the prone knee bend test is routinely done. Adding the slump test to the prone knee bend test in side-lying makes it possible to differentiate between pain derived from neural versus nonneural structures (Figure PT.2). For more detailed treatment techniques of the lumbar spine, hip, knee, and the feet, see Lewit[57] and Maitland.[58,59]

Patellar mobilization

This technique should be incorporated when shortening of the soft tissue is responsible for lateral glide or rotation of the patella. Passive mobilizations are classified in grades 1–1V:[58]

Grade I   Small-amplitude movement performed at the beginning of range.

Grade II Large-amplitude movement performed within the free range but not moving into any resistance or stiffness.

Grade III Large-amplitude movement performed up to the limit of range.

Grade IV Small-amplitude movement performed at the limit of range.

Passive mobilizations can be used to treat pain and resistance of the patellofemoral joint. The transverse–medial glide movement is often the most restricted movement. Medial gliding is the most commonly used technique. Different angles of flexion should be used, if joint irritability allows this (Figure PT.3). When pain is predominant, Grades I and II of passive mobilization should be applied (sometimes performed with distraction of the patella). When pain is the result of tight structures, Grades III and IV should be

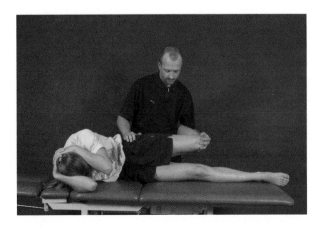

Figure PT.2 Prone knee-bend test (femoral nerve)

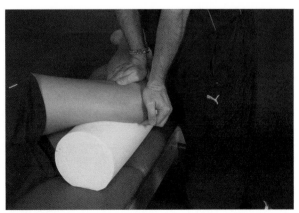

Figure PT.3 Medial gliding of the patella with the patient in side-lying position

used. These stronger techniques are more effective with the patient lying on the unaffected side. These techniques, combined with the prone knee bend test, allow patellar mobilization in the neuromeningeal prestretch position. (Figure PT.4). The therapist applies a force to the lateral border of the patella with the heel of the hand, thus producing a medial glide. If a lateral tilt is present, the force is applied to the anterior surface of the patella, medial to the midline, thus causing the lateral border of the patella to lift. To stretch the lateral structures more efficiently, the therapist can combine the applied force with passive lifting of the lateral border of the patella, a so-called 'shelling' technique (Figures PT.5, PT.6).

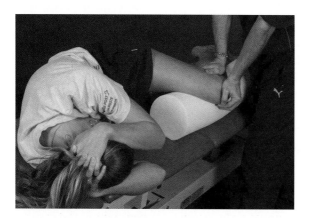

Figure PT.4   Medial gliding of the patella with the patient in slump position

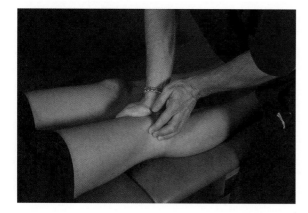

Figure PT.5   Test for the tightness of the lateral structures

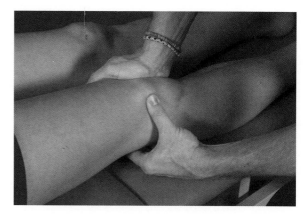

Figure PT.6   Treatment. 'Shelling' technique

The lateral structures of the knee are a common source of patellofemoral pain as a result of mechanical or chemical irritation.[60,61] Tightness is often present before the onset of any symptoms. Symptoms may be exacerbated later by joint overload or trauma.[60] Neural damage[62,63] of the lateral retinaculum is a potential source of patellofemoral pain in patients with retinaculum tightness. Repetitive irritation through malalignment or increased physical activity could generate pain from lateral and medial retinacula nerve endings.[60] Recognizing the tightness and potential of onset of symptoms prepares the physician and the therapist to initiate manual therapy as a preventive measure.

The most common abnormality causing patellofemoral pain occurs when the medial glide of the patella is restricted by the vastus lateralis, iliotibial band structures and tight lateral retinacula.[64] Shortening of the lateral retinacula with a chronic lateral patellar tilt, and the resultant chronic patellofemoral imbalance, may change the length: tension ratio of the vastus medialis obliquus muscle. This makes it more difficult for the lengthened vastus medialis obliquus muscle to generate a force against the resistance of shortened lateral retinacula. The greater part of the lateral retinaculum originates at the iliotibial band.[65,66] Thus, correcting the imbalance in the tight lateral retinaculum requires a combination of mobilization and stretching of both structures. Before stretching the lateral retinaculum, deep frictions in the region of the peripatellar retinacula (over the lateral femoral condyle) can be used for mobilization. Stretching of the lateral iliotibial band by the therapist is effectively performed when the patient is side-lying with the knee uppermost and in approximately 90° of flexion (or the position where the iliotibial band is the tightest). Using the heel of the hand, the therapist glides the patella medially for a sustained stretch. Self-mobilization by the patient is helpful as it can be performed frequently for short periods (5–10 seconds) throughout the day. The patient sits with the leg in full extension and uses an end-of-range mobilizing technique at the medial border of the patella, thus tilting the lateral patellar border anteriorly[67,68] (Figure PT.7).

The patient must be reassessed after the mobilization, before the treatment is continued. With decreased pain, more intensive passive movements of the patella can be applied in different directions and in varying degrees of patellar compression. Reassessment of progress will indicate whether or not to continue. It may be necessary to vary the degree of knee flexion, altering the contact area between patella and femur. Mobilization techniques to glide and tilt the patella medially can be performed by the patient several times per day. Patellar taping can be useful in providing an extended stretch.

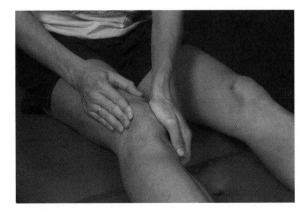

Figure PT.7   Self-treatment for lateral structures

Stretching muscles and soft tissues

Musculoskeletal problems, including muscle imbalance, are common during adolescence. Soft-tissue tightness is particularly prevalent in adolescents who are growing rapidly. This leads to decreased flexibility, which may cause altered stresses on the patellofemoral joint and may also compromise muscle control. Active 'knee alignment' requires flexible and strong muscles acting on and around the knee. Hamstrings and iliotibial band tightness are the most commonly involved structures in patellofemoral pain.

In this portion of the chapter, we describe stretching interventions for the hamstrings, iliotibial band, gastrocnemius and soleus muscles, the quadriceps, the hip muscles, and muscles controlling the pelvis.

Hamstrings muscle group

The hamstrings are forces that balance the patella by controlling the internal and external rotation of the tibia. Hamstrings and gastrocnemius tightness cause lateral tracking of the patella. Hamstrings tightness also leads to prolonged knee flexion at foot strike and midstance when walking. This results in a shortened stride, requiring more forceful quadriceps contraction in order to extend the knee. The tightness and forceful contraction can lead to increased osseous pressure on the patella.[69] The hamstrings are most frequently stretched with the leg straight while sitting or while lying supine with the hip in 90° of flexion and extending the knee (Figure PT.8). Stretching performed in the basic stepping position, if possible, would be more functional. Another way of testing and stretching the hamstrings, especially in patients with poor pelvic control, is to have the patient extend the knee while sitting with the hip flexed to 90°. Thus, the antagonist (quadriceps) stretches the hamstrings. During the stretching, the knee should extend to 10° for optimal length (Figure PT.9). Performing the same exercise on a

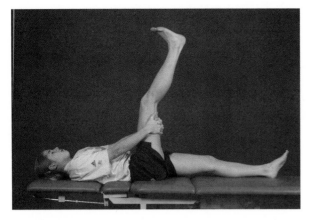

Figure PT.8 Stretching of the hamstrings in the supine position

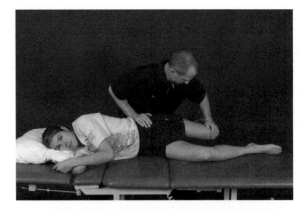

Figure PT.10 Test and treat for iliotibial band tightness

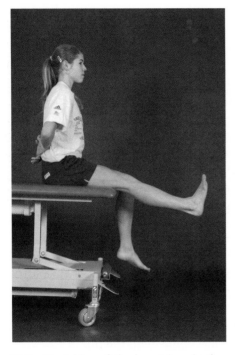

Figure PT.9 Stretching of the hamstrings in the seated position

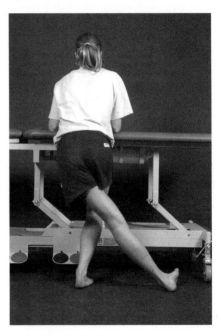

Figure PT.11 Iliotibial band stretching in a modified standing position

Swiss ball can make the stretching and balancing more challenging.

Iliotibial band

Tightness of the iliotibial band increases the lateral pull on the patella.[70] With knee flexion, the iliotibial band increases lateral compression of the patella by pulling its structure laterally.[71] Pain-free patients have less iliotibial band tightness (Figure PT.10). A patient with a shortened iliotibial band demonstrates excessive medial rotation of the hip during the stance phase of gait. This makes the pelvis on the opposite side drop (Trendelenburg sign). Stretching of the iliotibial band, especially the distal portion, is difficult (Figure PT.11). To achieve a more effective and

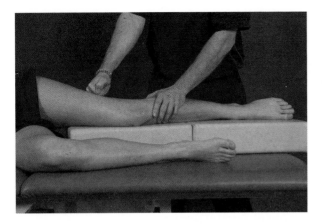

Figure PT.12 Soft tissue massage for iliotibial band tightness

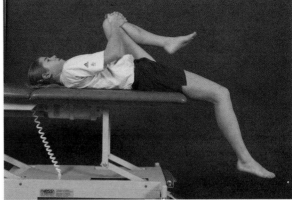

Figure PT.13 Test position for ventral hip and knee musculature

durable stretch of this lower portion, soft-tissue massage or myofascial release techniques can be used before stretching (Figure PT.12).

The gastrocnemius and soleus muscles

These reduce ankle dorsiflexion when they are tight. They also alter the gait cycle at mid-stance, causing a premature heel lift. Increased dynamic foot pronation may occur as compensation at the subtalar joint; this contributes to patellofemoral pain.[72] In a retrospective study, Gerrard[73] found that 80% of patients with unilateral patellofemoral pain had decreased ankle dorsiflexion on the affected side. Both the gastrocnemius and soleus muscles can be stretched by standing in the long-stepping position.

The quadriceps muscle

This has a significant correlation with the incidence of patellofemoral pain when it is shortened. Thus, stretching of the quadriceps muscle may help to unload painful structures (Figure PT.13). The quadriceps can be stretched by knee flexion lying prone, over the side of the bed while lying supine, or in standing. The leg must remain in the neutral position and not move not into abduction (Figure PT.14).

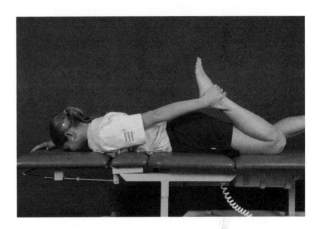

Figure PT.14 Rectus femoris stretching

Hip muscles

Hip muscles that limit hip rotation due to soft-tissue restriction can be caused by any or a combination of a tight anterior hip capsule, and short adductor, tensor fasciae latae, iliopsoas, or rectus femoris muscles. Pathological internal or external hip rotation may produce abnormal biomechanical stress on the patellofemoral joint. Limitation of hip rotation can be assessed in a figure-four position (reversed Faber's test) (Figure PT.15) when the patient is lying prone.

Restricted external rotation will require stretching of the hip musculature and retraining of the external rotators in a shortened position.[73]

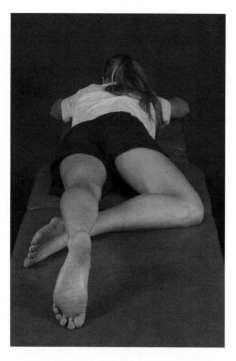

Figure PT.15   Figure four position

The problem is treated by stretching and strengthening of the glutei, hip abductors and adductors. This can be achieved through a combination of exercises with resistance, pelvic stabilization and proprioception training.

Myofascial trigger point treatment

This can be used with many interventions – stretch and spray, needling, injection, massage, compression, transcutaneous electrical nerve stimulation, laser and ultrasound. For patients with patellofemoral pain, trigger point treatment (stretching) can relieve pain and lengthen short overactive muscles, (e.g. hamstrings and tensor fascia latae).[74]

Massage

Massage can help to promote the repair process and restore normal function. The most effective form of massage therapy for patellofemoral pain seems to be the myofascial release technique.

Conclusion of interventions section

Successful nonoperative treatment of patello-femoral pain includes initial reduction of inflammation and pain using passive interventions, of which ice application and transcutaneous electrical nerve stimulation seem to be the most effective. Manual therapy may be appropriate after the passive interventions. An individual evaluation will lead to a specific training and exercise programme. Continuation of exercises (compliance) is vital to the successful outcome of the treatment programme.

Principles of training and rehabilitation

Patellofemoral disorders frequently cause dysfunction of the knee extensor muscles.[75,76] The goal of the rehabilitation, in combination with other modalities of physical therapy, is to restore the normal muscular function of the extensor apparatus and, with this, to improve load acceptance. The increase of loading must be managed according to the patient's symptoms and the selection of exercises must respect the Envelope of Function.[77] Exercises causing pain must be strictly avoided. Unphysiological loading of the patellofemoral joint delays or impedes normal healing of all the structures involved.[77] These principles of individual load acceptance must be respected during muscle rehabilitation. The common principles of training and rehabilitation include:

♦ Respect of the individual load acceptance of each patient.

♦ Individual load acceptance of each joint.

♦ Avoidance of exercises causing pain.

Biomechanics

Biomechanics of knee extension

Quadriceps force and compressive forces in the patellofemoral contact area change during flexion–extension movements. The amount of these forces depends on the tension of the quadriceps mechanism and the knee flexion angle.[78,79] Quadriceps force is greatest near full knee extension and decreases with more flexion. In full extension, the patella contacts the femur at a point just proximal to its apex.[80] As the knee proceeds into greater degrees of knee flexion, the contact area of the patellofemoral joint moves toward the proximal pole of the patella.[80] Because these conditions can change with the different types of exercises (e.g. open and closed kinetic chain exercises), they must be considered when choosing exercises for rehabilitation and training.[7,81]

The biomechanical aspects of open and closed kinetic chain exercises have been studied by numerous authors.[82–85] In an open kinetic chain exercise, the distal segment is free to move without any external resistance (e.g. seated knee extension). In a closed kinetic chain exercise, the feet are fixed from moving and are opposed with resistance.[86] Closed kinetic chain exercises replicate more functional activities, whereas open kinetic chain exercises are often used for isolated muscle strengthening.

Open kinetic chain exercises produce approximately 45% more rectus femoris activity than closed chain exercises. The lever arm of the knee joint increases with extension while it decreases forces on the patella.[87] Higher quadriceps strength for the final extension movement is necessary. Patients with quadriceps weakness have an extension deficit.[34]

Squats in closed kinetic chain exercises produce 40–50% more vastus medialis and lateralis activity.[86] When performing squats in the closed kinetic chain, quadriceps activity increases continuously with greater knee flexion and shows the greatest activity between 80° and 90°. Near full extension and in more than 90° of flexion, quadriceps activity with squats is low. Hamstrings activity is greatest during squats between 50° and 70° with the knee extending. The lateral parts of the hamstrings show greater activity than the medial part.[83] With closed kinetic chain exercises, the flexion moment arm increases with greater knee flexion. To resist these forces, greater quadriceps muscle activity is necessary; but this also increases the patellofemoral joint reaction forces. These forces are approximately half of the body weight during normal walking, three or four times the body weight when ascending or descending stairs, and seven to eight times the body weight when performing squats.[88] This explains why activities in loaded knee flexion are more painful.[34]

Witvrouw et al[29] prospectively studied the efficacy of open and closed kinetic chain exercises during nonoperative rehabilitation. Both treatment groups reported a significant decrease in pain, increase in muscle strength and increase in functional performance 3 months after rehabilitation. We encourage the least painful form of muscular training. The goal of the training is to improve the patient's objective findings and Envelope of Function in daily living activities. Training in the standing position improves the synergistic muscular interplay of the whole lower extremity. The form and intensity of the exercises are adapted based on the patient's subjective reports and clinical symptoms.

We train with open kinetic chain exercises from 90° to 40° of knee flexion at the beginning of rehabilitation. This range of motion provides the lowest amount of patellofemoral joint reaction forces while exhibiting the largest patellofemoral contact area.[34] But we replace the open kinetic chain as soon as possible with closed kinetic chain exercises in 0–30° or 0–60° of knee flexion.

Biomechanical faults of the lower extremity

These are believed to contribute to patellofemoral pain. Intrinsic structural factors (e.g. trochlear dysplasia, femoral anteversion) and extrinsic structural faults (e.g. muscular tightness, decreased flexibility, abnormal foot pronation) must be evaluated and considered when designing a rehabilitation programme. The joints of the ankle, knee, hip and pelvis form a functional unit. Injuries or pain may disturb and alter the normal functions of this unit. Gray[90] and Bizzini and Munzinger[89] have described an often-observed malfunctioning of this unit as 'medial collapse' in the one-leg-standing position with slight knee flexion. This insufficient active stabilization of the lower limb, and consequently of the whole body, is caused by noncoordinated synergistic muscular activity.

The abnormalities resulting in malfunction are noted, from distal to proximal, as follows:

♦ Flattened medial longitudinal plantar arch.

♦ Internal tibial torsion.

♦ Increased internally rotated tibia position.

♦ Internal femoral torsion.

♦ Increased internally rotated femur position.

♦ Externally rotated adducted (frequent) or abducted (rare) pelvic position.

♦ Mild scoliosis of the lumbar spine (concavity to the loaded side).

The lower limb exerts loads, especially in the medial capsular and ligamentous structures of the ankle and knee joints. The ipsilateral hip joint (in its posterolateral structures) and the ipsilateral sacroiliac joint, as well as the ipsilateral lumbar facets, are unilaterally compressed. Knee flexion is controlled by the quadriceps muscle, with resulting different patellofemoral joint reaction forces and activation patterns. The iliotibial tract, the biceps femoris and the lateral head of the gastrocnemius are synergistically active in controlling knee flexion. Therefore, structural overloading or overuse of the functional unit formed by the lower extremity, pelvis and lower back may occur. The 'medial collapse' in the one-leg-standing position is not only a typical observation in nonoperative or postoperative patients with different knee pathologies, but also in patients presenting with ankle and hip musculoskeletal problems. It can be observed in patients with an overall physical deconditioning or with generalized joint laxity. In cases of bony variances, such as femoral anteversion (excessive or diminished), tibial torsion (inwards or outwards) or knee varus or valgus, considerations about 'medial collapse' should be taken with caution. The presented therapeutic principles and exercises (see Motor control, below) can be applied in the rehabilitation of most patients with patellofemoral pain.

Biomechanical training principles include:

♦ Promoting and improving control and active stabilization of the lower limb, based on a biomechanical model.

♦ Promoting trunk and pelvis control and stabilization – a key element.

Quadriceps training techniques

Inhibition of the quadriceps muscle by pain and swelling leads to weakness and hypotrophy. The vastus medialis obliquus muscle shows the greatest amount of muscular inhibition compared to the vastus lateralis or rectus femoris muscles. Changes in the quadriceps muscle strongly influence the dynamics of the patellofemoral joint. To know that lack of equilibrium of strength and function of the quadriceps muscle is a significant problem is important for clinical practice. Restoration of strength and function of the quadriceps muscle is a key component of physical therapy.[7,19] A common strengthening programme of the quadriceps muscle is not the same as the muscular rehabilitation of a patient with patellofemoral pain. This rehabilitation requires a specific training of all components of strength according to a precise analysis of the deficit.

The vastus medialis obliquus muscle plays a significant, but not yet completely elucidated, role in the treatment of patients with patellofemoral pain. Powers[7] indicates that numerous authors have reported isolated insufficiency of the vastus medialis obliquus and asynchronous neuromuscular timing between the vastus medialis obliquus muscle and the vastus lateralis muscle. The vastus medialis obliquus muscle, with its distal fibres angled at approximately 55° from the longitudinal axis of the femur, is a medial stabilizer of the patella. It helps to prevent lateral subluxation.[91] The literature offers conflicting reports on the relative recruitment and neuromuscular timing of the vasti musculature.

Various forms of therapeutic exercises (open and closed kinetic chain), based on biomechanical principles, in combination with external support (taping, bracing), should be incorporated in the treatment programme, always individually adapted.

The rehabilitation programme consists of three different steps:

1. *Static exercises.* Isometric exercises are often the only possibility for strengthening the quadriceps in the acute phase of patellofemoral pain.[92] Painless improvement of the neuromuscular activation of the quadriceps must be achieved. Usually, exercises at 0–20° of knee flexion are pain-free (Figure PT.16). Hyperextension must be strictly avoided. The goals are to:

   ♦ Develop control and stabilization while standing on both legs.
   ♦ Develop control and stabilization while standing on one leg.

2. *Dynamic exercises.* These exercises are added as soon as possible. Strengthening exercises of the quadriceps are preferably performed with the patient seated at the end of a table. Exercises are performed against gravity, then weights may be added. To minimize the patellofemoral joint reaction forces, open kinetic chain exercises are allowed in a range of 90–40° of flexion. Patients should train in a pain-free manner and with reference to the individual Envelope of Function (Figures PT.17, PT.18). The goals are to:

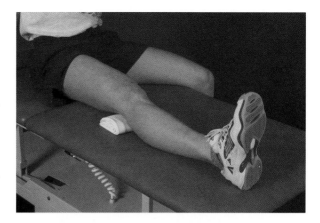

Figure PT.16 Isolated open kinetic chain static exercise for quadriceps muscle

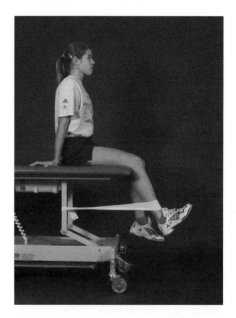

Figure PT.17 Isolated open kinetic chain dynamic exercise for quadriceps muscle against elastic resistance

♦ Develop control and stabilization with both knees flexed.
♦ Develop monopodal control and stabilization with the knee flexed.
♦ Use bodyweight (Figures PT.19, PT.20, PT.21), machines (Figure PT.22), and free weights (Figures PT.23, PT.24).

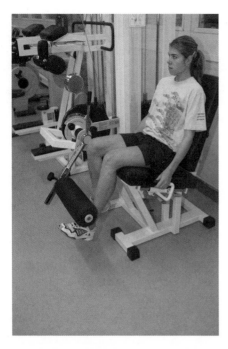

Figure PT.18 Isolated open kinetic chain dynamic exercise for quadriceps muscle with a weight-training machine

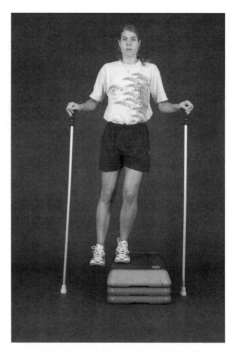

Figure PT.20 Dynamic closed kinetic chain exercise with body weight: single leg lateral step up

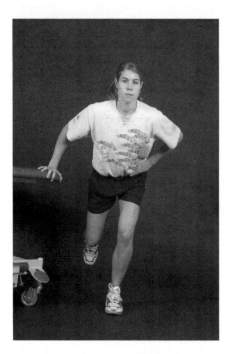

Figure PT.19 Dynamic closed kinetic chain exercise with body weight: single leg squat

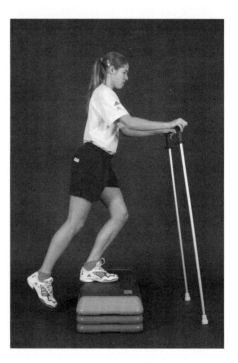

Figure PT.21 Dynamic closed kinetic chain exercise with body weight: single leg front step up

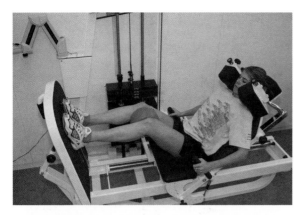

Figure PT.22 Dynamic closed kinetic chain exercise with weight-training machine: double leg squat, squeezing a soft ball to increase medial stabilization

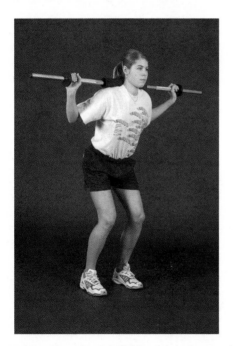

Figure PT.23 Dynamic closed kinetic chain exercise with free weight: double leg squat

3. *Reactive exercises.* (Figures PT.25a,b, PT.26, PT.27, PT.28, PT.29).

Patellar taping

The master plan of patellar taping in combination with functional exercises for the lower extremity was first described in 1986 by McConnell.[68]

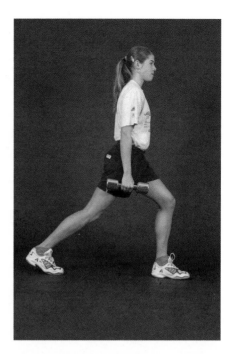

Figure PT.24 Dynamic closed kinetic chain exercise with free weights: front lunge

(a)

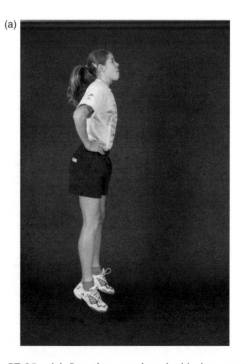

Figure PT.25 (a) Reactive exercise: double leg squat jump. (b) Reactive exercise: double leg squat jump (optimal landing)

(b)

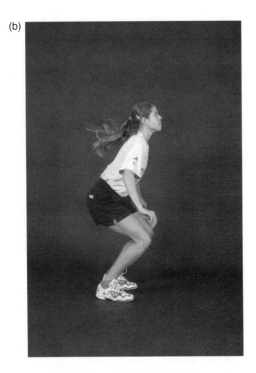

Figure PT.25 (*continued*)

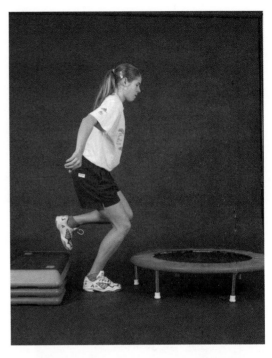

Figure PT.27 Reactive exercise: single leg plyometrics between step and trampoline

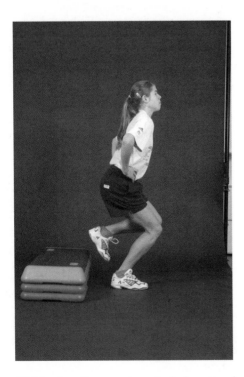

Figure PT.26 Reactive exercise: single leg step down jump (optimal landing)

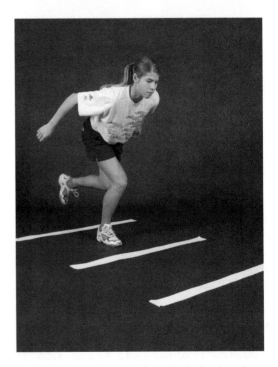

Figure PT.28 Reactive exercise: single leg hop for distance

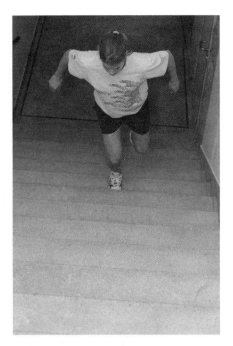

Figure PT.29   Reactive exercise: single leg hop upstairs

The primary goal of patellar taping is to improve patellar tracking and to change the patient's symptoms.[93] Patellar tape should facilitate functional muscle training and mobility exercises by reducing the pain.

Techniques of patellar taping

Precise assessment of the patellar position is mandatory for a successful outcome. Patellar taping is unique to each patient and to each disorder.[94] The exact direction and tension of the tape must be clear. After application of each piece of tape, the effect on pain reduction, load acceptance and the patient's symptoms must be reassessed. If the tape influences the patient's symptoms positively, training in the open and closed kinetic chain exercises can begin (Figures PT.30, PT.31, PT.32, PT.33).

Patellar taping examples

The different techniques can be used alone or combined in order to correct patellar position. Taping can facilitate gluteal and vastus

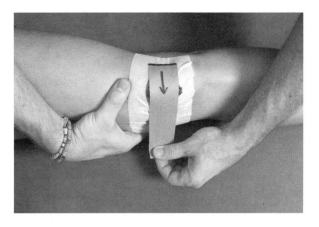

Figure PT.30   Patellar taping for medial glide correction

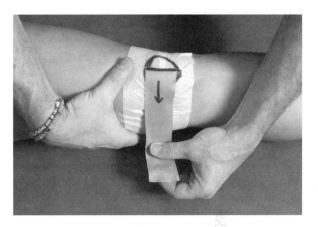

Figure PT.31   Patellar taping for tilt correction

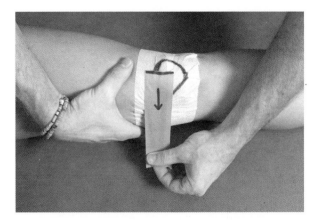

Figure PT.32   Patellar taping for glide and anterior–posterior correction

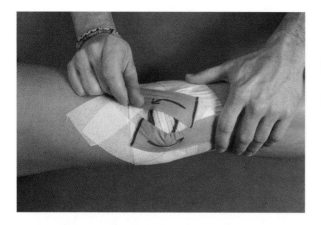

Figure PT.33   Patellar taping for rotational correction

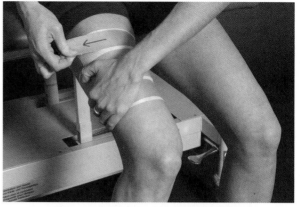

Figure PT.35   Patellar taping to facilitate vastus lateralis (application by the patient)

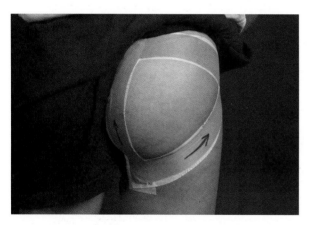

Figure PT.34   Patellar taping to facilitate gluteal activation

lateralis activation to unload the infrapatellar fat pad. Examples of taping are shown in Figures PT.34–PT.41.

Strengthening the whole lower extremity

Rehabilitation programmes designed for patients with patellofemoral pain must address the strengthening of the whole lower extremity, according to the individual's needs, such as hip rotators (Figures PT.42, PT.43), hip abductors and adductors (Figures PT.44, PT.45), hip extensors (Figures PT.46, PT.47), calf muscles (Figures PT.48, PT.49) and trunk musculature

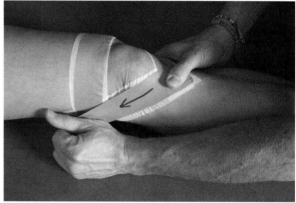

Figure PT.36   Patellar taping to unload the infrapatellar fat pad

for core stability (Figures PT.50, PT.51, PT.52, PT.53).

Electrical stimulation

Electrical muscle stimulation has been discussed in the previous pages of this chapter. It may be used in a static way when the musculature is stimulated at different angles of knee flexion, and later it may be combined with dynamic exercises (Figure PT.54).

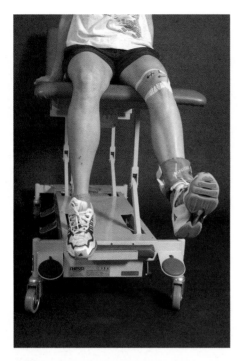

Figure PT.37 Patellar taping with dynamic open kinetic chain exercise using ankle weight

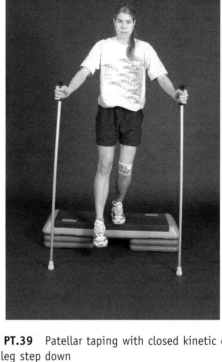

Figure PT.39 Patellar taping with closed kinetic chain single leg step down

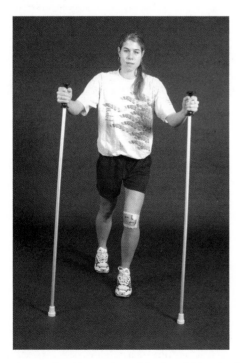

Figure PT.38 Patellar taping with closed kinetic chain single leg squat

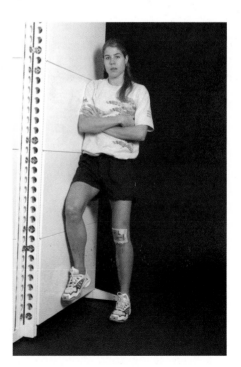

Figure PT.40 Patellar taping with a wall-supported closed kinetic chain single leg squat

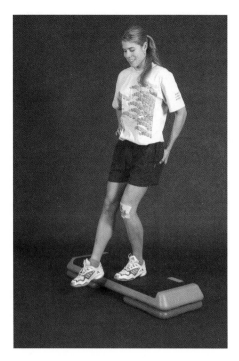

Figure PT.41 Patellar taping with a single leg step down (patient facilitating gluteal muscles)

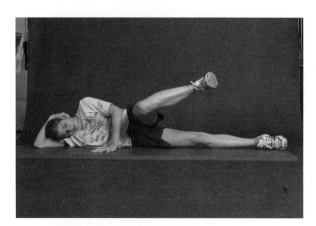

Figure PT.42 Hip rotators exercise

Biofeedback

The most frequently used biofeedback in physical therapy is electromyographic biofeedback. This simple application reveals visible and audible information about the patient's muscle activation.

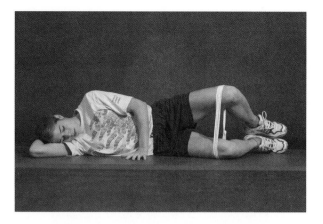

Figure PT.43 Hip rotators exercise with elastic resistance

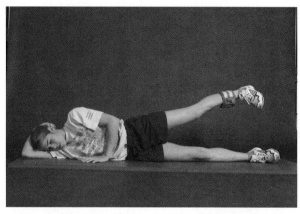

Figure PT.44 Hip abductors exercise with ankle weight

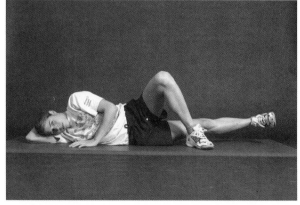

Figure PT.45 Hip adductors exercise

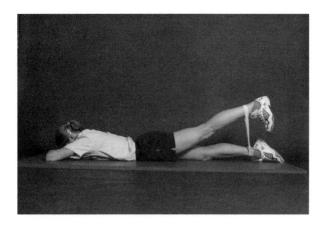

Figure PT.46 Hip extensors exercise with elastic resistance

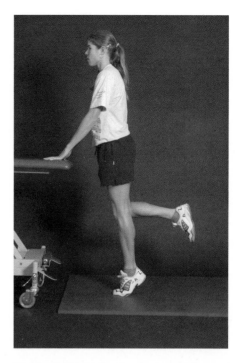

Figure PT.48 Calf muscles (gastrocnemius) exercise in standing position

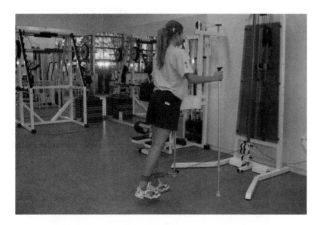

Figure PT.47 Hip extensors exercise with a free cable column

The patient must concentrate on neuromuscular control to activate the stimulated muscle.

Dursun et al[95] studied the effect of biofeedback in patients with patellofemoral pain. Musculature activation was improved after 4 weeks, but the clinical outcome did not change. McConnell et al[94] recommend biofeedback to improve activation and timing of the vastus medialis obliquus muscle and vastus lateralis to optimize patellar balancing.

We see biofeedback as an additional help to motivate the patient (Figure PT.55).

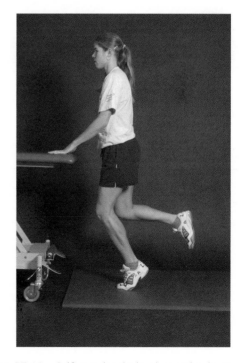

Figure PT.49 Calf muscles (soleus) exercise in standing position

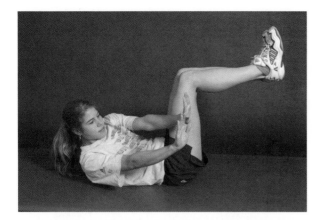

Figure PT.50　Lateral abdominal muscles exercise

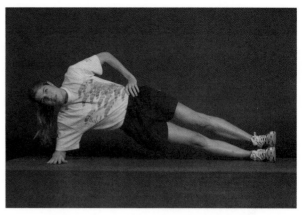

Figure PT.53　Core muscles stabilization exercise (lateral supported position)

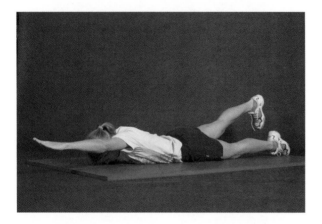

Figure PT.51　Back extensors muscle exercise in prone position

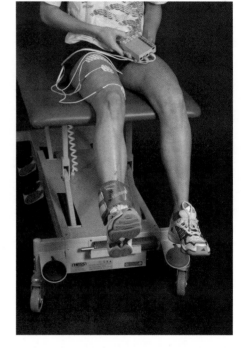

Figure PT.54　Quadriceps electrical stimulation in open kinetic chain exercise with ankle weight

Isokinetic testing and exercise

Isokinetic testing is helpful to analyse the different types of strength under dynamic conditions.[35] Isokinetic exercises include variable resistance or force adapted to recruitment of the muscle fibres. The angle velocity remains constant and the range

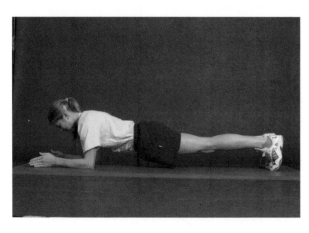

Figure PT.52　Core muscles stabilization exercise (ventral supported position)

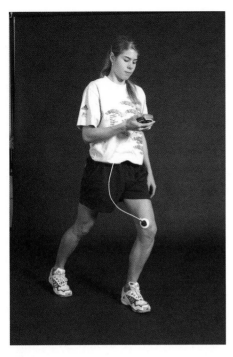

Figure PT.55 Vastus medialis biofeedback training in single leg stance

of motion is not decreased by fatigue. These types of exercises are called 'accommodating resistance' exercises.

Stiene et al[82] compared two groups of patients with patellofemoral dysfunctions who participated in different programmes – one with open kinetic chain exercises (isokinetic training) and the other with closed kinetic chain exercises (short squats). They evaluated them after 8 weeks of training and 1 year later. The results showed that both groups had significant improvement of isokinetic strength, but that only the group with closed kinetic chain training also improved in some other tests and in function.

Motor control

Poor quality of movement refers to the improper biomechanics of the lower extremities, trunk and arms during physical activities. It has been theorized that poor quality of movement may be one of the factors for the development of patellofemoral pain.

Numerous muscles altering the biomechanics of the knee joint have been implicated. These include weakness of the hip abductor and external rotator muscles. Structural or biomechanical alterations of the lower extremity, such as excessive foot pronation, excessive Q angle, static tibial external rotation and femoral anteversion, have been considered to be contributory factors in the development of patellofemoral pain.[96]

Numerous hypotheses abound, but the controversy about the cause of patellofemoral pain continues. Apparently, there is not one single cause for patellofemoral pain in all patients. This is abundantly clear in the Case Studies presented in this book.

Sensorimotor system

The sensorimotor system (Figure PT.56) represents the composite of the physiological systems

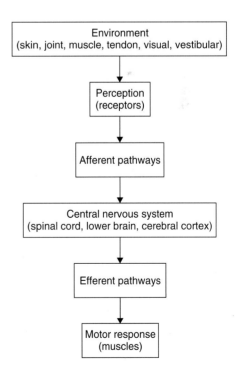

Figure PT.56 Sensorimotor system. Modified after Biedert[97,100]

of the complex neurosensory and neuromuscular process. 'Sensorimotor system' describes mechanisms involved in the acquisition of a sensory stimulus to a neural signal, along with transmission of the signal via afferent pathways to the central nervous system.[97] It describes processing and integration of the signal by the various centres of the central nervous system and central command generators, as well as the motor responses resulting in muscle activation for locomotion and the performance of functional tasks and joint stabilization.

The process by which afferent peripheral signals are used for motor control can be categorized into either feedback or feedforward mechanisms. *Feedback* is characterized by a reactive reflex to imposed forces on a joint; feedback neuromuscular control mechanisms are involved in maintaining posture and regulating slow movements.[98] *Feedforward* is characterized by preactivated muscle control in anticipation to loads or subsequent events; the feedforward mechanisms are used to evaluate results and to help programme future muscle-activation strategies. The idea is that preactivated (stiff) muscles recognize unexpected (destabilizing) joint loads quicker and can also facilitate feedback neuromuscular control.[98]

Motor learning

Motor learning, as defined by Schmidt and Lee,[99] is a series of internal processes that, combined with training and experience, lead to long-term adaptations or changes in motor skills. Three main stages of motor learning have been proposed. During the (verbal) cognitive phase, the patient learns the goals and the appropriate responses. In the motor stage (or intermediate phase), the patient focuses more on effective response strategies. In the last phase (autonomous phase), the patient's responses are automatic and executed on the subconscious level.

The motor learning literature indicates that nearly any variation that increases the availability of information feedback benefits performance; the practice phase increases the rate of improvement over trials. Motor learning strategies integrate the afferent (perceptive) and efferent functions of mind and body. These functions govern posture and movement. Optimal motor learning requires programmed activity for muscles that produce a desired movement and for muscles that stabilize the moving parts to ensure their correct position.[100]

Cognitive, perceptual and motor mechanisms are not independent elements, but are inseparable parts of the motor behaviour. A large amount of rehabilitation can be seen as a learning process, during which the patient must master new skills (e.g. walking with crutches) or must reacquire old skills (e.g. decelerating and stabilizing the knee after landing from a jump). The therapist is the designer of the learning situations. The physical therapist should not teach the patient how to master skills, but rather should give guidelines to the patient on how to regain skills, including loading and stabilizing the lower extremity. The patient must develop his/her own motor strategies.

Integrating the concepts of motor learning into rehabilitation occurs in the acute or subacute phase (*see* the discussion of rehabilitation phases in Rehabilitation protocols, above). The key points to guide the patient safely and effectively in the functional weight-bearing positions are:

♦ Respect the knee-joint status (pain, swelling).

♦ Respect the safe ranges of motion during exercises and activities.

♦ Allow only qualitative coordinated motion and stabilization strategies.

The third point is an important aspect in individual progression. When the patient can no longer control the body position, or if muscle shaking occurs while performing a motor task, the patient should stop training. These are the two first signs of neuromuscular fatigue.

During the chronic phase of rehabilitation, the individual progression can be intensified. The focus is set on specific goals of the patient (job, hobby and sport).

Principles of motor control and motor learning have been derived from research:[99]

♦ *Random practice.* The physical therapist randomizes the order in which exercises and activities are performed from session to session. This type of practice ensures long-term skill acquisition.

♦ *Variable practice.* The practice of exercises and activities takes place under varying degrees of difficulty, speed and environmental conditions. This helps the patient to develop his/her own motor control strategies during old and new tasks.

♦ *Summary feedback.* The physical therapist provides the patient, after some practice, with a performance summary (focusing on a few key points). This allows the patient to develop internal feedback mechanisms.[101]

Methods for sensorimotor training

Body position(s)

One of the keys in sensorimotor rehabilitation is to teach the patient how to stabilize his/her lower extremity and body. Bizzini[102] describes the following model, consisting of four steps:

1. *Ensure a stable basis.* The rearfoot and forefoot complex must be actively stabilized. Synergistic muscle activities, such as between the tibialis anterior and peroneus longus muscles, are necessary. If this is not possible, the use of orthotics, tape, or special shoes may be needed. These increase the stabilization of the tibia with a synergistic interplay between the tibialis posterior and soleus muscles, as an example (Figure PT.57a,b).

2. *Align the femur.* Correct alignment of the femur must be achieved in order to avoid excessive internal rotation. Stabilization by

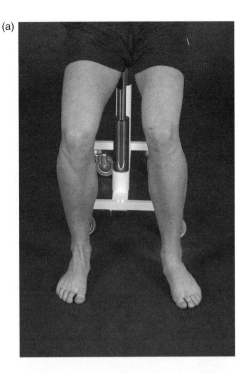

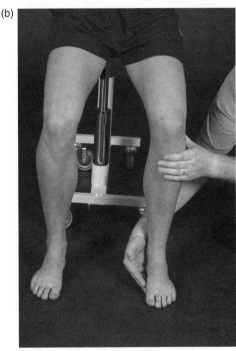

Figure PT.57 (a) Spontaneous poor active stabilization of the left leg in sitting position. (b) Tactile stimulation to improve position sense and active stabilization of the left leg in sitting position

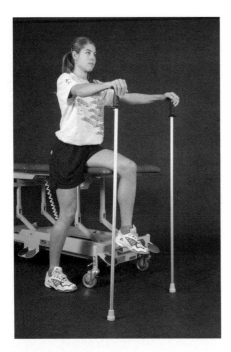

Figure PT.58 Exercise to improve position sense and active stabilization of the right leg in a stable sitting position (table)

the two-joint muscle groups, such as the pes anserinus group, are necessary (Figures PT.58, PT.59, PT.60a,b).

3. *Optimize the pelvis position.* The position of the pelvis can be stabilized by hip abductor and hip rotator muscle groups (Figure PT.61).

4. *Stabilize the spine and trunk.* Stabilization of the lumbar spine and the whole trunk is necessary (Figure PT.62).

Functional exercise progression

The patient should be able to master each motor task before progressing to the next motor task. This correlates with the third point of a criterion-based protocol. The stresses imposed by these activities must progress gradually to give the

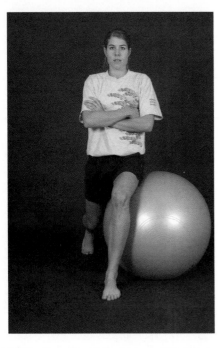

Figure PT.59 Exercise to improve position sense and active stabilization of the left leg in an unstable sitting position (Swiss ball)

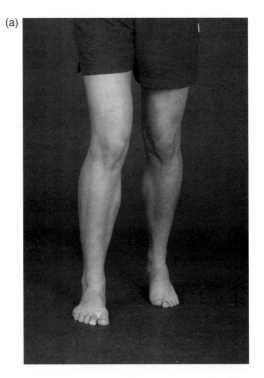

Figure PT.60 (a) Spontaneous poor active stabilization of the right leg in standing position. (b) Tactile stimulation to improve position sense and active stabilization of the right leg in standing position

(b)

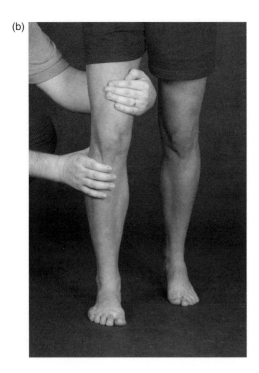

Figure PT.60 (*continued*)

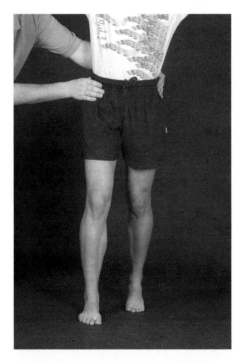

Figure PT.61 Tactile stimulation to improve position sense and active stabilization of the pelvis and right leg in standing position

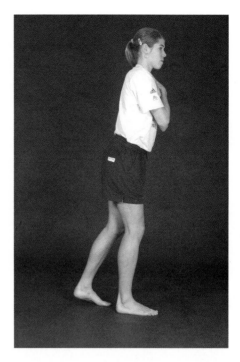

Figure PT.62 Acquired ability for active stabilization of the whole body in standing position

patient time to adapt to these loads. Bizzini[102] describes the following three-step progression:

1. Progress from double-leg to single-leg body positions (Figures PT.63, PT.64).

2. Progress from static to dynamic motor tasks (Figures PT.65, PT.66).

3. Progress from dynamic to reactive motor tasks; increase speed and intensity (Figures PT.67, PT.68, PT.69, PT.70).

Training devices

Numerous devices are used in functional progression to enhance the neuromuscular stabilization by increasing the muscular activations,[102] e.g:

♦ *Proprioceptive* (using the old terminology) devices (e.g. balance board).

♦ *External resistance* devices (e.g. physical therapist hands, Thera band).

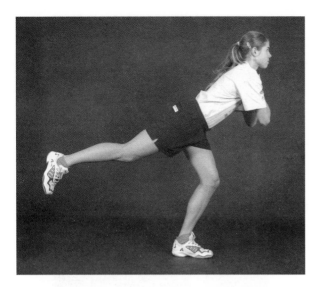

Figure PT.63   Challenging single leg active stabilization

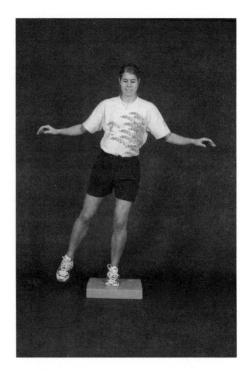

Figure PT.65   Single leg active stabilization on foam surface

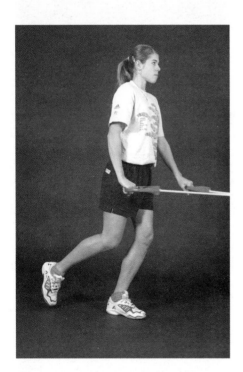

Figure PT.64   Single leg active stabilization against elastic resistance

♦ *Visual* devices (e.g. mirror).

♦ *Patient's own* devices (e.g. racquet by a tennis player).

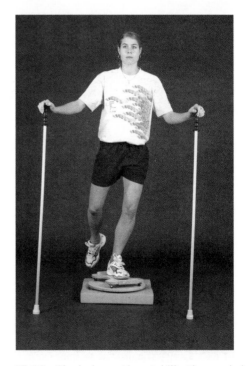

Figure PT.66   Single leg active stabilization on balance board

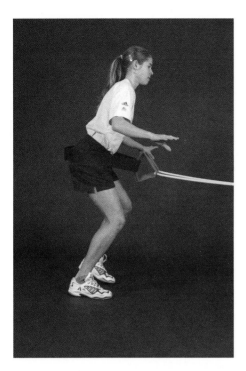

Figure PT.67 Reactive skippings against elastic resistance

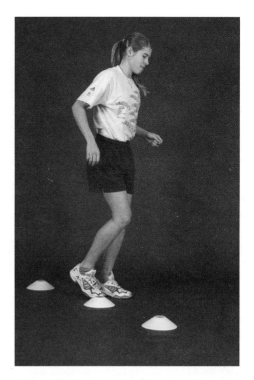

Figure PT.69 Reactive direction changings

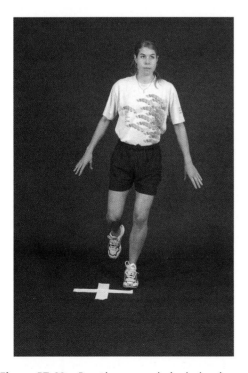

Figure PT.68 Reactive crossed single leg jumps

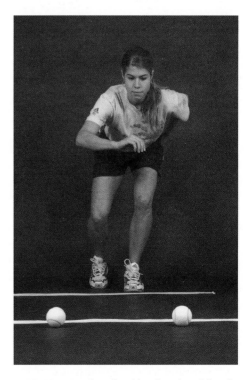

Figure PT.70 Acceleration/deceleration (shuttle-run)

Summary

In this concluding section of the chapter we have emphasized the principles of training and rehabilitation for patients with patellofemoral pain. The nonoperative treatment for these patients is individually designed (criterion-based) by the therapist. It promotes pain-free exercises, and works toward pain-free load acceptance. Based upon biomechanical principles, we promote a static exercise programme followed by a dynamic exercise programme to improve control and to help the patient stabilize the trunk, pelvis and lower limbs. We help the patient integrate the concepts of motor learning through biofeedback and sensorimotor learning. Rehabilitation consists of therapeutic interventions and a training programme, but the ultimate goal is to help the patient attain goals of choice (job, hobbies, sports) because the patient has learned the proper body mechanics.

References

1. Thomee R, Augustsson J, Karlsson J (1999) Patellofemoral pain syndrome: a review of current issues. *Sports Med* 28: 245–262
2. Sackett DL (2000) *Evidence-based Medicine: How to Practice and Teach EBM*, 2nd edn. New York, Churchill Livingstone
3. Dye SF (1996) The knee as a biologic transmission with an envelope of function: a theory. *Clin Orthop* 325: 10–18
4. Merchant AC (1988) Classification of patellofemoral disorders. *Arthroscopy* 4: 235–240
5. Wilk KE, Davies GJ, Mangine RE, Malone TR (1998) Patellofemoral disorders: a classification system and clinical guidelines for nonoperative rehabilitation. *J Orthop Sports Phys Ther* 28: 307–322
6. Engel GL (1977) The need for a new medical model: a challenge for biomedicine. *Science* 196: 129–136
7. Powers CM (1998) Rehabilitation of patellofemoral joint disorders: a critical review. *J Orthop Sports Phys Ther* 28: 345–354
8. Philadelphia P (2001) Philadelphia panel evidence-based clinical practice guidelines on selected rehabilitation interventions for knee pain. *Phys Ther* 81: 1675–1700
9. Bizzini M, Childs JD, Piva SR, Delitto A (2003) Systematic review of the quality of randomized controlled trials for patellofemoral pain syndrome. *J Orthop Sports Phys Ther* 33: 4–20
10. Antich TJ, Randall CC, Westbrook RA et al (1986) Physical therapy treatment of knee extensor mechanism disorders: comparison of four treatment modalities. *J Orthop Sports Phys Ther* 8: 255–259
11. Clark DI, Downing N, Mitchell J et al (2000) Physiotherapy for anterior knee pain: a randomised controlled trial. *Ann Rheum Dis* 59: 700–704
12. Eburne J, Bannister G (1996) The McConnell regimen versus isometric quadriceps exercises in the management of anterior knee pain. A randomised prospective controlled trial. *The Knee* 3: 151–153
13. Eng JJ, Pierrynowski MR (1993) Evaluation of soft foot orthotics in the treatment of patellofemoral pain syndrome. *Phys Ther* 73: 62–8; discussion 68–70
14. Finestone A, Radin EL, Lev B et al (1993) Treatment of overuse patellofemoral pain. Prospective randomized controlled clinical trial in a military setting. *Clin Orthop* 293: 208–210
15. Fulkerson JP, Folcik MA (1986) Comparison of diflunisal and naproxen for relief of anterior knee pain. *Clin Ther* 9 (suppl C): 59–61
16. Harrison EL, Sheppard MS, McQuarrie AM (1999) A randomized controlled trial of physical therapy treatment programs in patellofemoral pain syndrome. *Physiother Canada* Spring: 93–100
17. Jensen R, Gothesen O, Liseth K, Baerheim A (1999) Acupuncture treatment of patellofemoral pain syndrome. *J Alt Compl Med* 5: 521–527
18. Kannus P, Natri A, Niittymaki S, Jarvinen M (1992) Effect of intraarticular glycosaminoglycan polysulfate treatment on patellofemoral pain syndrome. A prospective, randomized double-blind trial comparing glycosaminoglycan polysulfate with placebo and quadriceps muscle exercises. *Arthritis Rheum* 35: 1053–1061

19. Kannus P, Natri A, Paakkala T, Jarvinen M (1999) An outcome study of chronic patellofemoral pain syndrome. Seven-year follow-up of patients in a randomized, controlled trial. *J Bone Joint Surg Am* **81**: 355–363

20. Kowall MG, Kolk G, Nuber GW et al (1996) Patellar taping in the treatment of patellofemoral pain. A prospective randomized study. *Am J Sports Med* **24**: 61–66

21. Miller MD, Hinkin DT, Wisnowski JW (1997) The efficacy of orthotics for anterior knee pain in military trainees. A preliminary report. *Am J Knee Surg* **10**: 10–13

22. Raatikainen T, Vaananen K, Tamelander G (1990) Effect of glycosaminoglycan polysulfate on chondromalacia patellae. A placebo-controlled 1-year study. *Acta Orthop Scand* **61**: 443–448

23. Rogvi-Hansen B, Ellitsgaard N, Funch M et al (1991) Low-level laser treatment of chondromalacia patellae. *Int Orthop* **15**: 359–361

24. Roush MB, Sevier TL, Wilson JK et al (2000) Anterior knee pain: a clinical comparison of rehabilitation methods. *Clin J Sport Med* **10**: 22–28

25. Rowlands BW, Brantingham JW (1999) The efficacy of patella mobilization in patients suffering from patellofemoral pain syndrome. *J Neuromusculoskeletal System* **7**: 142–149

26. Suter E, McMorland G, Herzog W, Bray R (2000) Conservative lower back treatment reduces inhibition in knee-extensor muscles: a randomized controlled trial. *J Manip Physiol Ther* **23**: 76–80

27. Timm KE (1998) Randomized controlled trial of Protonics on patellar pain, position, and function. *Med Sci Sports Exerc* **30**: 665–670

28. Thomee R (1997) A comprehensive treatment approach for patellofemoral pain syndrome in young women. *Phys Ther* **77**: 1690–1703

29. Witvrouw E, Lysens R, Bellemans J et al (2000) Open versus closed kinetic chain exercises for patellofemoral pain. A prospective, randomized study. *Am J Sports Med* **28**: 687–694

30. Nagy SZ (1991) Disability concepts revised: implications for prevention. In: Pope AM, Tarlov AR (eds), *Disability in America: Toward a National Agenda for Prevention.* Washington, DC, National Academy Press, pp 309–327

31. Shelbourne KD, Nitz P (1990) Accelerated rehabilitation after anterior cruciate ligament reconstruction. *Am J Sports Med* **18**: 292–299

32. Wilk KE, Andrews JR (1992) Current concepts in the treatment of anterior cruciate ligament disruption. *J Orthop Sports Phys Ther* **15**: 279–293

33. Mangine RE, Kremchek TE (1997) Evaluation-based protocol of the anterior cruciate ligament. *J Sports Rehab* **6**: 157–181

34. McGinty G, Irrgang JJ, Pezzullo D (2000) Biomechanical considerations for rehabilitation of the knee. *Clin Biomech (Bristol, Avon)* **15**: 160–166

35. Werner S (1995) An evaluation of knee extensor and knee flexor torques and EMGs in patients with patellofemoral pain syndrome in comparison with matched controls. *Knee Surg Sports Traumatol Arthrosc* **3**: 89–94

36. Irrgang JJ, Snyder-Mackler L, Wainner RS et al (1998) Development of a patient-reported measure of function of the knee. *J Bone Joint Surg Am* **80**: 1132–1145

37. Grana WA, Kriegshauser LA (1985) Scientific basis of extensor mechanism disorders. *Clin Sports Med* **4**: 247–257

38. Leroux A, Belanger M, Boucher JP (1995) Pain effect on monosynaptic and polysynaptic reflex inhibition. *Arch Phys Med Rehabil* **76**: 576–582

39. Cesarelli M, Bifulco P, Bracale M (2000) Study of the control strategy of the quadriceps muscles in anterior knee pain. *IEEE Trans Rehabil Eng* **8**: 330–341

40. Fulkerson JP, Shea KP (1990) Disorders of patellofemoral alignment. *J Bone Joint Surg Am* **72**: 1424–1429

41. Shelton GL (1992) Conservative management of patellofemoral dysfunction. *Prim Care* **19**: 331–350

42. Kowal MA (1983) Review of physiological effects of cryotherapy. *J Orthop Sports Phys Ther* **5**: 66–73

43. Knight KL, Londeree BR (1980) Comparison of blood flow in the ankle of uninjured subjects during therapeutic applications of heat, cold, and exercise. *Med Sci Sports Exerc* **12**: 76–80

44. Knight KL (1990) Cold as a modifier of sports-induced inflammation. In: Leadbetter WB, Buckwalter JA, Gordon SL (eds), *Sports-induced*

Inflammation. Chicago, American Academy of Orthopedic Furgeons, pp 463–477

45. Herrington L, Payton CJ (1983) Effects of corrective taping of the patella on patients with patellofemoral pain. *Physiotherapy* 83: 566–572

46. Hultman E, Sjoholm H, Jaderholm-Ek I, Krynicki J (1983) Evaluation of methods for electrical stimulation of human skeletal muscle *in situ*. *Pfluger's Arch* 398: 139–141

47. Godfrey CM, Jayawardena A, Welsh P (1979) Comparison of electro-stimulation and isometric exercise in strengthening the quadriceps muscle. *Physiother Canada* 31: 265–267

48. Williams RA, Morrisey MC, Brewster CE (1986) The effect of electrical stimulation on quadriceps strength and thigh circumference in meniscectomy patients. *J Orthop Sports Phys Ther* 8: 143–146

49. Trimble MH, Enoka RM (1991) Mechanisms underlying the training effects associated with neuromuscular electrical stimulation. *Phys Ther* 71: 273–280; discussion, 280–282

50. Coderre TJ, Katz J, Vaccarino AL, Melzack R (1993) Contribution of central neuroplasticity to pathological pain: review of clinical and experimental evidence. *Pain* 52: 259–285

51. Willer JC (1988) Relieving effect of TENS on painful muscle contraction produced by an impairment of reciprocal innervation: an electrophysiological analysis. *Pain* 32: 271–274

52. O'Brien WJ, Rutan FM, Sanborn C, Omer GE (1984) Effect of transcutaneous electrical nerve stimulation on human blood β-endorphin levels. *Phys Ther* 64: 1367–1374

53. Fargas-Babjak AM, Pomeranz B, Rooney PJ (1992) Acupuncture-like stimulation with codetron for rehabilitation of patients with chronic pain syndrome and osteoarthritis. *Acupunct Electrother Res* 17: 95–105

54. Jensen H, Zesler R, Christensen T (1991) Transcutaneous electrical nerve stimulation (TENS) for painful osteoarthritis of the knee. *Int J Rehab Res* 14: 356–358

55. Melzack R, Stillwell DM, Fox EJ (1977) Trigger points and acupuncture points for pain: correlations and implications. *Pain* 3: 3–23

56. Robertson VJ, Baker KG (2001) A review of therapeutic ultrasound: effectiveness studies. *Phys Ther* 81: 1339–1350

57. Lewit K (1997) *Manuelle Medizin*. Leipzig, Barth

58. Maitland GD (1977) *Peripheral Manipulation*, 2nd edn. London, Butterworth

59. Maitland GD (1986) *Vertebral Manipulation*, 5th edn. London, Butterworth

60. Biedert RM, Kernen V (2001) Neurosensory characteristics of the patellofemoral joint: what is the genesis of patellofemoral pain? *Sports Med Arthrosc Rev* 9: 295–300

61. Dye SF, Stäubli HU, Biedert RM, Vaupel GL (1999) The mosaic of pathophysiology causing patellofemoral pain: therapeutic implications. *Operative Tech Sports Med* 7: 46–54

62. Fulkerson JP (1982) Awareness of the retinaculum in evaluating patellofemoral pain. *Am J Sports Med* 10: 147–149

63. Sanchis-Alfonso V, Rosello-Sastre E (2000) Immunohistochemical analysis for neural markers of the lateral retinaculum in patients with isolated symptomatic patellofemoral malalignment. A neuroanatomic basis for anterior knee pain in the active young patient. *Am J Sports Med* 28: 725–731

64. Puniello MS (1993) Iliotibial band tightness and medial patellar glide in patients with patellofemoral dysfunction. *J Orthop Sports Phys Ther* 17: 144–148

65. Fulkerson JP, Hungerford DS (1990) *Disorders of the Patellofemoral Joint*, 2nd edn. Baltimore, MD, Williams & Wilkins

66. Terry GC, Hughston JC, Norwood LA (1986) The anatomy of the iliopatellar band and iliotibial tract. *Am J Sports Med* 14: 39–45

67. Thein J, Thein BL (1998) Nonoperative treatment for patellofemoral pain. *J Orthop Sports Phys Ther* 28: 336–344

68. McConnell J (1986) The management of chondromalacia patellae: a long-term solution. *Aust J Physiother* 32: 215–223

69. Witvrouw E, Lysens R, Bellemans J et al (2000) Intrinsic risk factors for the development of anterior knee pain in an athletic population. A two-year prospective study. *Am J Sports Med* 28: 480–489

70. Doucette SA, Goble EM (1992) The effect of exercise on patellar tracking in lateral patellar compression syndrome. *Am J Sports Med* 20: 434–440

71. Winslow J, Yoder E (1995) Patellofemoral pain in female ballet dancers: correlation with iliotibial band tightness and tibial external rotation. *J Orthop Sports Phys Ther* **22**: 18–21

72. Klingman RE, Liaos SM, Hardin KM (1997) The effect of subtalar joint posting on patellar glide position in subjects with excessive rearfoot pronation. *J Orthop Sports Phys Ther* **25**: 185–191

73. Gerrard B (1995) The patellofemoral complex. In: Zuluaga M, Briggs C, Carlisle J et al (eds), *Sports Physiotherapy: Applied Science and Practice*. Melbourne, Churchill Livingstone

74. Travell J, Simons D (1983) *Myofascial Pain and Dysfunction: The Trigger Point Manual*. Baltimore, MD, Williams & Wilkins

75. Callaghan MJ, Oldham JA (1996) The role of quadriceps exercise in the treatment of patellofemoral pain syndrome. *Sports Med* **21**: 384–391

76. Moller BN, Jurik AG, Tidemand-Dal C et al (1987) The quadriceps function in patellofemoral disorders. A radiographic and electromyographic study. *Arch Orthop Trauma Surg* **106**: 195–198

77. Dye SF (2001) Patellofemoral pain current concepts: an overview. *Sports Med Arthrosc Rev* **9**: 264–272

78. Hungerford DS, Barry M (1979) Biomechanics of the patellofemoral joint. *Clin Orthop* **144**: 9–15

79. Mansat C, Bonnel F, Jaeger JH (1982) *L'appareil Éxtenseur du Genou*. Paris, Masson

80. Müller W (1982) *Das Knie*. Heidelberg, Springer-Verlag

81. van Eijden TM, Kouwenhoven E, Weijs WA (1987) Mechanics of the patellar articulation. Effects of patellar ligament length studied with a mathematical model. *Acta Orthop Scand* **58**: 560–566

82. Stiene HA, Brosky T, Reinking MF et al (1996) A comparison of closed kinetic chain and isokinetic joint isolation exercise in patients with patellofemoral dysfunction. *J Orthop Sports Phys Ther* **24**: 136–141

83. Escamilla RF (2001) Knee biomechanics of the dynamic squat exercise. *Med Sci Sports Exerc* **33**: 127–141

84. Cohen ZA, Roglic H, Grelsamer RP et al. (2001) Patellofemoral stresses during open and closed kinetic chain exercises. An analysis using computer simulation. *Am J Sports Med* **29**: 480–487

85. Wallace DA, Salem GJ, Salinas R, Powers CM (2002) Patellofemoral joint kinetics while squatting with and without an external load. *J Orthop Sports Phys Ther* **32**: 141–148

86. Escamilla RF, Fleisig GS, Zheng N et al (1998) Biomechanics of the knee during closed kinetic chain and open kinetic chain exercises. *Med Sci Sports Exerc* **30**: 556–569

87. Grood ES, Suntay WJ (1983) A joint coordinate system for the clinical description of three-dimensional motions: application to the knee. *J Biomech Eng* **105**: 136–144

88. Reilly DT, Martens M (1972) Experimental analysis of the quadriceps muscle force and patellofemoral joint reaction force for various activities. *Acta Orthop Scand* **43**: 126–137

89. Bizzini M, Munzinger U (1998) Bewegungsanalyse der Einbeinkniebeuge. Beeinflussung der ventralen tibialen Translation durch eine definierte Korperstellung. Konsequenzen in der Kreuzbandrehabilitation. *Man Ther* **2**: 19–27

90. Gray G (1994) *Chain Reaction Plus. Successful Strategies for Closed Chain and Open Chain Testing and Rehabilitation*. Adrian, MI, Wynn Marketing

91. Cerny K (1995) Vastus medialis oblique/vastus lateralis muscle activity ratios for selected exercises in persons with and without patellofemoral pain syndrome. *Phys Ther* **75**: 672–683

92. Moller BN, Krebs B, Tidemand-Dal C, Aaris K (1986) Isometric contractions in the patellofemoral pain syndrome. An electromyographic study. *Arch Orthop Trauma Surg* **105**: 24–27

93. Grelsamer RP, McConnell J (1998) *The Patella. A Team Approach*. Gaithersburg, MD, Aspen

94. McConnell J (2002) The physical therapist's approach to patellofemoral disorders. *Clin Sports Med* **21**: 363–387

95. Dursun N, Dursun E, Kilic Z (2001) Electromyographic biofeedback-controlled exercise versus conservative care for patellofemoral pain syndrome. *Arch Phys Med Rehabil* **82**: 1692–1695

96. Eckhoff DG, Montgomery WK, Kilcoyne RF, Stamm ER (1994) Femoral morphometry and anterior knee pain. *Clin Orthop* **302**: 64–68

97. Biedert RM (2000) Contribution of the three levels of nervous system motor control: spinal cord,

lower brain, cerebral cortex. In: Lephart SM, Fu FH (eds), *Proprioception and Neuromuscular Control in Joint Stability*. Champaign, IL, Human Kinetics, pp 23–39

98. Lephart SM, Riemann BL, Fu FH (2001) Introduction to the sensorimotor system. In: Lephart SM, Fu FH (eds), *Proprioception and Neuromuscular Control in Joint Stability*. Champaign, IL, Human Kinetics

99. Schmidt RA, Lee TD (1999) *Motor Control and Learning. A Behavioral Emphasis*, 3rd edn. Champaign, IL, Human Kinetics

100. Biedert RM (1999) Sensory–Motor Function of the Knee Joint. Histologic, Anatomic, and Neurophysiologic Investigations. Thesis, University of Basel, Switzerland

101. Winstein CJ (1991) Knowledge of results and motor learning – implications for physical therapy. *Phys Ther* 71: 140–149

102. Bizzini M (2000) *Sensomotorische Rehabilitation nach Beinverletzungen*. Stuttgart, New York, Georg Thieme-Verlag

Suggested reading

Biedert RM (1999) Sensory–Motor Function of the Knee Joint. Histologic, Anatomic, and Neurophysiologic Investigations. Thesis, University of Basel, Switzerland

Biedert RM, Kernen V (2001) Neurosensory characteristics of the patellofemoral joint: what is the genesis of patellofemoral pain? *Sports Med Arthrosc Rev* 9: 295–300

Bizzini M (2000) *Sensomotorische Rehabilitation nach Beinverletzungen*. Stuttgart, New York, Georg Thieme-Verlag

Gray G (1994) *Chain Reaction Plus. Successful Strategies for Closed Chain and Open Chain Testing and Rehabilitation*. Adrian, MI, Wynn Marketing

McConnell J (2002) The physical therapist's approach to patellofemoral disorders. *Clin Sports Med* 21: 363–387

Thein J, Thein BL (1998) Nonoperative treatment for patellofemoral pain. *J Orthop Sports Phys Ther* 28: 336–344

Thomee R, Augustsson J, Karlsson J (1999) Patellofemoral pain syndrome: a review of current issues. *Sports Med* 28: 245–262

Werner S, Arvidsson H, Arvidsson I, Eriksson E (1993) Electrical stimulation of vastus medialis and stretching of lateral thigh muscles in patients with patellofemoral symptoms. *Knee Surg Sports Traumatol Arthrosc* 1: 85–92

Werner S, Eriksson E (1993) Isokinetic quadriceps training in patients with patellofemoral pain syndrome. *Knee Surg Sports Traumatol Arthrosc* 1: 162–168

Glossary

Active pathology   Interruption or interference with normal physiological processes and efforts of the organism to regain a normal state.[1,2]

Albee procedure   Surgical technique to reconstruct the lateral femur condyle, using a bone wedge from the tibia to elevate the lateral condyle in the treatment of habitual dislocation of the patella.[3–5]

Anterior knee pain   There is no consensus on a broader definition of anterior knee pain. It is not clearly defined.

Apprehension test   Test in which the examiner holds the relaxed knee in 30° of flexion and tries to subluxate the patella laterally. The patellar apprehension test may be so strongly positive that the patient withdraws the leg rapidly as the examiner approaches the knee with his/her hand, thus preventing any contact.[6]

Bandi procedure   *see* Maquet procedure.

Bayonet sign   Seen when a tibia vara of the proximal third causes a markedly increased Q angle. The alignment of quadriceps, patellar tendon and the tibial shaft resembles a French bayonet.[4]

Bernageau index   The only method to calculate the patellar height with reference to the trochlea. It is measured on a lateral radiograph with the leg in extension and the quadriceps muscle contracted. The distance between the superior line of the trochlea and the inferior edge of the articular surface is calculated. A patella alta is present if the distance is 6 mm or more; a patella baja is present if the distance is 6 mm or less.[7]

Blackburne–Peel index   Method to calculate the patellar height with reference to the tibia. The index by Blackburne–Peel[8] is represented by the ratio of the perpendicular line of the inferior pole of the articular surface of the patella to the tangent of the tibial plateau and the length of the articular surface of the patella.[3,8]

Blumensaat line   Line connecting the most anterior and posterior edges of the intercondylar notch roof. Used to measure the patellar height.[8]

Bump sign (trochlear bump)   Anterior translation of the trochlear floor measured on a true lateral radiograph. The 'bump sign' is a quantitative characteristic that is particularly significant in trochlear dysplasia. The trochlear bump increases with increasing severity of trochlear dysplasia. A bump of more than 3 mm is abnormal.[3,9]

Camel sign   Double hump seen from the side view; the hump is caused by a high-riding patella and uncovered infrapatellar fat pad.[4]

Catching   Transient, usually painful, interruptions in the normal gliding of the patella.[4]

Caton–Deschamps index   Method to calculate the patellar height with reference to the tibia. The index by Caton and Deschamps[10] is represented by the ratio of the distance between the distal edge of the articular surface of the patella and the anterosuperior angle of the tibia to the length of the articular surface of the patella.[11,12]

Patellofemoral Disorders: Diagnosis and Treatment.   Edited by Roland M. Biedert
© 2004 John Wiley & Sons, Ltd   ISBN: 0-470-85011-6

Congruence angle (Merchant angle) Angle to measure the patellofemoral joint congruence and to evaluate the patellar position; the only method that considers the orientation of the trochlea in the sagittal plane and quantitates, in degrees, the extent of lateralization. It is measured on a standard tangential (axial) radiograph of the patella with the knee in 45° of flexion and the X-ray beam projected at a 30° angle from the horizontal. This angle, which defines the relationship of the apex of the patella to the bisected femoral trochlea (bisected sulcus angle), must be less than 16° to be within the limits that Merchant defined as normal. The angle is positive if the patellar point is lateral to the bisector line (lateral subluxation).[13,14] The congruence reported by Schutzer[15] corresponds to the congruence angle described by Merchant to evaluate the patellar axial roentgenogram at 45° of knee flexion.

Crepitus Grating sensation caused by the dry synovial surfaces of a joint rubbing together. It is detected by examining the knee with the hand placed, palm downwards, upon the knee cap and with the joint flexed and extended. Crepitus may be both felt and heard, but is so regularly evident in asymptomatic knees that this feature is not of diagnostic value.[6]

Crossing sign A pathognomic factor of a dysplastic trochlea. The analysis is made with a lateral radiograph in 30° of knee flexion. The trochlear dysplasia is expressed by crossing of both condylar outlines (internal and external) with the outline of the trochlear floor. Three types of trochlear dysplasia can be defined, according to the level of crossing.[12] The dysplasia is more severe[3,9] when the point of crossing is more distal.

Cryokinetics Combination of ice application and exercise.[16,17]

Dejour sign Documentation of patella alta using CT scans. On CT scans through the femoral condyle, the notch has the form of a Roman arch; the patella is not visible in case of patella alta.

Disability Inability or limitation in performance of socially defined roles and tasks expected of an individual within a sociocultural and physical environment.[1,2]

Elmslie procedure (Roux–Elmslie–Trillat) Surgical technique in the treatment of habitual dislocation of the patella. Includes medial transfer of the tibial tuberosity on a periosteal hinge without anterior or posterior displacement. The tuberosity is fixed with a screw.[3,18]

Evidence-based medicine The conscientious, explicit, and judicious use of current best evidence in making decisions about the care of individual patients. The practice of evidence-based medicine means integrating individual clinical expertise with the best available external clinical evidence from systematic research.[19]

External tibial torsion Angle formed by the line tangent to the posterior aspect of the tibial plateau and the line through the bimalleolar axis.[9]

Femoral anteversion An angle formed by the intersection of a line joining the centre of the femoral head and femoral neck with a line tangential to the posterior aspects of the femoral condyles.[9]

Femoral sulcus depth index An index determined by a line drawn on a film. The line is drawn tangential to the posterior surface of the femoral condyles. The distances from this line to the most anterior points of the lateral and medial condyles and to the bottom of the sulcus are measured.[13]

Free nerve endings Type IVa: joint receptors which constitute the articular nociceptive system. They transmit information on pain and inflammation.[20,21] Type IVb: joint receptors which function as efferent vasomotors.[20]

Fulkerson procedure Surgical technique in the treatment of habitual dislocation of the patella. Includes anteromedial transposition of the tibial tuberosity.[18]

Functional limitation Limitation in performance at the level of the whole organism or person. Restriction in basic physical or emotional activities.[1,2]

Geometry Description of the shape, configuration and dimensions of an object or group of objects.

Giving-way Sudden weakness of the quadriceps muscle as a reflex to pain or to a feeling of the kneecap slipping over the lateral side of the trochlea, causing the knee to give way.[4]

Goldthwait procedure Surgical technique that involves the transfer of the lateral half of the patellar tendon behind the medial half. The lateral half is attached immediately adjacent to the remaining medial part of the patellar tendon.[22]

Green quadricepsplasty procedure Surgical technique to realign the deranged extensor mechanism proximally with concomitant lateral release and vastus medialis advancement.

Grelsamer index (Insall–Salvati index modified) see Insall–Salvati index modified.

Habitual dislocation Occasional repetitive dislocation of the patella to lateral or, rarely, to medial.

Hauser procedure Surgical technique with distal and medial transposition of the tibial tubercle.[4,18]

Height of the trochlea see Trochlear height.

Homeostasis Constant maintenance of normal physiological processes at all cellular and molecular levels, as well as the capability of restoring normal physiological processes after injury.[23–25]

Hunter's cap see Wiberg classification.

Impairment Loss or abnormality of an anatomical, physiological, mental or emotional ability.[1,2]

Index of trochlear height Index that corresponds to an angle defined by the crossing point

of reference of two straight lines. One is the tangential line of the posterior cortex of the femur, the other is a line from the most anterior point of the intercondylar groove. The angle is formed by these two lines. The measurement of this angle helps to define and to document dysplastic trochlea type 3 and more. see also Trochlear height and Chapter 6 – Radiographs.

Insall–Salvati index Method to calculate the patellar height with reference to the tibia. The index by Insall–Salvati is represented by the ratio of the length of the patellar tendon to the longest sagittal diameter of the patella.[26]

Insall–Salvati index modified (Grelsamer) Method to calculate the patellar height with reference to the tibia. It is represented by the ratio of the length of the patellar tendon to the length of the articular surface of the patella.[27]

J-sign Pathological patellar tracking during the beginning of knee flexion.[28] see Chapter 5 – Physical examination.

Krogius procedure Surgical technique advancing the vastus medialis obliquus muscle and the medial retinaculum together while loosening the lateral structures.[4]

Lateral patellar displacement Lateral transposition of the patella out of the trochlear groove, measured in millimeters on axial images.[13,29]

Lateral patellar tilt Angle between the line intersecting the widest part of the patella and the line tangential to the anterior surfaces of the femoral condyles.[13,29]

Lateral release Release of the oblique and superficial lateral retinaculum of the patellofemoral joint. It is performed by an open incision or arthroscopically.[3]

Laurin angle An angle that defines the patellar tilt. It is measured on axial views with 20° of knee flexion. The angle is formed by two lines, one joining the summits of the two trochlear slopes, the other tangential to the lateral slope of the patella. The Laurin angle can be positive (open laterally), null (lines parallel), or negative (open medially).[12,30,31] *see* Chapter 6 – Radiographs.

Laxity   Increased joint play caused by the constitutional quality of ligaments. The quality depends on collagen composition, age and gender.[32]

Locking   Sudden loss of full extension that might be relieved by manipulation of the knee. The locking may be intermittent or persistent. It must be distinguished from the often painful block caused by a torn meniscus or a loose body.[4,6]

Madigan procedure   Surgical technique transferring the vastus medialis muscle to lateral and distal with or without release of the lateral retinaculum.[33]

Maquet (Bandi) procedure   Surgical technique reducing the co-action of patella and trochlea. The tibial tuberosity is moved 2 cm anteriorly, with or without medialization or lateral release.[3]

Masse procedure   Reconstruction of the trochlea with deepening of the articular side, regaining the normal sulcus angle.[34]

Medial patellofemoral ligament   The most important medial soft-tissue stabilizer of the patella. The majority of this ligament originates at the medial epicondyle, just proximal to the insertion of the medial collateral ligament and distal to the insertion of the adductor magnus tendon. The lateral insertion is at the proximal two-thirds of the medial margin of the patella. It has a direct insertion and fibres joining the suprapatellar quadriceps fibres.[35]

Medial shelf   *see* Plica.

Merchant angle   *see* Congruence angle.

Motor control   An area of study dealing with the understanding of the neural, physical and behavioural aspects of movement.[36]

Motor learning   A set of internal processes associated with practice or experience, leading to relatively permanent changes in the capability for motor skill.[36]

Nail patellar syndrome   Autosomal dominant condition characterized by nail dysplasia, patellar aplasia–hypoplasia, arthrodysplasia of the elbows, iliac horns and nephropathy.

Nose of the patella   Most distal point of the patella.[37]

Overhang   Increased lateral or medial displacement of the patella over the femoral condyle.

Passive patellar tilt test   Test evaluating the tightness of the lateral retinaculum, by trying to lift off the lateral border of the patella. If the patella cannot be everted beyond the horizontal axis, lateral tightness is present.

Patella alta   Pathological proximalization of the patella measured with reference to the tibia[8,10,26] or with reference to the trochlea.[7] For the values, *see* Chapter 6 – Radiographs.

Patella baja   Pathological distalization of the patella measured with reference to the tibia[8,10,26] or with reference to the trochlea.[7] For the values, *see* Chapter 6 – Radiographs.

Patellar dislocation   Complete loss of contact between the patella and the trochlea (normally opposing articular surfaces). The mechanism can be direct (traumatic) or indirect (atraumatic).[32]

Patellar grind   The patellar posterior surface articulating against the femoral condyles. The compression or grinding causes discomfort.[6] To test for patellar grind, the patient lies supine with both knees extended. The examiner pushes the patella towards the trochlea while the patient contracts the quadriceps muscle.

Patellar height   Position of the patella with reference to the tibia or the trochlea. Calculated by using different indices[7,8,10,26] on a lateral radiograph in 30° of knee flexion.[12]

Patellar hypermobility   Increased patellofemoral joint play.

Patellar instability (objective and potential)
Patellofemoral joint condition characterized
by abnormally increased limits of motion or
displacement.[32] **Objective** patellar instability:
multifactorial pathological condition in association with instability factors. **Potential** patellar
instability: monofactorial pathological condition
characterized by the sole presence of trochlear
dysplasia with an abnormal anterior translation
of the floor of the trochlea.[38]

Patellar subluxation Partial loss of contact
between the patella and the trochlea with lateral
or medial displacement.

Patellar tilt Angle formed by the line through
the transverse axis of the patella and a line
tangential to the posterior aspect of the femoral
condyles.[9]

Patellar tilt test A test performed when the knee
is flexed 20°. The examiner's thumb attempts to
flip the lateral edge of the patella upwards. A
patient with an excessively tight lateral retinaculum will have almost no upward movement. Normally the patella can be lifted upwards above the
horizontal.

Patellar tracking The course of the patella
when flexing from extension or extending from
flexion. Tracking during active knee extension
is considered normal if only minimal lateral
displacement is noted when the patella exits the
femoral sulcus (absence of tilt). Abrupt lateral
translation of the patella is considered abnormal.

Patellar width Distance between the most
medial and most lateral part of the patella.[13]

Patellofemoral index *see* Laurin angle.

Patellofemoral pain syndrome A common diagnostic and treatment problem for the clinician.[39]
see Chapter 4 – Pathogenesis of patellofemoral
pain.

Patellofemoral joint play Multidirectional
mobility of the patellofemoral joint. It is measured with the knee flexed 30°. The patella is
divided into longitudinal quadrants. Joint play of

one to two quadrants is normal. A lateral glide
of three quadrants is suggestive of an incompetent medial restraint. A medial glide of less than
one quadrant is consistent with a tight lateral
restraint, while a medial glide of three quadrants
suggests a hypermobile patella.[40,41]

Patellolateral condyle index[30,40] An index measured from axial MR or CT images in 0° of knee
flexion. A line is drawn passing the anterior surfaces of the femoral condyles tangentially, and
another line is drawn perpendicular to the first
at the top of the lateral condyle. The latter line
usually crosses the patella, and the patellolateral
condyle index is the percentage of the patella lateral to the latter line.

Patellotrochlear index[42] Method of measuring patellar height on sagittal MRI. The index
describes the patella:trochlea articular cartilage
ratio and, with this, the real articular cartilage
relationship in the patellofemoral joint.

Plica Synovial structure remnant of the patellofemoral joint evolution. Suprapatellar, mediopatellar (medial shelf) and intercondylar forms can
occur.

Prominence of the trochlea To analyse the
trochlea on a true lateral radiographic view, a
straight line tangential to the anterior femoral
cortex along its distal-most 10 cm is drawn. The
floor of the trochlea is measured at the most
anterior point. According to the position of
this point, anterior, posterior or flush with this
anterior cortical line, the floor of the trochlea
can be positive, negative or zero, measured in
millimeters. A translation more than 3 mm is
considered as pathological (positive or negative
prominence). *see* Chapter 6 – Radiographs.

Prone knee bend test Test for any patient with
knee, anterior thigh and hip and upper lumbar
symptoms. The usual sensation is a pulling or
pain in the area of the quadriceps muscle.[43]

Q angle An angle that is usually measured using
two lines: one line is drawn from the middle of

the patella to the centre of the tibial tuberosity, and a second is drawn from the middle of the patella to the centre of the anterior superior iliac spine.[39] *see* Chapter 5 – Physical examination.

Quadriceps muscle dysplasia   A condition documented on an axial CT scan when the patellar tilt in extension is more than 20°.[9,44]

Randomized controlled clinical trial   A clinical trial in which a group of patients is randomized into an experimental group and a control group. These groups are followed up for the variables and outcomes designated in the study design.[19]

Recentring beak   The cortical beak of the trochlea on which the patella rests in extension. The recentring beak is where the common line of the trochlea ends after the crossing of the lines drawn on the radiograph.[9,45]

Re-Elmslie   A surgical technique bringing the medialized tibial tuberosity back to its original anatomical location.

Retinaculum   Soft tissue structure consisting of a lateral (superficial and oblique) and a medial part.[46]

Roman arch   Form of the notch in the proximal part of the trochlea. Important landmark in the axial CT scan to determine the height of the patella.[12]

Roux procedure   Surgical technique transferring the patellar tendon medially in combination with the release of the lateral retinaculum and implication of the medial retinaculum.[4,47]

Sensorimotor system   The system of sensory, motor, central integration, and processing components involved with maintaining joint homeostasis during functional activity.[48]

Simmons procedure   Surgical technique transposing the tibial tuberosity distally.[18]

Skills   Movements that are dependent on practice and experience for their execution, as opposed to being genetically defined.[36]

Slump test   Tension test to allow differentiation of nervous system involvement from non-nervous structures.[43]

Substance P   Neurotransmitter of nociceptive sensation.[49–52]

Sulcus angle (trochlear angle)   Angle between two lines drawn from the deepest point of the trochlea, one passing across the edge of the medial condyle and the other across the edge of the lateral condyle. The sulcus angle is measured on axial radiographs with 30° of knee flexion.[13]

Systematic review   A summary of the medical literature that uses explicit methods to perform a thorough literature search and critical appraisal of individual studies and that uses appropriate statistical techniques to combine the valid studies.[19]

Tibial tuberosity–trochlear groove distance   Distance between the anterior tibial tuberosity and the deepest point of the trochlear groove.[7] It quantifies objectively the valgus component of the extensor mechanism of the knee, which can be estimated clinically with the Q angle or the bayonet sign. On a radiograph, the tibial tuberosity–trochlear groove distance is calculated by the superimposition of two perpendicular cuts to the posterior bicondylar line – one tibial cut passing through the summit of the anterior tibial tuberosity, and one femoral cut passing through the deepest point of the trochlear groove where the intercondylar notch has the form of a Roman arch.[53] The tibial tuberosity–trochlear groove distance is measured in millimeters and gives information about the lateral positioning of the anterior tibial tuberosity and the external rotation of the knee, which are two individually variable values.

Trigger point   A focus of hyperirritability in a tissue that, when compressed, is locally tender and, if sufficiently hypersensitive, gives rise to referred pain and tenderness and sometimes to referred autonomic phenomena and distortion of proprioception.[54]

Trochlear angle (sulcus angle) *see* Sulcus angle.

Trochlear depth A measurement made on the true lateral radiograph of the knee; it is a quantitative criterion of trochlear dysplasia. The most anterior point of the trochlear floor corresponds with the lowest depth of the trochlea.[9,12] *see* Chapter 6 – Radiographs.

Trochlear dysplasia classification A new classification that consists of four degrees: A, B, C and D. It requires both standard radiological examination and evaluation with CT scans. The analysis with CT is performed following a first cut of reference at the level of the trochlea, where the cartilage begins. Rémy[55] validated the reproducibility of this new classification by analysing the two most important factors of trochlear dysplasia: the crossing sign and the recentring beak.

Trochlear groove Femoral part of the articulation of the patellofemoral joint that articulates with the patella backside during flexion–extension movements.[9]

Trochlear height *see* Index of trochlear height.

Trochlear length Individually variable distance between the most distal and most proximal point of the articular part of the trochlea.

Trochlearplasty *see* Masse procedure.[34]

Tubercle–sulcus angle Angle between the horizontal transepicondylar line and the axis of the patellar tendon measured in 90° of knee flexion. This angle should be 0°. An angle of more than 10° is pathological.[41]

Wiberg classification A classification that describes six types of patellae. This classification has not been demonstrated to correlate with clinical signs of patellofemoral pain.[56,57]

Abbreviations

ACL   Anterior cruciate ligament.
AKP   Anterior knee pain.
CA   Congruence angle (Merchant's angle).
CT   Computed tomography.
FNE   Free nerve endings.
MRI   Magnetic resonance imaging.
RCCT   Randomized controlled clinical trial.
ROM   Range of motion.

References

1. Nagy SZ (1991) Disability concepts revised: implications for prevention. In: Pope AM, Tarlov AR (eds), *Disability in America: Toward a National Agenda for Prevention*. Washington, DC, National Academy Press, pp 309–327

2. Jette AM (1994) Physical disablement concepts for physical therapy research and practice. *Phys Ther* **74**: 380–386

3. Dandy DJ (1996) Chronic patellofemoral instability. *J Bone Joint Surg Br* **78**: 328–335

4. Hughston JC, Walsh WM, Puddu G (1984) *Patellar Subluxation and Dislocation. Saunders Monographs in Clinical Orthopaedics*, volume V. Philadelphia, PA, WB Saunders

5. Albee FH (1915) The bone graft wedge in the treatment of habitual dislocation of the patella. *Med Rec* **88**: 257–259

6. Macnicol MF (1986) *The Problem Knee*. London, William Heinemann Medical Books

7. Bernageau J, Goutallier D, Debeyre J, Ferrane J (1969) Nouvelle technique d'exploration de l'articulation fémoro-patellaire. Incidinces axiales quadriceps contracté et décontracté. *Rev Chir Orthop Reparatrice Appar Mot* **61**(suppl 2): 286–290

8. Blackburne JS, Peel TE (1977) A new method of measuring patellar height. *J Bone Joint Surg Br* **59**: 241–242

9. Dejour H, Walch G, Nove-Josserand L, Guier C (1994) Factors of patellar instability: an anatomic radiographic study. *Knee Surg Sports Traumatol Arthrosc* **2**: 19–26

10. Caton J, Deschamps G, Chambat P et al (1982) [Patella infera. Apropos of 128 cases]. *Rev Chir Orthop Reparatrice Appar Mot* **68**: 317–325

11. Walch G, Dejour H (1989) [Radiology in femoro-patellar pathology]. *Acta Orthop Belg* **55**: 371–380

12. Galland O, Walch G, Dejour H, Carret JP (1990) An anatomical and radiological study of the

femoropatellar articulation. *Surg Radiol Anat* **12**: 119–125

13. Kujala UM, Osterman K, Kormano M et al (1989) Patellofemoral relationships in recurrent patellar dislocation. *J Bone Joint Surg Br* **71**: 788–792

14. Fulkerson JP, Shea KP (1990) Disorders of patellofemoral alignment. *J Bone Joint Surg Am* **72**: 1424–1429

15. Schutzer SF, Ramsby GR, Fulkerson JP (1986) Computed tomographic classification of patellofemoral pain patients. *Orthop Clin North Am* **17**: 235–248

16. Handling KA (1982) Rehabilitating athletic injuries with cryotherapy. *J Phys Educ Recreat Dance* **53**: 338–340

17. Knight KL, Londeree BR (1980) Comparison of blood flow in the ankle of uninjured subjects during therapeutic applications of heat, cold, and exercise. *Med Sci Sports Exerc* **12**: 76–80

18. Papagelopoulos PJ, Sim FH (1997) Patellofemoral pain syndrome: diagnosis and management. *Orthopedics* **20**: 148–157; quiz 158–159

19. Sackett DL (2000) *Evidence-based Medicine: How to Practice and Teach EBM*, 2nd edn. New York, Churchill Livingstone

20. Biedert RM, Stauffer E, Friederich NF (1992) Occurrence of free nerve endings in the soft tissue of the knee joint. A histologic investigation. *Am J Sports Med* **20**: 430–433

21. Kennedy JC, Alexander IJ, Hayes KC (1982) Nerve supply of the human knee and its functional importance. *Am J Sports Med* **10**: 329–335

22. Goldthwait JE (1904) Slipping or recurrent dislocation of the patella: with the report of eleven cases. *Boston Med Surg* **150**: 169

23. Dye SF, Chew MH (1993) The use of scintigraphy to detect increased osseous metabolic transmission with an envelope of function. *J Bone Joint Surg Am* **75**: 1388–1406

24. Guyton AC, Hall JE (1996) *Textbook of Medical Physiology*. Philadelphia, PA, WB Saunders

25. Dye SF, Stäubli HU, Biedert RM, Vaupel GL (1999) The mosaic of pathophysiology causing patellofemoral pain: therapeutic implications. *Operative Tech Sports Med* **7**: 46–54

26. Insall J, Salvati E (1971) Patella position in the normal knee joint. *Radiology* **101**: 101–104

27. Grelsamer RP, Meadows S (1992) The modified Insall–Salvati ratio for assessment of patellar height. *Clin Orthop* **282**: 170–176

28. Teitge RA, Faerber WW, Des Madryl P, Matelic TM (1996) Stress radiographs of the patellofemoral joint. *J Bone Joint Surg Am* **78**: 193–203

29. Martinez S, Korobkin M, Fondren FB et al (1983) Diagnosis of patellofemoral malalignment by computed tomography. *J Comput Assist Tomogr* **7**: 1050–1053

30. Biedert RM, Gruhl C (1997) Axial computed tomography of the patellofemoral joint with and without quadriceps contraction. *Arch Orthop Trauma Surg* **116**: 77–82

31. Laurin CA, Levesque HP, Dussault R et al (1978) The abnormal lateral patellofemoral angle: a diagnostic roentgenographic sign of recurrent patellar subluxation. *J Bone Joint Surg Am* **60**: 55–60

32. Jakob RP, Stäubli HU (1990) *The Knee and the Cruciate Ligaments*. Berlin, Heidelberg, Springer-Verlag

33. Madigan R, Wissinger HA, Donaldson WF (1975) Preliminary experience with a method of quadricepsplasty in recurrent subluxation of the patella. *J Bone Joint Surg Am* **57**: 600–607

34. Masse Y (1978) [Trochleoplasty. Restoration of the intercondylar groove in subluxations and dislocations of the patella]. *Rev Chir Orthop Reparatrice Appar Mot* **64**: 3–17

35. Tuxoe JI, Teir M, Winge S, Nielsen PL (2002) The medial patellofemoral ligament: a dissection study. *Knee Surg Sports Traumatol Arthrosc* **10**: 138–140

36. Schmidt RA, Lee TD (1999) *Motor Control and Learning. A Behavioral Emphasis*, 3rd edn. Champaign, IL, Human Kinetics

37. Servien E (2001) La luxation de rotule: étude rétrospectivede 190 cas opérés et analyse de la dysplasie fémorale-patellaire. Thesis, University of Lyon

38. Dejour H, Walch G, Nové-Josserand L, Guier CA (1994) *Diagnosis and treatment of ligament injuries about the knee*. In: Feagin JA Jr (ed), *The Crucial Ligaments*. New York, Churchill Livingstone, pp 361–367

39. Biedert RM, Warnke K (2001) Correlation between the Q angle and the patella position: a

clinical and axial computed tomography evaluation. *Arch Orthop Trauma Surg* **121**: 346–349

40. Pinar H, Akseki D, Karaoglan O, Genc I (1994) Kinematic and dynamic axial computed tomography of the patellofemoral joints in patients with anterior knee pain. *Knee Surg Sports Traumatol Arthrosc* **2**: 170–173

41. Kolowich PA, Paulos LE, Rosenberg TD, Farnsworth S (1990) Lateral release of the patella: indications and contraindications. *Am J Sports Med* **18**: 359–365

42. Biedert RM, Albrecht S (2003) Patellotrochlear index: another method of measuring patellar height on sagittal MRI. In: Proceedings of the International Patellofemoral Study Group, Naples, FL, USA

43. Butler DS (1991) *Mobilisation of the Nervous System*. London, Churchill Livingstone

44. Brattström H (1964) Shape of the intercondylar groove normally and in recurrent dislocation of the patella. *Acta Orthop Scand* **68**(suppl): 1–148

45. Tavernier T, Dejour D (2001) [Knee imaging: what is the best modality?]. *J Radiol* **82**: 387–405; 407–408

46. Ford DH, Post WR (1997) Open or arthroscopic lateral release. Indications, techniques, and rehabilitation. *Clin Sports Med* **16**: 29–49

47. Roux C (1888) Luxation habituelle de la rotule. *Rev Chir* **8**: 682

48. Lephart SM, Riemann BL, Fu FH (2001) Introduction to the sensorimotor system. In: Lephart SM, Fu FH (eds), *Proprioception and Neuromuscular Control in Joint Stability*. Champaign, IL, Human Kinetics

49. Sanchis-Alfonso V, Rosello-Sastre E, Monteagudo-Castro C, Esquerdo J (1998) Quantitative analysis of nerve changes in the lateral retinaculum in patients with isolated symptomatic patellofemoral malalignment. A preliminary study. *Am J Sports Med* **26**: 703–709

50. Sanchis-Alfonso V, Rosello-Sastre E (2000) Immunohistochemical analysis for neural markers of the lateral retinaculum in patients with isolated symptomatic patellofemoral malalignment. A neuroanatomic basis for anterior knee pain in the active young patient. *Am J Sports Med* **28**: 725–731

51. Walsh DA, Salmon M, Mapp PI et al (1993) Microvascular substance P binding to normal and inflamed rat and human synovium. *J Pharmacol Exp Ther* **267**: 951–960

52. Menkes CJ, Renoux M, Laoussadi S et al (1993) Substance P levels in the synovium and synovial fluid from patients with rheumatoid arthritis and osteoarthritis. *J Rheumatol* **20**: 714–717

53. Dejour H, Walch G (1987) La pathologie fémoro-patellaire. In: 6èmes Journées Lyonnaises de Chirurgie du Genou, University of Lyon

54. Travell J, Simons D (1983) *Myofascial Pain and Dysfunction: The Trigger Point Manual*. Baltimore, MD, Williams & Wilkins

55. Rémy F, Gougeon F, Ala Eddine T et al (2001) Reproductibilité de la nouvelle classification de la dysplasie de la trochlée fémorale selon Dejour et valeur prédictive sur la sévérité de l'instabilité fémoro-patellaire sur 47 genoux. *Rev Chir Orthop Reparatrice Appar Mot* **87** (suppl 2): 60

56. Grelsamer RP, Proctor CS, Bazos AN (1994) Evaluation of patellar shape in the sagittal plane. A clinical analysis. *Am J Sports Med* **22**: 61–66

57. Wiberg G (1941) Roentgenographic and anatomic studies on the femoropatellar joint. *Acta Orthop Scand* **12**: 319–410

Bibliography

Abe T, Morgan DA, Gutterman DD (1997) Protective role of nerve growth factor against postischemic dysfunction of sympathetic coronary innervation. *Circulation* **95**: 213–220

Abernethy PJ, Townsend PR, Rose RM, Radin EL (1978) Is chondromalacia patellae a separate clinical entity? *J Bone Joint Surg Br* **60**: 205–210

Abramson SB (2002) Et tu, acetaminophen? *Arthritis Rheum* **46**: 2831–2835

Aderinto J, Cobb AG (2002) Lateral release for patellofemoral arthritis. *Arthroscopy* **18**: 399–403

Aglietti P, Insall JN, Cerulli G (1983) Patellar pain and incongruence. I: measurements of incongruence. *Clin Orthop* **176**: 217–224

Ahmed AM, Burke DL, Hyder A (1987) Force analysis of the patellar mechanism. *J Orthop Res* **5**: 69–85

Alaca R, Yilmaz B, Goktepe AS et al (2002) Efficacy of isokinetic exercise on functional capacity and pain in patellofemoral pain syndrome. *Am J Phys Med Rehabil* **81**: 807–813

Albee FH (1915) The bone graft wedge in the treatment of habitual dislocation of the patella. *Med Rec* **88**: 257–259

American College of Rheumatology Subcommittee on Osteoarthritis Guidelines (2000) Recommendations for the medical management of osteoarthritis of the hip and knee. *Arthritis Rheum* **43**: 1905–1915

American Geriatrics Society Panel on Chronic Pain in Older Persons (1998) The management of chronic pain in older persons. Clinical practice guidelines. *J Am Geriatric Soc* **46**: 635–651

American Physical Therapy Association (2001) Philadelphia Panel evidence-based clinical practice guidelines on selected rehabilitation interventions for knee pain. *Phys Ther* **81**: 1675–1700

Amis AA, Farahmand F (1996) Biomechanics masterclass: extensor mechanism of the knee. *Curr Orthop* **10**: 102–109

Amis AA, Firer P, Mountney J et al (2003) Anatomy and biomechanics of the medial patellofemoral ligament. *The Knee* **10**: 215–220

Andersson SA, Hansson GEH, Renberg O (1976) Evaluation of the pain suppression effect of different frequencies of peripheral electrical stimulation in chronic pain conditions. *Acta Orthop Scand* **47**: 149–157

Andriacchi TP, Natarajan RN, Hurwitz DE (1991) Musculoskeletal dynamics, locomotion, and clinical applications. In: Mow VC, Hayes WC (eds), *Basic Orthopaedic Biomechanics*. New York, Raven, pp 51–92

Antich TJ, Randall CC, Westbrook RA et al (1986) Physical therapy treatment of knee extensor mechanism disorders: comparison of four treatment modalities. *J Orthop Sports Phys Ther* **8**: 255–259

Arcerio R, Toomey H (1988) Patellofemoral arthroplasty: a three- to nine-year follow-up study. *Clin Orthop* **236**: 60–71

Arendt EA, Fithian DC, Cohen E (2002) Current concepts of lateral patella dislocation. *Clin Sports Med* **21**: 499–519

Argenson JN, Guillaume JM, Aubaniac JM (1995) Is there a place for patellofemoral arthroplasty? *Clin Orthop* **321**: 162–167

Arnbjornsson A, Egund N, Rydling O et al (1992) The natural history of recurrent dislocation of the patella. Long-term results of conservative and operative treatment. *J Bone Joint Surg Br* **74**: 140–142

Arroll B, Ellis-Pegler E, Edwards A, Sutcliffe G (1997) Patellofemoral pain syndrome. A critical review of the clinical trials on nonoperative therapy. *Am J Sports Med* **25**: 207–212

Atkin DM, Fithian DC, Marangi KS et al (2000) Characteristics of patients with primary acute lateral patellar dislocation and their recovery within the first 6 months of injury. *Am J Sports Med* **28**: 472–479

Bahlsen A (1988) The etiology of running injuries: a longitudinal, prospective study. Thesis, University of Calgary, Calgary, Alberta, Canada

Balint G, Szebenyi B (1997) Non-pharmacological therapies in osteoarthritis. *Baillières Clin Rheumatol* **11**: 795–815

Bandi W (1972) [Chondromalacia patellae and femoro-patellar arthrosis, etiology, clinical aspects and therapy]. *Helv Chir Acta* **39** (suppl 11): 1–70

Bandi W (1977) [Operative treatment of chondromalacia patellae (author's transl)]. *Zentralbl Chir* **102**: 1297–1301

Barrack RL, Lund PJ, Skinner HB (1994) Knee joint proprioception revisited. *J Sports Rehab* **3**: 18–42

Barrack RL, Skinner HB (1990) The sensory function of knee ligaments. In: Daniel DM, Akeson WH, O'Connor JJ (eds), *Knee Ligaments: Structure, Function, Injury, and Repair*. New York, Raven, pp 95–114

Basbaum AI, Fields HL (1978) Endogenous pain control mechanisms: review and hypothesis. *Ann Neurol* **4**: 451–462

Bassett FH (1976) Acute dislocation of the patella, osteochondral fractures, and injuries to the extensor mechanism of the knee. *Instr Course Lect* **25**: 40–49

Bellelli A, Nardis P (1997) [Dynamic magnetic resonance of the knee. Considerations on techniques and anatomy with a magnetic resonance system with open magnet]. *Radiol Med (Torino)* **93**: 199–205

Bennett JG, Stauber WT (1986) Evaluation and treatment of anterior knee pain using eccentric exercise. *Med Sci Sports Exerc* **18**: 526–530

Bennett WF, Doherty N, Hallisey MJ (1993) Insertion orientation of terminal vastus lateralis obliquus and vastus medialis obliquus muscle fibers in human knees. *Clin Anat* **6**: 129–134

Bentley G (1970) Chondromalacia patellae. *J Bone Joint Surg Am* **52**: 221–232

Bentley G, Dowd G (1984) Current concepts of etiology and treatment of chondromalacia patellae. *Clin Orthop* **189**: 209–228

Bereiter H (2000) Die Trochleaplastik bei Trochleadysplasie zur Therapie der rezidivierenden Patellaluxation. In: Wirth CJ, Rudert M (eds), *Das Patellofemorale Schmerzsyndrom*. Darmstadt, Steinkopff-Verlag, pp 162–177

Bereiter H, Gautier E (1994) Die Trochleaplastik als chirurgische Therapie der rezidivierenden Patellaluxation bei Trochleadysplasie des Femurs. *Arthroskopie* **7**: 281–286

Bernageau J, Goutallier D, Debeyre J, Ferrane J (1969) Nouvelle technique d'exploration de l'articulation fémoro-patellaire. Incindinces axiales quadriceps contracté et décontracté. *Rev Chir Orthop Reparatrice Appar Mot* **61**(suppl 2): 286–290

Berry DJ, Rand JA (1993) Isolated patellar component revision of total knee arthroplasty. *Clin Orthop* **286**: 110–115

Betz RR, Magill JT III, Lonergan RP (1987) The percutaneous lateral retinacular release. *Am J Sports Med* **15**: 477–482

Beynnon BD, Fleming BC (1998) Anterior cruciate ligament strain *in vivo*: a review of previous work. *J Biomech* **31**: 519–525

Biedert R, Friederich N (1996) [Femoropatellar pain syndrome: which operation is still sensible?]. *Ther Umsch* **53**: 775–779

Biedert RM (1999) Sensory–Motor Function of the Knee Joint. Histologic, Anatomic, and Neurophysiologic Investigations. Thesis, University of Basel, Switzerland

Biedert RM (2000) A new perspective of patellofemoral pain. Where is the pain coming from? In: Symposia Handouts and Abstracts of the 67th Annual Meeting of the American Academy of Orthopaedic Surgeons, Orlando, FL, p 247

Biedert RM (2000) Is there an indication for lateral release and how I do it. In: Proceedings of the International Patellofemoral Study Group, Garmisch-Partenkirchen, Germany

Biedert RM (2000) Korrelation zwischen Q-Winkel und Patellaposition. In: Wirth CJ, Rudert M (eds), *Das patellofemorale Schmerzsyndrom*. Darmstadt, Steinkopff-Verlag

Biedert RM (2000) Contribution of the three levels of nervous system motor control: spinal cord, lower brain, cerebral cortex. In: Lephart SM, Fu FH (eds), *Proprioception and Neuromuscular Control in Joint Stability*. Champaign, IL, Human Kinetics, pp 23–39

Biedert RM (2000) 124 operations to treat 10 patients suffering from patellofemoral pain. What was wrong? In: Proceedings of the International Patellofemoral Study Group, Garmisch-Partenkirchen, Germany

Biedert RM (2003) Complicated case studies. In: Sanchis-Alfonso V (ed), *Anterior Knee Pain and Patellofemoral Instability in the Active Young. The Black Hole of Orthopaedics*. Medica Panamericana, Madrid, Spain, 287–301

Biedert RM (2002) Patellaluxation beim Kind und Jugendlichen. *Sportorthopädie-Sporttraumatologie* **18**: 164–168

Biedert RM, Albrecht S (2003) Patellotrochlear index: another method of measuring patellar height on sagittal MRI. In: Proceedings of the International Patellofemoral Study Group, Naples, FL, USA

Biedert RM, Elsig A (1984) Kniebeschwerden beim Sportler: Behandlungsmöglichkeiten durch Korrektur der Statik. *Schweiz Z Sportmed Sporttraumatol* **32**: 91–94

Biedert RM, Friederich NF (1994) Failed lateral retinacular release: clinical outcome. *J Sports Traumatol* **16**: 162–173

Biedert RM, Gruhl C (1997) Axial computed tomography of the patellofemoral joint with and without quadriceps contraction. *Arch Orthop Trauma Surg* **116**: 77–82

Biedert RM, Kernen V (2001) Neurosensory characteristics of the patellofemoral joint: what is the genesis of patellofemoral pain? *Sports Med Arthrosc Rev* **9**: 295–300

Biedert RM, Sanchis-Alfonso V (2002) Sources of anterior knee pain. *Clin Sports Med* **21**: 335–347

Biedert RM, Stauffer E, Friederich NF (1992) Occurrence of free nerve endings in the soft tissue of the knee joint. A histologic investigation. *Am J Sports Med* **20**: 430–433

Biedert RM, Vogel U, Friederich NF (1997) Chronic patellar tendonitis: a new surgical treatment. *Sports Exerc Injury* **3**: 150–154

Biedert RM, Warnke K (2001) Correlation between the Q angle and the patella position: a clinical and axial computed tomography evaluation. *Arch Orthop Trauma Surg* **121**: 346–349

Bijlsma JW (2002) Analgesia and the patient with osteoarthritis. *Am J Ther* **9**: 189–197

Bizzini M (2000) *Sensomotorische Rehabilitation nach Beinverletzungen*. Stuttgart, New York, Georg Thieme-Verlag

Bizzini M, Childs JD, Piva SR, Delitto A (2003) Systematic review of the quality of randomized controlled trials for patellofemoral pain syndrome. *J Orthop Sports Phys Ther* **33**: 4–20

Bizzini M, Munzinger U (1998) Bewegungsanalyse der Einbeinkniebeuge. Beeinflussung der ventralen tibialen Translation durch eine definierte Körperstellung. Konsequenzen in der Kreuzbandrehabilitation. *Man Ther* **2**: 19–27

Bizzini M, Munzinger U (1998) Motion analysis of the squat exercise. Influence of the body position on the anterior tibial shear in normal, ACL-deficient and ACL-reconstructed knees. In: *8th Congress of the European Society of Sports Traumatology, Knee Surgery, and Arthroscopy. Book of Abstracts*. Nice, European Society of Sports Traumatology, Knee Surgery, and Arthroscopy

Blackburne JS, Peel TE (1977) A new method of measuring patellar height. *J Bone Joint Surg Br* **59**: 241–242

Blazina ME, Fox JM, Del Pizzo W et al (1979) Patellofemoral replacement. *Clin Orthop* **144**: 98–102

Blazina ME, Kerlan RK, Jobe FW et al (1973) Jumper's knee. *Orthop Clin North Am* **4**: 665–678

Bockrath K, Wooden C, Worrell T et al (1993) Effects of patella taping on patella position and perceived pain. *Med Sci Sports Exerc* **25**: 989–992

Boden BP, Pearsall AW, Garrett WE Jr, Feagin JA Jr (1997) Patellofemoral instability: evaluation and management. *J Am Acad Orthop Surg* **5**: 47–57

Bosshard C, Stäubli HU, Rauschning W (1997) Konturinkongruenz von Gelenkknorpeloberflächen und subchondralem Knochen des Femoropatellargelenks in der sagittalen Ebene. *Arthroskopie* **10**: 72–76

Brandt KD (2000) The role of analgesics in the management of osteoarthritis pain. *Am J Ther* **7**: 75–90

Brattström H (1964) Shape of the intercondylar groove normally and in recurrent dislocation of the patella. *Acta Orthop Scand Suppl* **68**: 1–148

Brody LT, Thein JM (1998) Nonoperative treatment for patellofemoral pain. *J Orthop Sports Phys Ther* **28**: 336–344

Brooks V (1986) *The Neural Basis of Motor Control.* New York, Oxford Press

Brossmann J, Muhle C, Schroder C et al (1993) Patellar tracking patterns during active and passive knee extension: evaluation with motion-triggered cine MR imaging. *Radiology* **187**: 205–212

Brügger A (1980) *Die Erkrankungen des Bewegungsapparates und seines Nervensystems*, 2nd edn. Stuttgart, G. Fischer

Buchbinder MR, Napora NJ, Biggs EW (1979) The relationship of abnormal pronation to chondromalacia of the patella in distance runners. *J Am Podiatry Assoc* **69**: 159–162

Buechel FF Sr, Buechel FF Jr, Pappas MJ, D'Alessio J (2001) Twenty-year evaluation of meniscal bearing and rotating platform knee replacements. *Clin Orthop* **388**: 41–50

Buechel FF, Rosa RA, Pappas MJ (1989) A metal-backed, rotating-bearing patellar prosthesis to lower contact stress. An 11-year clinical study. *Clin Orthop* **248**: 34–49

Bull AM, Katchburian MV, Shih YF, Amis AA (2002) Standardisation of the description of patellofemoral motion and comparison between different techniques. *Knee Surg Sports Traumatol Arthrosc* **10**: 184–193

Burks RT, Desio SM, Bachus KN et al (1998) Biomechanical evaluation of lateral patellar dislocations. *Am J Knee Surg* **11**: 24–31

Busch MT, DeHaven KE (1989) Pitfalls of the lateral retinacular release. *Clin Sports Med* **8**: 279–290

Butler DS (1991) *Mobilisation of the Nervous System.* London, Churchill Livingstone

Callaghan MJ, Oldham JA (1996) The role of quadriceps exercise in the treatment of patellofemoral pain syndrome. *Sports Med* **21**: 384–391

Cameron ML, Frondoza CG, Holland C, Hungerford DS (1999) Expression of proinflammatory IL-1 and TNF by osteoarthritic chondrocytes in altered response to mechanical stress. Abstract. *Trans Orthop Res Soc* **24**: 606

Carillon Y, Dejour D, Tavernier T, Dejour H (1997) Aspect scannographique de la trochlée fémorale en cas d'instabilité rotulienne objective. In: *XXIV Groupe d'Etude et de Travail de l'Imagerie Osteoarticulatife*, University of Lyon, pp 215–225

Carson WG Jr, James SL, Larson RL et al (1984) Patellofemoral disorders: physical and radiographic evaluation. Part II: Radiographic examination. *Clin Orthop* **185**: 178–186

Cartier P, Sanouiller JL, Grelsamer R (1990) Patellofemoral arthroplasty. 2–12 year follow-up study. *J Arthroplasty* **5**: 49–55

Cash JD, Hughston JC (1988) Treatment of acute patellar dislocation. *Am J Sports Med* **16**: 244–249

Caton J, Deschamps G, Chambat P et al (1982) [Patella infera. Apropos of 128 cases]. *Rev Chir Orthop Reparatrice Appar Mot* **68**: 317–325

Caylor D, Fites R, Worrell TW (1993) The relationship between quadriceps angle and anterior knee pain syndrome. *J Orthop Sports Phys Ther* **17**: 11–16

Ceder LC, Larson RL (1979) Z-plasty lateral retinacular release for the treatment of patellar compression syndrome. *Clin Orthop* **144**: 110–113

Cerny K (1995) Vastus medialis oblique/vastus lateralis muscle activity ratios for selected exercises in persons with and without patellofemoral pain syndrome. *Phys Ther* **75**: 672–683

Cesarelli M, Bifulco P, Bracale M (2000) Study of the control strategy of the quadriceps muscles in anterior knee pain. *IEEE Trans Rehabil Eng* **8**: 330–341

Chadwick P (1987) The significance of spinal joint signs in the management of groin strain and patellofemoral pain by manual techniques. *Physiotherapy* **73**: 507–513

Clark DI, Downing N, Mitchell J et al (2000) Physiotherapy for anterior knee pain: a randomised controlled trial. *Ann Rheum Dis* **59**: 700–704

Coderre TJ, Katz J, Vaccarino AL, Melzack R (1993) Contribution of central neuroplasticity to pathological pain: review of clinical and experimental evidence. *Pain* **52**: 259–285

Cohen ZA, Roglic H, Grelsamer RP et al (2001) Patellofemoral stresses during open and closed kinetic chain exercises. An analysis using computer simulation. *Am J Sports Med* **29**: 480–487

Conlan T, Garth WP Jr, Lemons JE (1993) Evaluation of the medial soft-tissue restraints of the extensor mechanism of the knee. *J Bone Joint Surg Am* **75**: 682–693

Cooke TD, Price N, Fisher B, Hedden D (1990) The inward-pointing knee. *Clin Orthop* **260**: 56–60

Coppes MH, Marani E, Thomeer RT, Groen GJ (1997) Innervation of 'painful' lumbar discs. *Spine* **22**: 2342–2349; discussion 2349–2350

Cowan SM, Bennell KL, Hodges PW et al (2001) Delayed onset of electromyographic activity of vastus medialis obliquus relative to vastus lateralis in subjects with patellofemoral pain syndrome. *Arch Phys Med Rehabil* 82: 183–189

Cowan SM, Hodges PW, Bennell KL, Crossley KM (2002) Altered vastii recruitment when people with patellofemoral pain syndrome complete a postural task. *Arch Phys Med Rehabil* 83: 989–995

Crossley K, Bennell K, Green S, McConnell J (2001) A systematic review of physical interventions for patellofemoral pain syndrome. *Clin J Sport Med* 11: 103–110

Crossley K, Cowan SM, Bennell KL, McConnell J (2000) Patellar taping: is clinical success supported by scientific evidence? *Man Ther* 5: 142–150

Currier DP, Ray JM, Nyland J et al (1993) Effects of electrical and electromagnetic stimulation after anterior cruciate ligament reconstruction. *J Orthop Sports Phys Ther* 17: 177–184

Cutbill JW, Ladly KO, Bray RC et al (1997) Anterior knee pain: a review. *Clin J Sport Med* 7: 40–45

Dandy DJ (1996) Chronic patellofemoral instability. *J Bone Joint Surg Br* 78: 328–335

Davies AP, Costa ML, Shepstone L et al (2000) The sulcus angle and malalignment of the extensor mechanism of the knee. *J Bone Joint Surg Br* 82: 1162–1166

de Andrade JR, Grant C, Dixon ASTJ (1965) Joint distension and reflex muscle inhibition in the knee. *J Bone Joint Surg Am* 47: 313–322

de Winter WE, Feith R, van Loon CJ (2001) The Richards type II patellofemoral arthroplasty: 26 cases followed for 1–20 years. *Acta Orthop Scand* 72: 487–490

DeHaven KE, Collins HR (1975) Diagnosis of internal derangements of the knee. The role of arthroscopy. *J Bone Joint Surg Am* 57: 802–810

Dejour D, Nové-Josserand L, Walch G (1994) Patellofemoral disorders: classification and an approach to operative treatment for instability. In: Chan KM, Fu FH (eds), *Controversies in Orthopaedic Sports Medicine*. Hong Kong, Williams & Wilkins Asia-Pacific Ltd, pp 235–244

Dejour H, Walch G (1987) La pathologie fémoro-patellaire. In: *6èmes Journées Lyonnaises de Chirurgie du Genou*, University of Lyon

Dejour H, Walch G, Neyret P, Adeleine P (1990) [Dysplasia of the femoral trochlea]. *Rev Chir Orthop Reparatrice Appar Mot* 76: 45–54

Dejour H, Walch G, Nove-Josserand L, Guier C (1994) Factors of patellar instability: an anatomic radiographic study. *Knee Surg Sports Traumatol Arthrosc* 2: 19–26

Dejour H, Walch G, Nové-Josserand L, Guier CA (1994) Diagnosis and treatment of ligament injuries about the knee. In: Feagin JA Jr (ed), *The Crucial Ligaments*. New York, Churchill Livingstone, pp 361–367

Delgado-Martins H (1979) A study of the position of the patella using computerised tomography. *J Bone Joint Surg Br* 61: 443–444

Delitto A, Rose SJ, McKowen JM et al (1988) Electrical stimulation versus voluntary exercise in strengthening thigh musculature after anterior cruciate ligament surgery. *Phys Ther* 68: 660–663

Desio SM, Burks RT, Bachus KN (1998) Soft tissue restraints to lateral patellar translation in the human knee. *Am J Sports Med* 26: 59–65

Deutsch AL, Mink JH, Shellock FG (1990) Magnetic resonance imaging of injuries to bone and articular cartilage. Emphasis on radiographically occult abnormalities. *Orthop Rev* 19: 66–75

Dienst M, Blauth M (2000) Bone bruise of the calcaneus. A case report. *Clin Orthop* 378: 202–205

Doucette SA, Goble EM (1992) The effect of exercise on patellar tracking in lateral patellar compression syndrome. *Am J Sports Med* 20: 434–440

Draper V, Ballard L (1991) Electrical stimulation versus electromyographic biofeedback in the recovery of quadriceps femoris muscle function following anterior cruciate ligament surgery. *Phys Ther* 71: 455–461; discussion 461–464

Duffey MJ, Martin DF, Cannon DW et al (2000) Etiologic factors associated with anterior knee pain in distance runners. *Med Sci Sports Exerc* 32: 1825–1832

Dupont JY (1998) [Patellofemoral pain]. *Rev Prat* 48: 1781–1786

Dursun N, Dursun E, Kilic Z (2001) Electromyographic biofeedback-controlled exercise versus conservative care for patellofemoral pain syndrome. *Arch Phys Med Rehabil* 82: 1692–1695

Dye SF (1993) Patellofemoral anatomy. In: Fox JM, Del Pizzo W (eds), *The Patellofemoral Joint*. New York, McGraw-Hill, pp 1–12

Dye SF (1994) Functional anatomy and biomechanics of the patellofemoral joint. In: Scott JE (ed), *The Knee*. St. Louis, Mosby, pp 381–389

Dye SF (1996) The knee as a biologic transmission with an envelope of function: a theory. *Clin Orthop* **325**: 10–18

Dye SF (1999) Invited commentary on Watson CJ, Propps M, Galt W, Redding A, Dobbs D. Reliability of McConnell's classification of patellar orientation in symptomatic and asymptomatic subjects. *J Orthop Sports Phys Ther* **29**: 378–393

Dye SF (2001) Therapeutic implications of a tissue homeostasis approach to patellofemoral pain. *Sports Med Arthritis Rev* **9**: 306–311

Dye SF (2001) Patellofemoral pain current concepts: an overview. *Sports Med Arthritis Rev* **9**: 264–272

Dye SF, Boll DA (1986) Radionuclide imaging of the patellofemoral joint in young adults with anterior knee pain. *Orthop Clin North Am* **17**: 249–262

Dye SF, Boll DH (1985) An analysis of objective measurements including radionuclide imaging in young patients with patellofemoral pain. *Am J Sports Med* **13**(abstr): 432

Dye SF, Chew MH (1993) The use of scintigraphy to detect increased osseous metabolic transmission with an envelope of function. *J Bone Joint Surg Am* **75**: 1388–1406

Dye SF, Peartree PK (1989) Sequential radionuclide imaging of the patellofemoral joint in symptomatic young adults. *Am J Sports Med* **17**: 727

Dye SF, Stäubli HU, Biedert RM, Vaupel GL (1999) The mosaic of pathophysiology causing patellofemoral pain: therapeutic implications. *Operative Tech Sports Med* **7**: 46–54

Dye SF, Vaupel GL (1994) The pathophysiology of patellofemoral pain. *Sports Med Arthritis Rev* **2**: 203–210

Dye SF, Vaupel GL, Dye CC (1998) Conscious neurosensory mapping of the internal structures of the human knee without intraarticular anesthesia. *Am J Sports Med* **26**: 773–777

Dye SF, Wojtys EM, Fu FH et al (1999) Factors contributing to function of the knee joint after injury or reconstruction of the anterior cruciate ligament. *Instr Course Lect* **48**: 185–198

Dzioba RB (1990) Diagnostic arthroscopy and longitudinal open lateral release. A four-year follow-up study to determine predictors of surgical outcome. *Am J Sports Med* **18**: 343–348

Eburne J, Bannister G (1996) The McConnell regimen versus isometric quadriceps exercises in the management of anterior knee pain. A randomised prospective controlled trial. *The Knee* **3**: 151–153

Eckhoff DG, Brown AW, Kilcoyne RF, Stamm ER (1997) Knee version associated with anterior knee pain. *Clin Orthop* **339**: 152–155

Eckhoff DG, Burke BJ, Dwyer TF et al (1996) The Ranawat Award. Sulcus morphology of the distal femur. *Clin Orthop* **331**: 23–28

Eckhoff DG, Montgomery WK, Kilcoyne RF, Stamm ER (1994) Femoral morphometry and anterior knee pain. *Clin Orthop* **302**: 64–68

Eifert-Mangine M, Brewster C, Wong M et al (1992) Patellar tendinitis in the recreational athlete. *Orthopedics* **15**: 1359–1367

Elftman H (1966) Biomechanics of muscle with particular application to studies of gait. *J Bone Joint Surg Am* **48**: 363–377

el-Khoury GY, Wira RL, Berbaum KS et al (1992) MR imaging of patellar tendinitis. *Radiology* **184**: 849–854

Ellis MI, Seedhom BB, Wright V, Dowson D (1980) An evaluation of the ratio between the tensions along the quadriceps tendon and patellar ligament. *Eng Med* **9**: 189–194

Eng JJ, Pierrynowski MR (1993) Evaluation of soft foot orthotics in the treatment of patellofemoral pain syndrome. *Phys Ther* **73**: 62–8; discussion 68–70

Engel GL (1977) The need for a new medical model: a challenge for biomedicine. *Science* **196**: 129–136

Ernst GP, Kawaguchi J, Saliba E (1999) Effect of patellar taping on knee kinetics of patients with patellofemoral pain syndrome. *J Orthop Sports Phys Ther* **29**: 661–667

Escamilla RF (2001) Knee biomechanics of the dynamic squat exercise. *Med Sci Sports Exerc* **33**: 127–141

Escamilla RF, Fleisig GS, Zheng N et al (1998) Biomechanics of the knee during closed kinetic chain and open kinetic chain exercises. *Med Sci Sports Exerc* **30**: 556–569

Fairbank JC, Pynsent PB, van Poortvliet JA, Phillips H (1984) Mechanical factors in the incidence of knee pain in adolescents and young adults. *J Bone Joint Surg Br* **66**: 685–693

Farahmand F, Senavongse W, Amis AA (1998) Quantitative study of the quadriceps muscles and trochlear groove geometry related to instability of the patellofemoral joint. *J Orthop Res* **16**: 136–143

Fargas-Babjak AM, Pomeranz B, Rooney PJ (1992) Acupuncture-like stimulation with codetron for rehabilitation of patients with chronic pain syndrome and osteoarthritis. *Acupunct Electrother Res* **17**: 95–105

Federico DJ, Reider B (1997) Results of isolated patellar debridement for patellofemoral pain in patients with normal patellar alignment. *Am J Sports Med* **25**: 663–669

Feller JA, Feagin JA Jr, Garrett WE (1993) The medial patellofemoral ligament revisited. An anatomical study. *Knee Surg Sports Traumatol Arthrosc* **1**: 184–186

Ficat P (1970) *Pathologie Fémorale-Patellaire*. Paris, Masson

Fields JL, Basbaum AI (1984) Endogenous pain control mechanisms. In: Will PD, Melzack R (eds), *Textbook of Pain*. Edinburgh, Churchill Livingstone

Finestone A, Radin EL, Lev B et al (1993) Treatment of overuse patellofemoral pain. Prospective randomized controlled clinical trial in a military setting. *Clin Orthop* **293**: 208–210

Fitzgerald GK, McClure PW (1995) Reliability of measurements obtained with four tests for patellofemoral alignment. *Phys Ther* **75**: 84–90; discussion 90–92

Fontaine C (1983) L'innervation de la rotule. *Acta Orthop Belg* **49**: 425–436

Ford DH, Post WR (1997) Open or arthroscopic lateral release. Indications, techniques, and rehabilitation. *Clin Sports Med* **16**: 29–49

Fredericson M, Powers CM (2002) Practical management of patellofemoral pain. *Clin J Sport Med* **12**: 36–38

Freeman MA, Wyke B (1967) The innervation of the knee joint. An anatomical and histological study in the cat. *J Anat* **101**: 505–532

Freemont AJ, Peacock TE, Goupille P et al (1997) Nerve ingrowth into diseased intervertebral disc in chronic back pain. *Lancet* **350**: 178–181

Fulkerson JP (1982) Awareness of the retinaculum in evaluating patellofemoral pain. *Am J Sports Med* **10**: 147–149

Fulkerson JP, Arendt EA (2000) Anterior knee pain in females. *Clin Orthop* **372**: 69–73

Fulkerson JP, Folcik MA (1986) Comparison of diflunisal and naproxen for relief of anterior knee pain. *Clin Ther* **9** (suppl C): 59–61

Fulkerson JP, Gossling HR (1980) Anatomy of the knee joint lateral retinaculum. *Clin Orthop* **153**: 183–188

Fulkerson JP, Hungerford DS (1990) *Disorders of the Patellofemoral Joint*, 2nd edn. Baltimore, MD, William & Wilkins

Fulkerson JP, Schutzer SF, Ramsby GR, Bernstein RA (1987) Computerized tomography of the patellofemoral joint before and after lateral release or realignment. *Arthroscopy* **3**: 19–24

Fulkerson JP, Shea KP (1990) Disorders of patellofemoral alignment. *J Bone Joint Surg Am* **72**: 1424–1429

Fulkerson JP, Tennant R, Jaivin JS, Grunnet M (1985) Histologic evidence of retinacular nerve injury associated with patellofemoral malalignment. *Clin Orthop* **197**: 196–205

Galland O, Walch G, Dejour H, Carret JP (1990) An anatomical and radiological study of the femoropatellar articulation. *Surg Radiol Anat* **12**: 119–125

Gambardella RA (1999) Technical pitfalls of patellofemoral surgery. *Clin Sports Med* **18**: 897–903

Gentile A (1987) Skill acquisition: action, movement, and neuromotor processes. In: Carr JH, Shepherd RB, Gordon J (eds), *Movement Science: Foundations for Physical Therapy in Rehabilitation*. Rockville, MD, Aspen, pp 93–154

Gerber BE, Maenza F (1998) [Shift and tilt of the bony patella in total knee replacement]. *Orthopade* **27**: 629–636

Gerrard B (1989) The patellofemoral pain syndrome: a clinical trial of the McConnell Programme. *Aust J Physiother* **35**: 71–80

Gerrard B (1995) The patellofemoral complex. In: Zuluaga M, Briggs C, Carlisle J et al (eds), *Sports Physiotherapy, Applied Science and Practice*. Melbourne, Churchill Livingstone

Gilleard W, McConnell J, Parsons D (1998) The effect of patellar taping on the onset of vastus medialis obliquus and vastus lateralis muscle activity in persons with patellofemoral pain. *Phys Ther* **78**: 25–32

Gillquist J (1996) Knee ligaments and proprioception. *Acta Orthop Scand* **67**: 533–535

Godfrey CM, Jayawardena A, Welsh P (1979) Comparison of electro-stimulation and isometric exercise in strengthening the quadriceps muscle. *Physiother Canada* **31**: 265–267

Golden BD, Abramson SB (1999) Selective cyclo-oxygenase-2 inhibitors. *Rheum Dis Clin North Am* **25**: 359–378

Goldring MB (2000) The role of the chondrocyte in osteoarthritis. *Arthritis Rheum* **43**: 1916–1926

Goldthwait JE (1904) Slipping or recurrent dislocation of the patella: with the report of eleven cases. *Boston Med Surg* **150**: 169

Goodfellow J, Hungerford DS, Woods C (1976) Patellofemoral joint mechanics and pathology. 2. Chondromalacia patellae. *J Bone Joint Surg Br* **58**: 291–299

Goodfellow J, Hungerford DS, Zindel M (1976) Patellofemoral joint mechanics and pathology. 1. Functional anatomy of the patellofemoral joint. *J Bone Joint Surg Br* **58**: 287–290

Goutallier D, Beaufils P, Bernageau J et al (1999) Pathologie fémoro-patellaire. In: *Le Cahiers d'Enseignement de la Société Française de Chirurgie Orthopedique et Traumatologie (SOFCOT) 1999 Concernant la Pathologie Fémoro-patellaire*, Paris

Goutallier D, Bernageau J (1997) Intérêt pratique de la TA-GT. Le genou traumatique et dégênératif. In: *XXIV Groupe d'Etude et de Travail de l'Imagerie Osteo-articulatife*, pp 259–270

Goutallier D, Bernageau J, Lecudonnec B (1978) [The measurement of the tibial tuberosity. Patella groove distanced technique and results (author's transl)]. *Rev Chir Orthop Reparatrice Appar Mot* **64**: 423–428

Grabiner MD, Koh TJ, Draganich LF (1994) Neuromechanics of the patellofemoral joint. *Med Sci Sports Exerc* **26**: 10–21

Grammont P (1985) [Influence of the patella on the equilibrium of the knee joint. Mutual effects of patellar and femorotibial arthrosis]. *Orthopade* **14**: 193–202

Grana WA, Hinkley B, Hollingsworth S (1984) Arthroscopic evaluation and treatment of patellar malalignment. *Clin Orthop* **186**: 122–128

Grana WA, Kriegshauser LA (1985) Scientific basis of extensor mechanism disorders. *Clin Sports Med* **4**: 247–257

Gray G (1994) *Chain Reaction Plus. Successful Strategies for Closed Chain and Open Chain Testing and Rehabilitation*. Adrian, MI, Wynn Marketing

Grelsamer RP (2000) Patellar malalignment. *J Bone Joint Surg Am* **82**: 1639–1650

Grelsamer RP, McConnell J (1998) *The Patella. A Team Approach*. Gaithersburg, MD, Aspen

Grelsamer RP, Meadows S (1992) The modified Insall–Salvati ratio for assessment of patellar height. *Clin Orthop* **282**: 170–176

Grelsamer RP, Proctor CS, Bazos AN (1994) Evaluation of patellar shape in the sagittal plane. A clinical analysis. *Am J Sports Med* **22**: 61–66

Grimmer K (1992) A controlled double-blind study comparing the effects of strong burst-mode TENS and high-rate TENS on painful osteoarthritic knees. *Aust J Physiother* **38**: 49–56

Grood ES, Suntay WJ (1983) A joint coordinate system for the clinical description of three-dimensional motions: application to the knee. *J Biomech Eng* **105**: 136–144

Grood ES, Suntay WJ, Noyes FR, Butler DL (1984) Biomechanics of the knee-extension exercise. Effect of cutting the anterior cruciate ligament. *J Bone Joint Surg Am* **66**: 725–734

Guyton AC, Hall JE (1986) *Textbook of Medical Physiology*. Philadelphia, PA, WB Saunders

Guzzanti V, Gigante A, Di Lazzaro A, Fabbriciani C (1994) Patellofemoral malalignment in adolescents. Computerized tomographic assessment with or without quadriceps contraction. *Am J Sports Med* **22**: 55–60

Hallisey MJ, Doherty N, Bennett WF, Fulkerson JP (1987) Anatomy of the junction of the vastus lateralis tendon and the patella. *J Bone Joint Surg Am* **69**: 545–549

Han JS, Chen XH, Sun SL et al (1991) Effect of low- and high-frequency TENS on Met-enkephalin-Arg-Phe and dynorphin A immunoreactivity in human lumbar CSF. *Pain* **47**: 295–298

Handfield TKJ (2000) Effect of McConnell taping on perceived pain and knee extensor torques during isokinetic exercise performed by patients with patellofemoral pain syndrome. *Physiother Canada* **4**: 39–44

Handling KA (1982) Rehabilitating athletic injuries with cryotherapy. *J Phys Educ Recreat Dance* **53**: 338–340

Hanten WP, Schulthies SS (1990) Exercise effect on electromyographic activity of the vastus medialis oblique and vastus lateralis muscles. *Phys Ther* **70**: 561–565

Harrison EL, Sheppard MS, McQuarrie AM (1999) A randomized controlled trial of physical therapy treatment programs in patellofemoral pain syndrome. *Physiother Canada* Spring: 93–100

Hauselmann HJ (2001) Nutripharmaceuticals for osteoarthritis. *Best Pract Res Clin Rheumatol* **15**: 595–607

Hautamaa PV, Fithian DC, Kaufman KR et al (1998) Medial soft tissue restraints in lateral patellar instability and repair. *Clin Orthop* **349**: 174–182

Hedberg A, Messner K, Persliden J, Hildebrand C (1995) Transient local presence of nerve fibres at onset of secondary ossification in the rat knee joint. *Anat Embryol (Berl)* **192**: 247–255

Heegaard J, Leyvraz PF, Van Kampen A et al (1994) Influence of soft structures on patellar three-dimensional tracking. *Clin Orthop* **299**: 235–243

Hehne HJ (1990) Biomechanics of the patellofemoral joint and its clinical relevance. *Clin Orthop* **258**: 73–85

Henry JH, Goletz TH, Williamson B (1986) Lateral retinacular release in patellofemoral subluxation. Indications, results, and comparison to open patellofemoral reconstruction. *Am J Sports Med* **14**: 121–129

Herrington L, Payton CJ (1983) Effects of corrective taping of the patella on patients with patellofemoral pain. *Physiotherapy* **83**: 566–572

Hille E, Schulitz KP, Henrichs C, Schneider T (1985) Pressure and contact-surface measurements within the femoropatellar joint and their variations following lateral release. *Arch Orthop Trauma Surg* **104**: 275–282

Hillsgrove DC, Paulos L (1995) Complications of patellofemoral surgery. In: *The Patella*. Berlin, Springer-Verlag, pp 277–290

Hirsch E, Moye D, Dimon JH III (1995) Congenital indifference to pain: long-term follow-up of two cases. *South Med J* **88**: 851–857

Hochberg MC, Altman RD, Brandt KD et al (1995) Guidelines for the medical management of osteoarthritis. Part I. Osteoarthritis of the hip. *Arthritis Rheum* **38**: 1535–1540

Hochberg MC, Dougados M (2001) Pharmacological therapy of osteoarthritis. *Best Pract Res Clin Rheumatol* **15**: 583–593

Hodges PW, Richardson CA (1993) The influence of isometric hip adduction on quadriceps femoris activity. *Scand J Rehabil Med* **25**: 57–62

Holmes PF, Henry JH (1989) The results of extensor mechanism realignment following failed lateral retinacular releases. *Clin Sports Med* **8**: 291–296

Hruska R (1998) Pelvic stability influences lower-extremity kinematics. *Biomechanics* **5**: 23–29

Hsieh LF, Guu CS, Liou HJ, Kung HC (1992) Isokinetic and isometric testing of knee musculature in young female patients with patellofemoral pain syndrome. *J Formos Med Assoc* **91**: 199–205

Huang MH, Chen CH, Chen TW (2000) The effects of weight reduction on the rehabilitation of patients with knee osteoarthritis and obesity. *Arthritis Care Research* **13**: 398–405

Hubbard JK, Sampson HW, Elledge JR (1997) Prevalence and morphology of the vastus medialis oblique muscle in human cadavers. *Anat Rec* **249**: 135–142

Hubbard JK, Sampson HW, Elledge JR (1998) The vastus medialis oblique muscle and its relationship to patellofemoral joint deterioration in human cadavers. *J Orthop Sports Phys Ther* **28**: 384–391

Huberti HH, Hayes WC (1984) Patellofemoral contact pressures. The influence of Q-angle and tendofemoral contact. *J Bone Joint Surg Am* **66**: 715–724

Hughes GS Jr, Lichstein PR, Whitlock D, Harker C (1984) Response of plasma β-endorphins to transcutaneous electrical nerve stimulation in healthy subjects. *Phys Ther* **64**: 1062–1066

Hughston JC (1968) Subluxation of the patella. *J Bone Joint Surg Am* **50**: 1003–1026

Hughston JC, Deese M (1988) Medial subluxation of the patella as a complication of lateral retinacular release. *Am J Sports Med* **16**: 383–388

Hughston JC, Walsh WM, Puddu G (1984) *Patellar Subluxation and Dislocation. Saunders Monographs in Clinical Orthopaedics*, volume V. Philadelphia, PA, WB Saunders

Hultman E, Sjoholm H, Jaderholm-Ek I, Krynicki J (1983) Evaluation of methods for electrical stimulation of human skeletal muscle *in situ*. *Pfluger's Arch* **398**: 139–141

Hungerford DS, Barry M (1979) Biomechanics of the patellofemoral joint. *Clin Orthop* **144**: 9–15

Hungerford DS, Lennox DW (1983) Rehabilitation of the knee in disorders of the patellofemoral joint:

relevant biomechanics. *Orthop Clin North Am* **14**: 397–402

Hunziker EB, Stäubli HU, Jakob RP (1992) Surgical anatomy of the knee joint. In: Jakob RP, Stäubli HU (eds), *The Knee and the Cruciate Ligaments*. Heidelberg, Springer-Verlag, pp 31–47

Hurley M, Walsh N (2001) Physical, functional and other nonpharmacological interventions for osteoarthritis. *Best Pract Res Clin Rheumatol* **15**: 569–581

Hurley MV, Jones BW, Wilson D, Newham DJ (1992) Rehabilitation of quadriceps inhibited due to isolates rupture to the anterior cruciate ligament. *J Orthop Rheumatol* **5**: 145–154

Hutchinson MR, Ireland ML (1995) Patella dislocation. *Physician Sportsmed* **23**: 53–60

Hvid I (1983) The stability of the human patellofemoral joint. *Eng Med* **12**: 55–59

Inoue M, Shino K, Hirose H, Horibe S, Ono K (1988) Subluxation of the patella. Computed tomography analysis of patellofemoral congruence. *J Bone Joint Surg Am* **70**: 1331–1337

Insall J (1979) 'Chondromalacia patellae': patellar malalignment syndrome. *Orthop Clin North Am* **10**: 117–127

Insall J (1982) Current Concepts Review: patellar pain. *J Bone Joint Surg Am* **64**: 147–152

Insall J, Falvo KA, Wise DW (1976) Chondromalacia patellae. A prospective study. *J Bone Joint Surg Am* **58**: 1–8

Insall J, Goldberg V, Salvati E (1972) Recurrent dislocation and the high-riding patella. *Clin Orthop* **88**: 67–69

Insall J, Salvati E (1971) Patella position in the normal knee joint. *Radiology* **101**: 101–104

Insall JN (1984) *Surgery of the Knee*. New York, Churchill Livingstone

Irrgang JJ, Snyder-Mackler L, Wainner RS et al (1998) Development of a patient-reported measure of function of the knee. *J Bone Joint Surg Am* **80**: 1132–1145

Isaacson LG, Crutcher KA (1995) The duration of sprouted cerebrovascular axons following intracranial infusion of nerve growth factor. *Exp Neurol* **131**: 174–179

Ishii H, Tanaka H, Katoh K et al (2002) Characterization of infiltrating T cells and Th1/Th2-type cytokines in the synovium of patients with osteoarthritis. *Osteoarthr Cartilage* **10**: 277–281

Jakob RP, Stäubli HU (1990) *The Knee and the Cruciate Ligaments*. Berlin, Heidelberg, Springer-Verlag

Javadpour DP, Finegan PJ, O'Brien M (1991) The anatomy of the extensor mechanism and its clinical relevance. *Clin J Sport Med* **1**: 229–235

Jensen H, Zesler R, Christensen T (1991) Transcutaneous electrical nerve stimulation (TENS) for painful osteoarthritis of the knee. *Int J Rehab Res* **14**: 356–358

Jensen R, Gothesen O, Liseth K, Baerheim A (1999) Acupuncture treatment of patellofemoral pain syndrome. *J Altern Compl Med* **5**: 521–527

Jerosch J, Prymka M (1996) Knee joint proprioception in patients with posttraumatic recurrent patella dislocation. *Knee Surg Sports Traumatol Arthrosc* **4**: 14–18

Jette AM (1994) Physical disablement concepts for physical therapy research and practice. *Phys Ther* **74**: 380–386

Johansson H, Sjolander P, Sojka P (1991) Receptors in the knee joint ligaments and their role in the biomechanics of the joint. *Crit Rev Biomed Eng* **18**: 341–368

Johnson DL, Bealle DP, Brand JC Jr et al (2000) The effect of a geographic lateral bone bruise on knee inflammation after acute anterior cruciate ligament rupture. *Am J Sports Med* **28**: 152–155

Johnson DP, Wakeley C (2002) Reconstruction of the lateral patellar retinaculum following lateral release: a case report. *Knee Surg Sports Traumatol Arthrosc* **10**: 361–363

Johnson LL, van Dyk GE, Green JR III et al (1998) Clinical assessment of asymptomatic knees: comparison of men and women. *Arthroscopy* **14**: 347–359

Julliard R (1989) Diagnostic radiographique de l'instabilité rotulienne. Les défilés en rotation externe. *J Chir* **3**: 169–175

Kadaba MP, Ramakrishnan HK, Wootten ME et al (1989) Repeatability of kinematic, kinetic, and electromyographic data in normal adult gait. *J Orthop Res* **7**: 849–860

Kannus P, Natri A, Niittymaki S, Jarvinen M (1992) Effect of intraarticular glycosaminoglycan polysulfate treatment on patellofemoral pain syndrome. A prospective, randomized double-blind trial comparing glycosaminoglycan polysulfate with placebo and quadriceps muscle exercises. *Arthritis Rheum* **35**: 1053–1061

Kannus P, Natri A, Paakkala T, Jarvinen M (1999) An outcome study of chronic patellofemoral pain syndrome. Seven-year follow-up of patients in a randomized, controlled trial. *J Bone Joint Surg Am* **81**: 355–363

Kannus P, Niittymaki S (1994) Which factors predict outcome in the nonoperative treatment of patellofemoral pain syndrome? A prospective follow-up study. *Med Sci Sports Exerc* **26**: 289–296

Karlsson J, Thomee R, Sward L (1996) Eleven-year follow-up of patellofemoral pain syndrome. *Clin J Sport Med* **6**: 22–26

Karrholm J, Brandsson S, Freeman MA (2000) Tibiofemoral movement 4: changes of axial tibial rotation caused by forced rotation at the weight-bearing knee studied by RSA. *J Bone Joint Surg Br* **82**: 1201–1203

Karst GM, Jewett PD (1993) Electromyographic analysis of exercises proposed for differential activation of medial and lateral quadriceps femoris muscle components. *Phys Ther* **73**: 286–295; discussion 295–299

Karst GM, Willett GM (1995) Onset timing of electromyographic activity in the vastus medialis oblique and vastus lateralis muscles in subjects with and without patellofemoral pain syndrome. *Phys Ther* **75**: 813–823

Katchburian MV, Bull AM, Shih YF et al (2003) Review article: measurement of patellar tracking: assessment and analysis of the literature. *Clin Orthop* **412**: 241–259

Kaufer H (1971) Mechanical function of the patella. *J Bone Joint Surg Am* **53**: 1551–1560

Kawaja MD (1998) Sympathetic and sensory innervation of the extracerebral vasculature: roles for p75NTR neuronal expression and nerve growth factor. *J Neurosci Res* **52**: 295–306

Keene GCR, Marans HJ (1993) Osteotomy for patellofemoral dysplasia. In: Fox JM, Del Pizzo W (eds), *The Patellofemoral Joint*. New York, McGraw-Hill, pp 169–175

Kendall FP, McCreary EK, Provance PG (1993) *Muscles: Testing and Function*, 4th edn. Baltimore, MD, Williams & Wilkins

Kennedy JC, Alexander IJ, Hayes KC (1982) Nerve supply of the human knee and its functional importance. *Am J Sports Med* **10**: 329–335

Kettelkamp DB (1981) Management of patellar malalignment. *J Bone Joint Surg Am* **63**: 1344–1348

Kimball ES (1991) *Cytokines and Inflammation*. Boca Raton, FL, CRC Press

King J (2000) Patellar dislocation and lesions of the patella tendon. *Br J Sports Med* **34**: 467–470

King JB, Perry DJ, Mourad K, Kumar SJ (1990) Lesions of the patellar ligament. *J Bone Joint Surg Br* **72**: 46–48

Kitai TA, Sale DG (1989) Specificity of joint angle in isometric training. *Eur J Appl Physiol Occup Physiol* **58**: 744–748

Klein-Vogelabch S (1990) *Ballgymnastik zur funktionellen Bewegungslehre*. Berlin, Springer-Verlag

Klingman RE, Liaos SM, Hardin KM (1997) The effect of subtalar joint posting on patellar glide position in subjects with excessive rearfoot pronation. *J Orthop Sports Phys Ther* **25**: 185–191

Knight KL (1990) Cold as a modifier of sports-induced inflammation. In: Leadbetter WB, Buckwalter JA, Gordon SL (eds), *Sports-induced Inflammation*. Chicago, American Academy of Orthopedic Surgeons, pp 463–477

Knight KL, Londeree BR (1980) Comparison of blood flow in the ankle of uninjured subjects during therapeutic applications of heat, cold, and exercise. *Med Sci Sports Exerc* **12**: 76–80

Koel G (1991) *Transcutane Elektrische Neuro Stimulatie (TENS)*. Lochem, The Netherlands, De Tijdstroom

Kolowich PA, Paulos LE, Rosenberg TD, Farnsworth S (1990) Lateral release of the patella: indications and contraindications. *Am J Sports Med* **18**: 359–365

Koshino T (1991) Stage classifications, types of joint destruction, and bone scintigraphy in Charcot joint disease. *Bull Hosp Jt Dis Orthop Inst* **51**: 205–217

Kowal MA (1983) Review of physiological effects of cryotherapy. *J Orthop Sports Phys Ther* **5**: 66–73

Kowall MG, Kolk G, Nuber GW et al (1996) Patellar taping in the treatment of patellofemoral pain. A prospective randomized study. *Am J Sports Med* **24**: 61–66

Krajca-Radcliffe JB, Coker TP (1996) Patellofemoral arthroplasty. A 2- to 18-year follow-up study. *Clin Orthop* **330**: 143–151

Kramers-de Quervain IA, Biedert R, Stüssi E (1997) Quantitative gait analysis in patients with medial patellar instability following lateral retinacular release. *Knee Surg Sports Traumatol Arthrosc* **5**: 95–101

Krenn V, Hensel F, Kim HJ et al (1999) Molecular IgV(H) analysis demonstrates highly somatic mutated B cells in synovialitis of osteoarthritis: a degenerative disease is associated with a specific, not locally generated immune response. *Lab Invest* **79**: 1377–1384

Krenn V, Hofmann S, Engel A (1990) First description of mechanoreceptors in the corpus adiposum infrapatellare of man. *Acta Anat (Basel)* **137**: 187–188

Kujala UM, Kormano M, Osterman K et al (1992) Magnetic resonance imaging analysis of patellofemoral congruity in females. *Clin J Sports Med* **2**: 21–26

Kujala UM, Osterman K, Kormano M et al (1989) Patellar motion analyzed by magnetic resonance imaging. *Acta Orthop Scand* **60**: 13–16

Kujala UM, Osterman K, Kormano M et al (1989) Patellofemoral relationships in recurrent patellar dislocation. *J Bone Joint Surg Br* **71**: 788–792

Kvist M, Kujala UM, Heinonen OJ et al (1989) Sports-related injuries in children. *Int J Sports Med* **10**: 81–86

Lapra C, Lecoultre B, Ait Si Selmi T, Neyret P (1997) Le tendon rotulien dans l'instabilité rotulienne: étude IRM. In: *XXIV Groupe d'Etude et de Travail de l'Imagerie Osteo-articulatife*, pp 227–231

Laprade J, Culham E, Brouwer B (1998) Comparison of five isometric exercises in the recruitment of the vastus medialis oblique in persons with and without patellofemoral pain syndrome. *J Orthop Sports Phys Ther* **27**: 197–204

Larson RL, Cabaud HE, Slocum DB et al (1978) The patellar compression syndrome: surgical treatment by lateral retinacular release. *Clin Orthop* **134**: 158–167

Laskin RS, van Steijn M (1999) Total knee replacement for patients with patellofemoral arthritis. *Clin Orthop* **367**: 89–95

Laurin CA, Levesque HP, Dussault R et al (1978) The abnormal lateral patellofemoral angle: a diagnostic roentgenographic sign of recurrent patellar subluxation. *J Bone Joint Surg Am* **60**: 55–60

Lazzarini KM, Troiano RN, Smith RC (1997) Can running cause the appearance of marrow edema on MR images of the foot and ankle? *Radiology* **202**: 540–542

Le Veau BF, Rogers C (1980) Selective training of the vastus medialis muscle using EMG biofeedback. *Phys Ther* **60**: 1410–1415

Lee TH, Kato H, Kogure K, Itoyama Y (1996) Temporal profile of nerve growth factor-like immunoreactivity after transient focal cerebral ischemia in rats. *Brain Res* **713**: 199–210

Leonard C (1998) *The Neuroscience of Human Movement*. St. Louis, MO, Mosby-Year Book

Lephart SM, Riemann BL, Fu FH (2001) Introduction to the sensorimotor system. In: Lephart SM, Fu FH (eds), *Proprioception and Neuromuscular Control in Joint Stability*. Champaign, IL, Human Kinetics

Leroux A, Belanger M, Boucher JP (1995) Pain effect on monosynaptic and polysynaptic reflex inhibition. *Arch Phys Med Rehabil* **76**: 576–582

Levine J (1979) Chondromalacia patellae. *Phys Sportsmed* **7**: 41–49

Lewis B, Lewis D, Cumming G (1994) The comparative analgesic efficacy of transcutaneous electrical nerve stimulation and a non-steroidal anti-inflammatory drug for painful osteoarthritis. *Br J Rheumatol* **33**: 455–460

Lewit K (1997) *Manuelle Medizin*. Leipzig, Barth

Lieber RL, Kelly MJ (1991) Factors influencing quadriceps femoris muscle torque using transcutaneous neuromuscular electrical stimulation. *Phys Ther* **71**: 715–721; discussion 722–723

Lieber RL, Silva PD, Daniel DM (1996) Equal effectiveness of electrical and volitional strength training for quadriceps femoris muscles after anterior cruciate ligament surgery. *J Orthop Res* **14**: 131–138

Lisignoli G, Toneguzzi S, Pozzi C et al (1999) Proinflammatory cytokines and chemokine production and expression by human osteoblasts isolated from patients with rheumatoid arthritis and osteoarthritis. *J Rheumatol* **26**: 791–799

Lorentzon R (1989) Ursache von Sportverletzungen. Innere Faktoren. In: Dirix A, Knuttgen HG, Tittel K (eds), *Olympia-Buch der Sportmedizen*. Cologne, Deutscher Ärzte Verlag

Lubinus HH (1979) Patella glide bearing replacement. *Orthopaedics* **2**: 119–127

Lutz GE, Palmitier RA, An KN, Chao EY (1993) Comparison of tibiofemoral joint forces during open-kinetic-chain and closed-kinetic-chain exercises. *J Bone Joint Surg Am* 75: 732–739

Macnicol MF (1986) *The Problem Knee*. London, William Heinemann Medical Books

Madigan R, Wissinger HA, Donaldson WF (1975) Preliminary experience with a method of quadricepsplasty in recurrent subluxation of the patella. *J Bone Joint Surg Am* 57: 600–607

Mäenpää H, Matti U, Lehto UK (1997) Patellar dislocation. The long-term results of nonoperative management in 100 patients. *Am J Sports Med* 25: 213–217

Maffiuletti NA, Martin A (2001) Progressive versus rapid rate of contraction during 7 weeks of isometric resistance training. *Med Sci Sports Exerc* 33: 1220–1227

Maitland GD (1977) *Peripheral Manipulation*, 2nd edn. London, Butterworth

Maitland GD (1980) The hypothesis of adding compression when examining and treating synovial joints. *J Orthop Sports Phys Ther* 2: 7–14

Maitland GD (1986) *Vertebral Manipulation*, 5th edn. London, Butterworth

Maitland GD, Corrigan B (1983) *Practical Orthopaedic Medicine*. London, Butterworth

Mak MK, Levin O, Mizrahi J, Hui-Chan CW (2003) Joint torques during sit-to-stand in healthy subjects and people with Parkinson's disease. *Clin Biomech (Bristol, Avon)* 18: 197–206

Malcangio M, Garrett NE, Cruwys S, Tomlinson DR (1997) Nerve growth factor- and neurotrophin-3-induced changes in nociceptive threshold and the release of substance P from the rat isolated spinal cord. *J Neurosci* 17: 8459–8467

Maldague B, Malghem J (1985) [Significance of the radiograph of the knee profile in the detection of patellar instability. Preliminary report]. *Rev Chir Orthop Reparatrice Appar Mot* 71 (suppl 2): 5–13

Malone T, Davies G, Walsh WM (2002) Muscular control of the patella. *Clin Sports Med* 21: 349–362

Mangine RE, Kremchek TE (1997) Evaluation-based protocol of the anterior cruciate ligament. *J Sports Rehab* 6: 157–181

Mansat C, Bonnel F, Jaeger JH (1982) *L'appareil Éxtenseur du Genou*. Paris, Masson

Martinez S, Korobkin M, Fondren FB et al (1983) Diagnosis of patellofemoral malalignment by computed tomography. *J Comput Assist Tomogr* 7: 1050–1053

Marumoto JM, Jordan C, Akins R (1995) A biomechanical comparison of lateral retinacular releases. *Am J Sports Med* 23: 151–155

Marx RG, Jones EC, Allen AA et al (2001) Reliability, validity, and responsiveness of four knee outcome scales for athletic patients. *J Bone Joint Surg Am* 83: 1459–1469

Masse Y (1978) [Trochleoplasty. Restoration of the intercondylar groove in subluxations and dislocations of the patella]. *Rev Chir Orthop Reparatrice Appar Mot* 64: 3–17

Mayer TG, Gatchel RJ (1988) *Functional Restoration for Spinal Disorders. The Sports Medicine Approach*. Philadelphia, PA, Lea & Febiger

McAlindon TE, LaValley MP, Gulin JP, Felson DT (2000) Glucosamine and chondroitin for treatment of osteoarthritis: a systematic quality assessment and meta-analysis. *J Am Med Assoc* 283: 1469–1475

McConnell J (1986) The management of chondromalacia patellae: a long-term solution. *Aust J Physiother* 32: 215–223

McConnell J (2002) The physical therapist's approach to patellofemoral disorders. *Clin Sports Med* 21: 363–387

McConnell J, Fulkerson JP (1996) The knee: patellofemoral and soft tissue injuries. In: Zachazewski JE, Magee DJ, Quillen WS (eds), *Athletic Injuries and Rehabilitation*. Philadelphia, PA, WB Saunders, pp 693–728

McGinty G, Irrgang JJ, Pezzullo D (2000) Biomechanical considerations for rehabilitation of the knee. *Clin Biomech (Bristol, Avon)* 15: 160–166

McGinty JB, McCarthy JC (1981) Endoscopic lateral retinacular release: a preliminary report. *Clin Orthop* 158: 120–125

McGoey BV, Deitel M, Saplys RJ, Kliman ME (1990) Effect of weight loss on musculoskeletal pain in the morbidly obese. *J Bone Joint Surg Br* 72: 322–323

McNeal DR, Baker LL (1988) Effects of joint angle, electrodes and waveform on electrical stimulation of the quadriceps and hamstrings. *Ann Biomed Eng* 16: 299–310

McPoil TG, Knecht HG (1985) A survey of foot types in normal females between the ages of 18 and 30 years. *J Orthop Sports Phys Ther* 9: 406–409

Meglan DA (1991) Enhanced Analysis of Human Locomotion. Thesis, Ohio State University, Columbus, OH

Melzack R (1976) Relief from chronic pain: taking the mystery out of acupuncture. *Physiother Canada* 28: 106–148

Melzack R, Stillwell DM, Fox EJ (1977) Trigger points and acupuncture points for pain: correlations and implications. *Pain* 3: 3–23

Melzack R, Wall PD (1965) Pain mechanisms: a new theory. *Science* 150: 971–979

Melzack R, Wall PD (1982) *The Challenge of Pain.* New York, Penguin USA

Menkes CJ, Renoux M, Laoussadi S et al (1993) Substance P levels in the synovium and synovial fluid from patients with rheumatoid arthritis and osteoarthritis. *J Rheumatol* 20: 714–717

Merchant AC (1988) Classification of patellofemoral disorders. *Arthroscopy* 4: 235–240

Merchant AC (2001) Patellofemoral imaging. *Clin Orthop* 389: 15–21

Merchant AC, Mercer RL, Jacobsen RH, Cool CR (1974) Roentgenographic analysis of patellofemoral congruence. *J Bone Joint Surg Am* 56: 1391–1396

Messier SP, Davis SE, Curl WW et al (1991) Etiologic factors associated with patellofemoral pain in runners. *Med Sci Sports Exerc* 23: 1008–1015

Metcalf RW (1982) An arthroscopic method for lateral release of subluxating or dislocating patella. *Clin Orthop* 167: 9–18

Miller JP, Sedory D, Croce RV (1997) Vastus medialis obliquus and vastus lateralis activity in patients with and without patellofemoral pain syndrome. *J Sports Rehab* 6: 1–10

Miller MD, Hinkin DT, Wisnowski JW (1997) The efficacy of orthotics for anterior knee pain in military trainees. A preliminary report. *Am J Knee Surg* 10: 10–13

Miller PR, Klein RM, Teitge RA (1991) Medial dislocation of the patella. *Skeletal Radiol* 20: 429–431

Minns RJ, Birnie AJ, Abernethy PJ (1979) A stress analysis of the patella, and how it relates to patellar articular cartilage lesions. *J Biomech* 12: 699–711

Moller BN, Jurik AG, Tidemand-Dal C et al (1987) The quadriceps function in patellofemoral disorders. A radiographic and electromyographic study. *Arch Orthop Trauma Surg* 106: 195–198

Moller BN, Krebs B, Tidemand-Dal C, Aaris K (1986) Isometric contractions in the patellofemoral pain syndrome. An electromyographic study. *Arch Orthop Trauma Surg* 105: 24–27

Mont MA, Haas S, Mullick T, Hungerford DS (2002) Total knee arthroplasty for patellofemoral arthritis. *J Bone Joint Surg Am* 84: 1977–1981

Moos V, Fickert S, Muller B et al (1999) Immunohistological analysis of cytokine expression in human osteoarthritic and healthy cartilage. *J Rheumatol* 26: 870–879

Moos V, Sieper J, Herzog W, Müller B (2001) Regulation of expression of cytokines and growth factors in osteoarthritic cartilage explants. *Clin Rheumatol* 20: 353–358.

Mori Y, Fujimoto A, Okumo H, Kuroki Y (1991) Lateral retinaculum release in adolescent patellofemoral disorders: its relationship to peripheral nerve injury in the lateral retinaculum. *Bull Hosp Jt Dis Orthop Inst* 51: 218–229

Mori Y, Kuroki Y, Yamamoto R et al (1991) Clinical and histological study of patellar chondropathy in adolescents. *Arthroscopy* 7: 182–197

Morrish GM, Woledge RC (1997) A comparison of the activation of muscles moving the patella in normal subjects and in patients with chronic patellofemoral problems. *Scand J Rehabil Med* 29: 43–48

Morscher E (1978) Osteotomy of the patella in chondromalacia. Preliminary report. *Arch Orthop Trauma Surg* 92: 139–147

Mulder T (1991) A process-oriented model of human motor behavior: toward a theory-based rehabilitation approach. *Phys Ther* 71: 157–164

Müller W (1982) *Das Knie.* Heidelberg, Springer-Verlag

Müller W, Wirz D (2000) Anatomie, Biomechanik und Dynamik des Patellofemoralgelenks. In: Wirth CJ, Rudert M (eds), *Das Patellofemorale Schmerzsyndrom.* Darmstadt, Steinkopff-Verlag, pp 3–19

Murray MP, Mollinger LA, Gardner GM, Sepic SB (1984) Kinematic and EMG patterns during slow, free and fast walking. *J Orthop Res* 2: 272–280

Myers JB, Lephart SM (2002) Sensorimotor deficits contributing to glenohumeral instability. *Clin Orthop* **400**: 98–104

Nagamine R, Otani T, White SE et al (1995) Patellar tracking measurement in the normal knee. *J Orthop Res* **13**: 115–122

Nagy SZ (1991) Disability concepts revised: implications for prevention. In: Pope AM, Tarlov AR (eds), *Disability in America: Toward a National Agenda for Prevention*. Washington, DC, National Academy Press, pp 309–327

Natri A, Kannus P, Jarvinen M (1998) Which factors predict the long-term outcome in chronic patellofemoral pain syndrome? A 7-year prospective follow-up study. *Med Sci Sports Exerc* **30**: 1572–1577

Nelson RM, Hayes KW, Currier DP (1999) *Clinical Electrotherapy*. Stamford, CT, Appleton & Lange

Neptune RR, Wright IC, van den Bogert AJ (2000) The influence of orthotic devices and vastus medialis strength and timing on patellofemoral loads during running. *Clin Biomech (Bristol, Avon)* **15**: 611–618

Newell KM (1976) Knowledge of results and motor learning. *Exerc Sport Sci Rev* **4**: 195–228

Neyret P, Dejour D, Ait Si Selmi T (2000) *Die trochleare Dysplasie. Das patellofemorale Schmerzsyndrom*. Darmstadt, Verlag-Steinkopff

Neyret P, Robinson AH, Le Coultre B et al (2002) Patellar tendon length – the factor in patellar instability? *The Knee* **9**: 3–6

Nigg BM, Cole GK, Nachbauer W (1993) Effects of arch height of the foot on angular motion of the lower extremities in running. *J Biomech* **26**: 909–916

Ninos JC, Irrgang JJ, Burdett R, Weiss JR (1997) Electromyographic analysis of the squat performed in self-selected lower extremity neutral rotation and 30 degrees of lower extremity turnout from the self-selected neutral position. *J Orthop Sports Phys Ther* **25**: 307–315

Nonweiler DE, DeLee JC (1994) The diagnosis and treatment of medial subluxation of the patella after lateral retinacular release. *Am J Sports Med* **22**: 680–686

Nove-Josserand L, Dejour D (1995) [Quadriceps dysplasia and patellar tilt in objective patellar instability]. *Rev Chir Orthop Reparatrice Appar Mot* **81**: 497–504

Nyland J, Brosky T, Currier D et al (1994) Review of the afferent neural system of the knee and its contribution to motor learning. *J Orthop Sports Phys Ther* **19**: 2–11

O'Brien WJ, Rutan FM, Sanborn C, Omer GE (1984) Effect of transcutaneous electrical nerve stimulation on human blood β-endorphin levels. *Phys Ther* **64**: 1367–1374

O'Neill DB, Micheli LJ, Warner JP (1992) Patellofemoral stress. A prospective analysis of exercise treatment in adolescents and adults. *Am J Sports Med* **20**: 151–156

O'Reilly S, Doherty M (2001) Lifestyle changes in the management of osteoarthritis. *Best Pract Res Clin Rheumatol* **15**: 559–568

O'Sullivan SB, Schmitz TJ (1998) *Physical Rehabilitation: Assessment and Treatment*, 2nd edn. Philadelphia, PA, F. A. Davis

Owings TM, Grabiner MD (2002) Motor control of the vastus medialis oblique and vastus lateralis muscles is disrupted during eccentric contractions in subjects with patellofemoral pain. *Am J Sports Med* **30**: 483–487

Paar O, Schneider B (1989) [Comparative clinical and arthroscopic study of the knee joint in chondromalacia patellae]. *Aktuelle Traumatol* **19**: 142–146

Palmitier RA, An KN, Scott SG, Chao EY (1991) Kinetic chain exercise in knee rehabilitation. *Sports Med* **11**: 402–413

Palumbo PM Jr (1981) Dynamic patellar brace: a new orthosis in the management of patellofemoral disorders. A preliminary report. *Am J Sports Med* **9**: 45–49

Pandolfi S, Exer P, Schwarz HA (2002) [Viscosupplementation in arthrosis]. *Ther Umsch* **59**: 545–549

Panni AS, Biedert RM, Maffulli N et al (2002) Overuse injuries of the extensor mechanism in athletes. *Clin Sports Med* **21**: 483–498

Papagelopoulos PJ, Sim FH (1997) Patellofemoral pain syndrome: diagnosis and management. *Orthopedics* **20**: 148–157; quiz 158–159

Paulos L, Rusche K, Johnson C, Noyes FR (1980) Patellar malalignment: a treatment rationale. *Phys Ther* **60**: 1624–1632

Pendleton A, Arden N, Dougados M et al (2000) European League Against Rheumatism (EULAR) recommendations for the management of knee osteoarthritis: report of a task force of the Standing

Committee for International Clinical Studies Including Therapeutic Trials (ESCISIT). *Ann Rheum Dis* **59**: 936–944

Percy EC, Strother RT (1985) Patellalgia. *Physician Sportsmed* **13**: 43–59

Pidoriano AJ, Weinstein RN, Buuck DA, Fulkerson JP (1997) Correlation of patellar articular lesions with results from anteromedial tibial tubercle transfer. *Am J Sports Med* **25**: 533–537

Pinar H, Akseki D, Karaoglan O, Genc I (1994) Kinematic and dynamic axial computed tomography of the patellofemoral joint in patients with anterior knee pain. *Knee Surg Sports Traumatol Arthrosc* **2**: 170–173

Poole AR (1995) Imbalances of anabolism and catabolism of cartilage matrix components in osteoarthritis. In: Kuettner KE, Goldberg VM (eds), *Osteoarthritic Disorders*. Rosemont, IL, American Academy of Orthopaedic Surgeons, pp 247–260

Powers CM (1998) Rehabilitation of patellofemoral joint disorders: a critical review. *J Orthop Sports Phys Ther* **28**: 345–354

Powers CM (2000) Patellar kinematics, Part I: the influence of vastus muscle activity in subjects with and without patellofemoral pain. *Phys Ther* **80**: 956–964

Powers CM, Landel R, Perry J (1996) Timing and intensity of vastus muscle activity during functional activities in subjects with and without patellofemoral pain. *Phys Ther* **76**: 946–955; discussion 956–967

Powers CM, Landel R, Sosnick T et al (1997) The effects of patellar taping on stride characteristics and joint motion in subjects with patellofemoral pain. *J Orthop Sports Phys Ther* **26**: 286–291

Powers CM, Maffucci R, Hampton S (1995) Rearfoot posture in subjects with patellofemoral pain. *J Orthop Sports Phys Ther* **22**: 155–160

Powers CM, Mortenson S, Nishimoto D, Simon D (1999) Criterion-related validity of a clinical measurement to determine the medial/lateral component of patellar orientation. *J Orthop Sports Phys Ther* **29**: 372–377

Powers CM, Perry J, Hsu A, Hislop HJ (1997) Are patellofemoral pain and quadriceps femoris muscle torque associated with locomotor function? *Phys Ther* **77**: 1063–1075; discussion 1075–1078

Powers CM, Shellock FG, Pfaff M (1998) Quantification of patellar tracking using kinematic MRI. *J Magn Reson Imaging* **8**: 724–732

Puniello MS (1993) Iliotibial band tightness and medial patellar glide in patients with patellofemoral dysfunction. *J Orthop Sports Phys Ther* **17**: 144–148

Raatikainen T, Vaananen K, Tamelander G (1990) Effect of glycosaminoglycan polysulfate on chondromalacia patellae. A placebo-controlled 1-year study. *Acta Orthop Scand* **61**: 443–448

Rabita G, Perot C, Lensel-Corbeil G (2000) Differential effect of knee extension isometric training on the different muscles of the quadriceps femoris in humans. *Eur J Appl Physiol* **83**: 531–538

Radin EL (1979) A rational approach to the treatment of patellofemoral pain. *Clin Orthop* **144**: 107–109

Reid DC (1993) The myth, mystique, and frustration of anterior knee pain. *Clin J Sport Med* **3**: 139–143

Reider B, Marshall JL, Ring B (1981) Patellar tracking. *Clin Orthop* **157**: 143–148

Reider B, Marshall JL, Warren RF (1981) Clinical characteristics of patellar disorders in young athletes. *Am J Sports Med* **9**: 270–274

Reilly DT, Martens M (1972) Experimental analysis of the quadriceps muscle force and patellofemoral joint reaction force for various activities. *Acta Orthop Scand* **43**: 126–137

Reimann I, Christensen SB (1977) A histological demonstration of nerves in subchondral bone. *Acta Orthop Scand* **48**: 345–352

Reischl SF, Powers CM, Rao S, Perry J (1999) Relationship between foot pronation and rotation of the tibia and femur during walking. *Foot Ankle Int* **20**: 513–520

Rémy F, Gougeon F, Ala Eddine T et al (2001) Reproductibilité de la nouvelle classification de la dysplasie de la trochlée fémorale selon Dejour et valeur prédictive sur la sévérité de l'instabilité fémorale-patellaire sur 47 genoux. *Rev Chir Orthop Reparatrice Appar Mot* **87**(suppl 2): 60

Rillmann P, Dutly A, Kieser C, Berbig R (1998) Modified Elmslie–Trillat procedure for instability of the patella. *Knee Surg Sports Traumatol Arthrosc* **6**: 31–35

Rizzo TD (1991) Getting a leg up on anterior knee pain. *Phys Sportsmed* **19**: 147–148

Robertson VJ, Baker KG (2001) A review of therapeutic ultrasound: effectiveness studies. *Phys Ther* 81: 1339–1350

Rogvi-Hansen B, Ellitsgaard N, Funch M et al (1991) Low-level laser treatment of chondromalacia patellae. *Int Orthop* 15: 359–361

Roush MB, Sevier TL, Wilson JK et al (2000) Anterior knee pain: a clinical comparison of rehabilitation methods. *Clin J Sport Med* 10: 22–28

Roux C (1888) Luxation habituelle de la rotule. *Rev Chir* 8: 682

Rowlands BW, Brantingham JW (1999) The efficacy of patella mobilization in patients suffering from patellofemoral pain syndrome. *J Neuromusculoskel Syst* 7: 142–149

Sackett DL (2000) *Evidence-based Medicine: How to Practice and Teach EBM*, 2nd edn. New York, Churchill Livingstone

Sahrmann S (2002) *Diagnosis and Treatment of Movement Impairment Syndromes*. St. Louis, Philadelphia, C. V. Mosby

Sala D, Silvestre A, Gomar-Sancho F (1999) Intraosseous hyperpressure of the patella as a cause of anterior knee pain. *Medscape Orth Sports Med* 3: 1–8

Sallay PI, Poggi J, Speer KP, Garrett WE (1996) Acute dislocation of the patella. A correlative pathoanatomic study. *Am J Sports Med* 24: 52–60

Salsich GB, Brechter JH, Farwell D, Powers CM (2002) The effects of patellar taping on knee kinetics, kinematics, and vastus lateralis muscle activity during stair ambulation in individuals with patellofemoral pain. *J Orthop Sports Phys Ther* 32: 3–10

Sanchis-Alfonso V, Roselló-Sastre E (2000) Immunohistochemical analysis for neural markers of the lateral retinaculum in patients with isolated symptomatic patellofemoral malalignment. A neuroanatomic basis for anterior knee pain in the active young patient. *Am J Sports Med* 28: 725–731

Sanchis-Alfonso V, Roselló-Sastre E (1998) [Hyperinnervation and ischemia]. *Rev Patol Rodilla* 3: 60–63

Sanchis-Alfonso V, Roselló-Sastre E, Martinez-Sanjuan V (1999) Pathogenesis of anterior knee pain syndrome and functional patellofemoral instability in the active young. *Am J Knee Surg* 12: 29–40

Sanchis-Alfonso V, Roselló-Sastre E, Monteagudo-Castro C, Esquerdo J (1998) Quantitative analysis of nerve changes in the lateral retinaculum in patients with isolated symptomatic patellofemoral malalignment. A preliminary study. *Am J Sports Med* 26: 703–709

Sanchis-Alfonso V, Roselló-Sastre E, Revert F (2001) Neural growth factor expression in the lateral retinaculum in painful patellofemoral malalignment. *Acta Orthop Scand* 72: 146–149

Sanchis-Alfonso V, Roselló-Sastre E, Subias-López A (1999) Mechanisms of pain in jumper's knee. A histological and immunohistological study. *J Bone Joint Surg Br* 81(suppl 82)

Sasaki T, Yagi T (1986) Subluxation of the patella. Investigation by computerized tomography. *Int Orthop* 10: 115–120

Schmidt RA, Lee TD (1999) *Motor Control and Learning. A Behavioral Emphasis*, 3rd edn. Champaign, IL, Human Kinetics

Schneider U, Graf J, Thomsen M, Wenz W, Niethard FU (1997) Das Hypertensionssyndrom der Patella: Nomenklatur, Diagnostik, und Therapie. *Z Orthop Ihre Grenzgeb* 135: 187–188

Schutzer SF, Ramsby GR, Fulkerson JP (1986) Computed tomographic classification of patellofemoral pain patients. *Orthop Clin North Am* 17: 235–248

Scott JE, Taor WS (1979) The 'small patella' syndrome. *J Bone Joint Surg Br* 61: 172–175

Seil R, Muller B, Georg T et al (2000) Reliability and interobserver variability in radiological patellar height ratios. *Knee Surg Sports Traumatol Arthrosc* 8: 231–236

Senavongse W, Farahmand F, Jones J et al (2003) Quantitative measurement of patellofemoral joint stability: force-displacement behavior of the human patella *in vitro*. *J Orthop Res* 21: 780–786

Servien E (2001) La luxation de rotule: étude rétrospective de 190 cas opérés et analyse de la dysplasie fémorale-patellaire. Thesis, University of Lyon

Shelbourne KD, Nitz P (1990) Accelerated rehabilitation after anterior cruciate ligament reconstruction. *Am J Sports Med* 18: 292–299

Shellock FG, Mink JH, Deutsch A et al (1990) Evaluation of patients with persistent symptoms after lateral retinacular release by kinematic magnetic resonance imaging of the patellofemoral joint. *Arthroscopy* 6: 226–234

Shellock FG, Mink JH, Deutsch AL et al (1993) Patellofemoral joint: identification of abnormalities with active-movement, 'unloaded' versus 'loaded' kinematic MR imaging techniques. *Radiology* **188**: 575–578

Shelton GL (1992) Conservative management of patellofemoral dysfunction. *Prim Care* **19**: 331–350

Shelton GL, Thigpen LK (1991) Rehabilitation of patellofemoral dysfunction: a review of the literature. *J Orthop Sports Phys Ther* **14**: 243–249

Simon LS (1999) Viscosupplementation therapy with intra-articular hyaluronic acid. Fact or fantasy? *Rheum Dis Clin North Am* **25**: 345–357

Sinacore DR, Delitto A, King DS, Rose SJ (1990) Type II fiber activation with electrical stimulation: a preliminary report. *Phys Ther* **70**: 416–422

Skoglund S (1973) Joint receptors and kinesthesis. In: *Handbook of Sensory Physiology*, volume I. New York, Springer-Verlag, pp 111–136

Sledge SL (2001) Microfracture techniques in the treatment of osteochondral injuries. *Clin Sports Med* **20**: 365–377

Smidt GL (1994) Current open and closed kinetic chain concepts – clarifying or confusing? *J Orthop Sports Phys Ther* **20**: 235

Smith AD, Stroud L, McQueen C (1991) Flexibility and anterior knee pain in adolescent elite figure skaters. *J Pediatr Orthop* **11**: 77–82

Smith AD, Tao SS (1995) Knee injuries in young athletes. *Clin Sports Med* **14**: 629–650

Smith AM, Peckett WR, Butler-Manuel PA et al (2002) Treatment of patellofemoral arthritis using the Lubinus patellofemoral arthroplasty: a retrospective review. *The Knee* **9**: 27–30

Smith MD, Triantafillou S, Parker A et al (1997) Synovial membrane inflammation and cytokine production in patients with early osteoarthritis. *J Rheumatol* **24**: 365–371

Snyder-Mackler L, Delitto A, Stralka SW, Bailey SL (1994) Use of electrical stimulation to enhance recovery of quadriceps femoris muscle force production in patients following anterior cruciate ligament reconstruction. *Phys Ther* **74**: 901–907

Snyder-Mackler L, Ladin Z, Schepsis AA, Young JC (1991) Electrical stimulation of the thigh muscles after reconstruction of the anterior cruciate ligament. Effects of electrically elicited contraction of the quadriceps femoris and hamstring muscles on gait and on strength of the thigh muscles. *J Bone Joint Surg Am* **73**: 1025–1036

Soderberg GL, Cook TM (1983) An electromyographic analysis of quadriceps femoris muscle setting and straight leg raising. *Phys Ther* **63**: 1434–1438

Somes S, Worrell TW, Corey B, Ingersoll CD (1997) Effects of patellar taping on patellar position in the open and closed kinetic chain: A preliminary study. *J Sports Rehab* **6**: 299–308

Souza DR, Gross MT (1991) Comparison of vastus medialis obliquus: vastus lateralis muscle integrated electromyographic ratios between healthy subjects and patients with patellofemoral pain. *Phys Ther* **71**: 310–316; discussion 317–320

Sowers MF, Lachance L (1999) Vitamins and arthritis. The roles of vitamin A, C, D, and E. *Rheum Dis Clin North Am* **25**: 315–332

Spencer JD, Hayes KC, Alexander IJ (1984) Knee joint effusion and quadriceps reflex inhibition in man. *Arch Phys Med Rehabil* **65**: 171–177

Stäubli HU, Bollmann C, Kreutz R et al (1999) Quantification of intact quadriceps tendon, quadriceps tendon insertion, and suprapatellar fat pad: MR arthrography, anatomy, and cryosections in the sagittal plane. *Am J Roentgenol* **173**: 691–698

Stäubli HU, Dürrenmatt U, Porcellini B, Rauschning W (1999) Anatomy and surface geometry of the patellofemoral joint in the axial plane. *J Bone Joint Surg Br* **81**: 452–458

Stäubli HU, Dürrenmatt U, Rauschning W (1997) Zur Frage der Kongruenz von Gelenkknorpeloberflächen und subchondralem Knochen des Femoropatellargelenks in der axialen Ebene. *Arthroskopie* **10**: 66–71

Steadman JR, Rodkey WG, Rodrigo JJ (2001) Microfracture: surgical technique and rehabilitation to treat chondral defects. *Clin Orthop* **391**(suppl): 362–369

Steindler A (1935) *Mechanics of Normal and Pathological Locomotion in Man*. Springfield, IL, Thomas

Steindler A (1955) *Kinesiology of the Human Body under Normal and Pathological Conditions*. Springfield, IL, Thomas

Steinkamp LA, Dillingham MF, Markel MD et al (1993) Biomechanical considerations in patellofemoral joint rehabilitation. *Am J Sports Med* **21**: 438–444

Stiene HA, Brosky T, Reinking MF et al (1996) A comparison of closed kinetic chain and isokinetic joint isolation exercise in patients with patellofemoral dysfunction. *J Orthop Sports Phys Ther* 24: 136–141

Stoller DW (1993) *Magnetic Resonance Imaging in Orthopaedics and Sports Medicine.* Philadelphia, PA, JB Lippincott

Suter E (1998) Inhibition of the quadriceps muscle in patients with anterior knee pain. *J Appl Biomech* 14: 360–373

Suter E, McMorland G, Herzog W, Bray R (2000) Conservative lower back treatment reduces inhibition in knee-extensor muscles: a randomized controlled trial. *J Manipulative Physiol Ther* 23: 76–80

Takai S, Sakakida K, Yamashita F et al (1985) Rotational alignment of the lower limb in osteoarthritis of the knee. *Int Orthop* 9: 209–215

Tang SF, Chen CK, Hsu R et al (2001) Vastus medialis obliquus and vastus lateralis activity in open and closed kinetic chain exercises in patients with patellofemoral pain syndrome: an electromyographic study. *Arch Phys Med Rehabil* 82: 1441–1445

Tardieu C, Dupont JY (2001) [The origin of femoral trochlear dysplasia: comparative anatomy, evolution, and growth of the patellofemoral joint]. *Rev Chir Orthop Reparatrice Appar Mot* 87: 373–383

Tauro B, Ackroyd CE, Newman JH, Shah NA (2001) The Lubinus patellofemoral arthroplasty. A five- to ten-year prospective study. *J Bone Joint Surg Br* 83: 696–701

Tavernier T, Dejour D (2001) [Knee imaging: what is the best modality?]. *J Radiol* 82: 387–405; 407–408

Taylor DC, Brooks DE, Ryan JB (1997) Viscoelastic characteristics of muscle: passive stretching versus muscular contractions. *Med Sci Sports Exerc* 29: 1619–1624

Teitge RA, Faerber WW, Des Madryl P, Matelic TM (1996) Stress radiographs of the patellofemoral joint. *J Bone Joint Surg Am* 78: 193–203

Terry GC (1989) The anatomy of the extensor mechanism. *Clin Sports Med* 8: 163–177

Terry GC, Hughston JC, Norwood LA (1986) The anatomy of the iliopatellar band and iliotibial tract. *Am J Sports Med* 14: 39–45

Thein J, Thein BL (1998) Nonoperative treatment for patellofemoral pain. *J Orthop Sports Phys Ther* 28: 336–344

Thomee R (1997) A comprehensive treatment approach for patellofemoral pain syndrome in young women. *Phys Ther* 77: 1690–1703

Thomee R, Augustsson J, Karlsson J (1999) Patellofemoral pain syndrome: a review of current issues. *Sports Med* 28: 245–262

Thomee R, Renstrom P, Karlsson J, Grimby G (1995) Patellofemoral pain syndrome in young women. I. A clinical analysis of alignment, pain parameters, common symptoms, and functional activity level. *Scand J Med Sci Sports* 5: 237–244

Tiberio D (1987) Evaluation of functional ankle dorsiflexion using subtalar neutral position. A clinical report. *Phys Ther* 67: 955–957

Tiberio D (1987) The effect of excessive subtalar pronation on patellofemoral mechanics; a theoretical model. *J Orthop Sports Phys Ther* 9: 160–165

Timm KE (1998) Randomized controlled trial of Protonics on patellar pain, position, and function. *Med Sci Sports Exerc* 30: 665–670

Travell J, Simons D (1983) *Myofascial Pain and Dysfunction: The Trigger Point Manual.* Baltimore, MD, Williams & Wilkins

Trillat A, Dejour H, Couette A (1964) Diagnostic et traitement des subluxations récidivantes de la rotule. *Rev Chir Orthop Reparatrice Appar Mot* 50: 813–824

Trimble MH, Enoka RM (1991) Mechanisms underlying the training effects associated with neuromuscular electrical stimulation. *Phys Ther* 71: 273–280; discussion 280–282

Tuxoe JI, Teir M, Winge S, Nielsen PL (2002) The medial patellofemoral ligament: a dissection study. *Knee Surg Sports Traumatol Arthrosc* 10: 138–140

Ushiyama T, Chano T, Inoue K, Matsusue Y (2003) Cytokine production in the infrapatellar fat pad: another source of cytokines in knee synovial fluids. *Ann Rheum Dis* 62: 108–112

Vainionpää S, Laasonen E, Silvennoinen T et al (1990) Acute dislocation of the patella. A prospective review of operative treatment. *J Bone Joint Surg Br* 72: 366–369

van den Berg F (2001) *Angewandte Physiologie 3 Therapie, Training, Tests.* Stuttgart, Thieme

van den Berg WB (1999) The role of cytokines and growth factors in cartilage destruction in osteoarthritis and rheumatoid arthritis. *Z Rheumatol* **58**: 136–141

van der Wal JC (1998) The Organization of the Substrate of Proprioception in the Elbow Region of the Rat. Thesis, Rijksuniversiteit Limburg, Maastrich, The Netherlands

van Eijden TM, de Boer W, Weijs WA (1985) The orientation of the distal part of the quadriceps femoris muscle as a function of the knee flexion–extension angle. *J Biomech* **18**: 803–809

van Eijden TM, Kouwenhoven E, Weijs WA (1987) Mechanics of the patellar articulation. Effects of patellar ligament length studied with a mathematical model. *Acta Orthop Scand* **58**: 560–566

Van Kampen A (1987) The Three-dimensional Tracking Pattern of the Patella. Thesis, University of Nijmegen, The Netherlands

van Kampen A, Huiskes R (1990) The three-dimensional tracking pattern of the human patella. *J Orthop Res* **8**: 372–382

Velluti C, Salvi M, Porcella C et al (1988) The clinical and radiological picture of the femoropatellar joint in sportsmen. *Ital J Sports Traumatol* **4**: 243–250

Voight ML, Wieder DL (1991) Comparative reflex response times of vastus medialis obliquus and vastus lateralis in normal subjects and subjects with extensor mechanism dysfunction. An electromyographic study. *Am J Sports Med* **19**: 131–137

Waisbrod H, Treiman N (1980) Intra-osseous venography in patellofemoral disorders. A preliminary report. *J Bone Joint Surg Br* **62**: 454–456

Walch G, Dejour H (1989) [Radiology in femoropatellar pathology]. *Acta Orthop Belg* **55**: 371–380

Wallace DA, Salem GJ, Salinas R, Powers CM (2002) Patellofemoral joint kinetics while squatting with and without an external load. *J Orthop Sports Phys Ther* **32**: 141–148

Walsh DA, Salmon M, Mapp PI et al (1993) Microvascular substance P binding to normal and inflamed rat and human synovium. *J Pharmacol Exp Ther* **267**: 951–960

Walsh WM, Huurman WW, Shelton GL (1985) Overuse injuries of the knee and spine in girls' gymnastics. *Orthop Clin North Am* **16**: 329–350

Warren LF, Marshall JL (1979) The supporting structures and layers on the medial side of the knee: an anatomical analysis. *J Bone Joint Surg Am* **61**: 56–62

Watson CJ, Leddy HM, Dynjan TD, Parham JL (2001) Reliability of the lateral pull test and tilt test to assess patellar alignment in subjects with symptomatic knees: student raters. *J Orthop Sports Phys Ther* **31**: 368–374

Watson CJ, Propps M, Galt W et al (1999) Reliability of McConnell's classification of patellar orientation in symptomatic and asymptomatic subjects. *J Orthop Sports Phys Ther* **29**: 378–385; discussion 386–393

Werner S (1995) An evaluation of knee extensor and knee flexor torques and EMGs in patients with patellofemoral pain syndrome in comparison with matched controls. *Knee Surg Sports Traumatol Arthrosc* **3**: 89–94

Werner S, Arvidsson H, Arvidsson I, Eriksson E (1993) Electrical stimulation of vastus medialis and stretching of lateral thigh muscles in patients with patellofemoral symptoms. *Knee Surg Sports Traumatol Arthrosc* **1**: 85–92

Werner S, Eriksson E (1993) Isokinetic quadriceps training in patients with patellofemoral pain syndrome. *Knee Surg Sports Traumatol Arthrosc* **1**: 162–168

Westacott CI, Barakat AF, Wood L et al (2000) Tumor necrosis factor α can contribute to focal loss of cartilage in osteoarthritis. *Osteoarthr Cartilage* **8**: 213–221

Whelton A (2001) Renal aspects of treatment with conventional nonsteroidal antiinflammatory drugs versus cyclooxygenase-2-specific inhibitors. *Am J Med* **110** (suppl 3A): 33–42

Wiberg G (1941) Roentgenographic and anatomic studies on the femoropatellar joint. *Acta Orthop Scand* **12**: 319–410

Wigerstad-Lossing I, Grimby G, Jonsson T et al (1988) Effects of electrical muscle stimulation combined with voluntary contractions after knee ligament surgery. *Med Sci Sports Exerc* **20**: 93–98

Wilk KE, Andrews JR (1992) Current concepts in the treatment of anterior cruciate ligament disruption. *J Orthop Sports Phys Ther* **15**: 279–293

Wilk KE, Davies GJ, Mangine RE, Malone TR (1998) Patellofemoral disorders: a classification system and clinical guidelines for nonoperative rehabilitation. *J Orthop Sports Phys Ther* **28**: 307–322

Wilk KE, Escamilla RF, Fleisig GS et al (1996) A comparison of tibiofemoral joint forces and electromyographic activity during open and closed kinetic chain exercises. *Am J Sports Med* **24**: 518–527

Wilk KE, Reinholf MM (2001) Principles of patellofemoral rehabilitation. *Sports Med Arthrosc Rev* **9**: 325–336

Willer JC (1988) Relieving effect of TENS on painful muscle contraction produced by an impairment of reciprocal innervation: an electrophysiological analysis. *Pain* **32**: 271–274

Williams RA, Morrisey MC, Brewster CE (1986) The effect of electrical stimulation on quadriceps strength and thigh circumference in meniscectomy patients. *J Orthop Sports Phys Ther* **8**: 143–146

Winslow J, Yoder E (1995) Patellofemoral pain in female ballet dancers: correlation with iliotibial band tightness and tibial external rotation. *J Orthop Sports Phys Ther* **22**: 18–21

Winstein CJ (1991) Knowledge of results and motor learning – implications for physical therapy. *Phys Ther* **71**: 140–149

Witonski D (2002) Dynamic magnetic resonance imaging. *Clin Sports Med* **21**: 403–415

Witonski D, Wagrowska-Danielewicz M (1999) Distribution of substance P nerve fibers in the knee joint in patients with anterior knee pain syndrome. A preliminary report. *Knee Surg Sports Traumatol Arthrosc* **7**: 177–183

Witvrouw E, Lysens R, Bellemans J et al (2002) Which factors predict outcome in the treatment program of anterior knee pain? *Scand J Med Sci Sports* **12**: 40–46

Witvrouw E, Lysens R, Bellemans J, Cambier D, Vanderstraeten G (2000) Intrinsic risk factors for the development of anterior knee pain in an athletic population. A two-year prospective study. *Am J Sports Med* **28**: 480–489

Witvrouw E, Lysens R, Bellemans J et al (2000) Open versus closed kinetic chain exercises for patellofemoral pain. A prospective, randomized study. *Am J Sports Med* **28**: 687–694

Wojtys EM, Beaman DN, Glover RA, Janda D (1990) Innervation of the human knee joint by substance P fibers. *Arthroscopy* **6**: 254–263

Woodall W, Welsh J (1990) A biomechanical basis for rehabilitation programs involving the patellofemoral joint. *J Sports Phys Ther* **11**: 535–542

Woolf CJ, Allchorne A, Safieh-Garabedian B, Poole S (1997) Cytokines, nerve growth factor, and inflammatory hyperalgesia: the contribution of tumour necrosis factor α. *Br J Pharmacol* **121**: 417–424

Worrell TW, Ingersoll CD, Farr J (1994) Effect of patellar taping and bracing on patellar position: an MRI case study. *J Sports Rehab* **3**: 146–153

Yoshioka Y, Cooke TD (1987) Femoral anteversion: assessment based on function axes. *J Orthop Res* **5**: 86–91

Yoshioka Y, Siu D, Cooke TD (1987) The anatomy and functional axes of the femur. *J Bone Joint Surg Am* **69**: 873–880

Yoshioka Y, Siu DW, Scudamore RA, Cooke TD (1989) Tibial anatomy and functional axes. *J Orthop Res* **7**: 132–137

Zakaria D, Harburn KL, Kramer JF (1997) Preferential activation of the vastus medialis oblique, vastus lateralis, and hip adductor muscles during isometric exercises in females. *J Orthop Sports Phys Ther* **26**: 23–28

Zavatsky AB, O'Connor JJ (1993) Ligament forces at the knee during isometric quadriceps contractions. *Proc Inst Mech Eng [H]* **207**: 7–18

Zeiss J, Saddemi SR, Ebraheim NA (1992) MR imaging of the quadriceps tendon: normal layered configuration and its importance in cases of tendon rupture. *Am J Roentgenol* **159**: 1031–1034

Zimmermann M (1979) Peripheral and central nervous mechanisms of nociception, pain, and pain therapy: facts and hypotheses. In: Bonica JJ (ed), *Advances in Pain Research and Therapy*, volume 3. New York, Raven, pp 3–32

Index